Health inequalities:
Lifecourse approaches

Edited by George Davey Smith

The POLICY PRESS

First published in Great Britain in July 2003 by

The Policy Press
Fourth Floor, Beacon House
Queen's Road
Bristol BS8 1QU
UK

Tel +44 (0)117 331 4054
Fax +44 (0)117 331 4093
e-mail tpp-info@bristol.ac.uk
www.policypress.org.uk

© George Davey Smith 2003

British Library Cataloguing in Publication Data
A catalogue record for this book is available from the British Library

ISBN 1 86134 322 1 paperback
A hardcover version of this book is also available

George Davey Smith is Professor of Clinical Epidemiology at the Department of Social Medicine, University of Bristol.

Cover design by Qube Design Associates, Bristol
Front cover: photographs kindly supplied by Mary Shaw (www.social-medicine.com/photogallery/)

The right of George Davey Smith to be identified as editor of this work has been asserted by him in accordance with the 1988 Copyright, Designs and Patents Act.

The publishers would like to thank the following for permission to reproduce George Davey Smith's works:

American Journal of Epidemiology (Chapter 21)
American Journal of Public Health (Chapters 5, 6, 19, 25), with permission from the American Public Health Association
British Journal of General Practice (Chapter 30)
British Medical Journal (Chapters 9, 10, 11, 15, 17, 27, 28, 29, 31, 32 34, 35, 38, Afterword))
Critical Public Health (Chapters 24, 36)
RSM Press, London (Chapter 37)   2 003 004 319
Health Economics (Chapter 39)
International Journal of Epidemiology (Chapter 14), with permission from Oxford University Press
Journal of Epidemiology and Community Health (Chapters 1, 3, 4, 7, 12, 16, 20, 22, 23)
Journal of the American Medical Association (Chapter 18)
Lancet (Chapters 2, 8, 26)
Routledge, London, a member of the Taylor & Francis Group (Chapter 33)
Social Science and Medicine (Chapter 13), with permission from Elsevier Science

The statements and opinions contained within this publication are solely those of the editor and contributors and not of The University of Bristol or The Policy Press. The University of Bristol and The Policy Press disclaim responsibility for any injury to persons or property resulting from any material published in this publication.

The Policy Press works to counter discrimination on grounds of gender, race, disability, age and sexuality.

Printed and bound in Great Britain by Hobbs the Printers Ltd, Southampton.

Contents

List of co-authors

Yoav Ben-Shlomo, Department of Social Medicine, University of Bristol

David Blane, Division of Neurosciences, Imperial College of Science, Technology and Medicine, London

Brenda Bonnett, Department of Ruminant Medicine and Epidemiology, Swedish University of Agricultural Sciences, Uppsala, Sweden

Douglas Carroll, Department of Health Psychology, Birmingham University

Nish Chaturvedi, Department of Primary Health Care and General Practice, Imperial College of Science, Technology and Medicine, London

Daniel Dorling, School of Geography, University of Leeds

Shah Ebrahim, Department of Social Medicine, University of Bristol

Matthias Egger, Department of Social Medicine, University of Bristol

Peter Elwood, Department of Social Medicine, University of Bristol

Stephen Frankel, Department of Social Medicine, University of Bristol

Charles Gillis, Department of Public Health, University of Glasgow

David Gordon, School for Policy Studies, University of Bristol

Rosemary Greenwood, Department of Social Medicine, University of Bristol

David Gunnell, Department of Social Medicine, University of Bristol

Seeromanie Harding, MRC Social and Public Health Sciences Unit, Glasgow

Carole Hart, Department of Public Health, University of Glasgow

Victor Hawthorne, School of Public Health, Department of Epidemiology, University of Michigan, Ann Arbor, US

David Hole, Department of Public Health, University of Glasgow

Diana Kuh, Department of Epidemiology and Public Health, University College London

David Leon, Department of Epidemiology and Population Sciences, London School of Hygiene and Tropical Medicine, London

Peter McCarron, Department of Social Medicine, University of Bristol

James McEwen, Department of Public Health, University of Glasgow

Pauline MacKinnon, Department of Public Health, University of Glasgow

Richard Mitchell, Research Unit in Health, Behaviour and Change, University of Edinburgh

James Nazroo, Epidemiology and Public Health, University College, London

James D. Neaton, Division of Biostatistics, School of Public Health, University of Minnesota, Minneapolis, US

Mona Okasha, Department of Social Medicine, University of Bristol

Scott Orford, Department of City and Regional Planning, Cardiff University

Sandra Rankin, Department of Psychology, Glasgow Polytechnic

The late **Geoffrey Rose**, formerly of the Department of Epidemiology and Population Sciences, London School of Hygiene and Tropical Medicine, London

David Rowan, Department of Psychology, Glasgow Polytechnic

Mary Shaw, Department of Social Medicine, University of Bristol

Martin J. Shipley, Department of Epidemiology and Population Sciences, London School of Hygiene and Tropical Medicine, London

Jeremiah Stamler, Department of Preventive Medicine, Northwestern University Medical School, Chicago, US

The late **Rose Stamler**, formerly of the Department of Preventive Medicine, Northwestern University Medical School, Chicago, US

Peter Sweetnam, Cardiff

Mark Upton, Department of General Practice, University of Glasgow

Graham Watt, Department of General Practice, University of Glasgow

Deborah Wentworth, Division of Biostatistics, School of Public Health, University of Minnesota, Minneapolis, US

Elise Whitley, Department of Social Medicine, University of Bristol

Rory Williams, MRC Social and Public Health Sciences Unit, Glasgow

John Yarnell, Department of Epidemiology and Public Health Medicine, Queen's University of Belfast

Acknowledgements

My principal acknowledgement and thanks is to all the co-authors of the papers reproduced in this book, many of whom were either already – or became – friends. The collaboration involved in writing these papers has been the most stimulating and enjoyable part of my working life. Mary Shaw has helped enormously with this volume, having organised the photographs (several of which she also took), helped with proof reading, assembled much of the material in Chapter 36 and generally contributed more than it is reasonable to hope for. Danny Dorling and Stephen Frankel are particularly thanked for allowing me to reproduce papers on which they were first authors. Besides the co-authors, I am indebted to Mel Bartley, Eric Brunner, Jane Ferrie, Nancy Krieger, Helen Lambert, Debbie Lawlor, John Lynch, John Macleod, Michael Marmot, Rich Mitchell, Jerry Morris, Jake Najman, Neil Pearce, Chris Power, Stephen Stansfeld and Richard Wilkinson, with whom I have discussed and debated many of the topics covered in this book over the years (sometimes with considerable disagreement). Angela Neale, Marie-Claire Hamilton, Claire Snadden and Anne Rennie typed (or re-typed) many of the papers in a way which belied the disorganisation of the material given to them. Dawn Rushen and Karen Bowler from The Policy Press were more tolerant of my laxity and general indolence than I deserved.

I was a Robert Wood Johnson Foundation Fellow ('An individual and population lifecourse approach to the determinants of health') during the assembly of this book and the writing of the Introduction.

Note on the text

These articles are reprinted as they originally appeared (although with correction of typographical errors) with the exception of Chapter 26. This was greatly shortened for publication in the *Lancet*; the version here is considerably longer. There is some duplication of the description of the methods of those studies that contribute to more than one chapter. This, however, does not greatly lengthen the book and it allows the individual chapters to be read independently. There is one notable piece of textual duplication, with the first paragraph of Chapter 24 and of Chapter 25 being very similar. I guess the only excuse for this is that I was plagiarising myself. I have resisted the temptation to revise some of the discussion sections of earlier articles where they contradict views I now hold, which leads to occasional (but perhaps informative) discrepancies in interpretation.

Photographic credits

Cover and pages 111, 357, 437 and 451: Mary Shaw
Page 269: Mark Power (from the series 'The shipping forecast')
Pages 1 and 87: Wellcome History of Medicine Photographic Library
Page 151: Wolf Suschitzsky
Page 219: John Pemberton
Pages 388 and 392: Robert Perry
Page 522: Gerald Welsby

For
Zachary Davey Lambert
born 19 April 2002

Introduction: lifecourse approaches to health inequalities

Discussions of health inequalities often begin with the statement that such inequalities are ubiquitous: the less affluent have always had worse health, they have worse health wherever they live, and they suffer more from all forms of ill-health. I entered the field thinking along these lines, but, as with most generalisations, a more than superficial acquaintance with empirical studies revealed that there were important exceptions; indeed it seemed to me that we could perhaps learn more about the processes generating inequalities in health by considering the exceptions, rather than carrying out more and more studies to prove the rule.

The lifecourse perspective offered one way of moving beyond simple generalisations about health inequalities. In Britain a major stimulus for embracing lifecourse approaches within epidemiology was the work of David Barker and colleagues on the early-life origins of adult disease. To me, and perhaps to other contemporary readers, Barker's initial 1986 *Lancet* publication in this area[1] appeared to develop the earlier ideas of Anders Forsdahl on how adverse environmental conditions in infancy and early childhood could increase the risk of cardiovascular disease in late adult life[2,3]. Forsdahl was concerned with the high mortality in the Norwegian county of Finnmark, and drew attention to a possible cause "which has not been discussed earlier, namely that the considerably high mortality today is a late consequence of the adverse circumstances to which a large part of the population was exposed during their childhood and adolescence"[2]. He showed that the main contributor to this high mortality was coronary heart disease (CHD) and that the current pattern of conventional risk factors – such as smoking and diet in adulthood – did not seem to account for this[4]. He then analysed data across the whole of Norway and demonstrated that infant mortality rates early in the 20th century correlated strongly with CHD mortality rates 70 years later[3] (Figure 1). Forsdahl speculated that permanent damage could be caused by nutritional deficit in early life that rendered individuals less able to tolerate particular forms of fat in their adult diet, a hypothesis he went on to test[5].

In their initial studies building on the work of Forsdahl, Barker and colleagues interpreted their findings as indicating an influence

Figure 1: Correlation between mortality from arteriosclerotic heart disease (1964-67), in men aged 40 to 69 years (standardised rates/100,000 population) and infant mortality rates (1896-1925)[3]

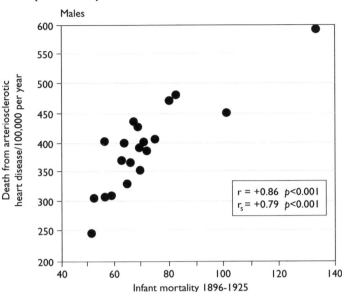

Note: r = product-moment correlation coefficient; r_s = Spearman's rank correlation coefficient.

of childhood nutrition[1], but the focus of the studies quickly came to rest on the pre-natal environment, in particular *in utero* fetal nutrition[6]. Only after a decade of almost exclusive concentration on this period of development did these studies again embrace the potentially modifying influence of experiences acting in later life[7,8]. However, to many researchers in the health inequalities field, and to some epidemiologists working on the aetiology of particular diseases, the 'fetal origins of adult disease' hypothesis stimulated thinking about how influences acting from before birth and then right through the lifecourse could influence patterns of disease. In 1997 a book edited by Diana Kuh and Yoav Ben-Shlomo, *A life course approach to chronic disease epidemiology*[9], collected together contributions from across the disciplinary and disease spectra, and for many researchers established lifecourse thinking as central to the epidemiological endeavour.

A key problem with the initial studies in the fetal origins field was that when relating socially patterned early-life exposures (such as birthweight) to socially patterned health outcomes (such as heart disease) many decades later, the intervening social trajectories of individuals born into poor circumstances would tend to be less favourable than those of individuals who entered the world as members of more affluent families. Different social trajectories across the lifecourse would thus lead to the differential accumulation of negative exposures among those who started life in less affluent circumstances. In other words, negative exposures in early life would tend to be correlated with negative exposures right across the lifecourse. Yoav Ben-Shlomo and I demonstrated this potential problem with respect to the studies that have correlated past infant mortality rates with present day mortality rates[10]. We initially replicated the findings of Forsdahl and Barker, showing that areas with high levels of infant

Figure 2: Infant mortality rates (1905-08), and female Ischaemic heart disease mortality age 65-74 in 1969-73 before control for measures of adult deprivation[10]

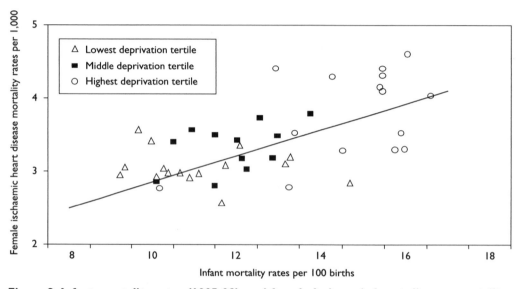

Figure 3: Infant mortality rates (1905-08), and female Ischaemic heart disease mortality age 65-74 in 1969-73 after control for measures of adult deprivation[10]

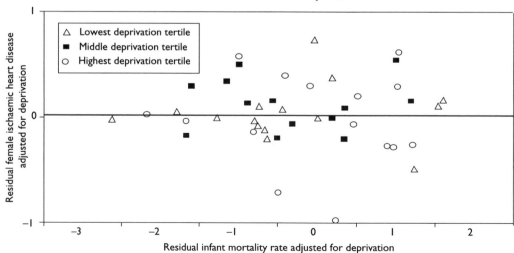

mortality in the early part of the 20th century had high CHD mortality among elderly adults in the 1980s (Figure 2). We then demonstrated that statistical adjustment for an area-based measure of current socioeconomic disadvantage abolished this association (Figure 3). We did not conclude that our findings demonstrated that early-life factors were unimportant, but that it "is unhelpful to consider an either/or model, which would exclude the possible interaction and cumulative effect of factors acting early and later in life. These ecological associations, however, do clearly point out the importance of considering a life course approach to disease aetiology"[10].

The implication of these findings for epidemiology was that detailed data for periods covering the entire lifecourse were required to identify the contribution of exposures acting at particular time periods. Researchers in the health inequality field were among the first to take up this challenge and attempt to better characterise the relative importance of influences acting at different stages of life to the generation of inequalities in health in adulthood. In this introduction I will attempt to sketch how the developing interest in lifecourse epidemiology influenced the work of myself and my colleagues over the period during which the papers reprinted in this book were written.

Explanations for inequalities in health: the legacy of the Black Report

The Black Report on inequalities in health was published in Britain in 1980[11] and its handling by the Conservative government that replaced the Labour administration which originally commissioned the report caused considerable controversy[12]. The recommendations in the Black Report focused particularly on the alleviation of child poverty, and implicitly suggested that this would have long-term effects on reducing inequalities in health, in line with some earlier research of one of the Black Committee members, Jerry Morris[13]. In the chapter of the Black Report on 'explanations for inequalities in health' there was some limited discussion of the potential contribution of early-life influences to later health. For example, it was suggested that social class differences in low birthweight "can have, except under the most advantageous conditions, long-term implications for the health and development of the young child". A general framework with four categories of explanation was put forward by the Black Committee: artefact, social selection, behavioural/cultural influences and aspects of the material conditions of life[11]. In the attention that the Black Report received after its release the recommendations on how to reduce inequalities in health received the most attention. Initially the approach of the Black Committee to explanation received little comment, although an influential review by David Blane in 1985 began to redress this neglect[14]. David, Mel Bartley and I published an evaluation of the explanatory categories in the *BMJ* in 1990, to mark the 10th anniversary of the publication of the Black Report[15], and this reassessment was expanded in a series of papers over the subsequent few years[16,17,18,19].

In brief we concluded in these reviews that the magnitude of health inequalities was probably underestimated (rather than overestimated) because of artefacts in data collection and analysis; that unfavourable social circumstances led to adverse health outcomes (rather than poor health leading to less favourable social locations); and that the origins of health inequalities could not be reduced in any simple way to the unconstrained adoption of insalubrious lifestyle choices. Developing the focus pioneered by David Blane on the contribution of lifetime exposure patterns to the generation of social class differences in adulthood health[20], we considered that the clustering of advantage and disadvantage across the lifecourse was key:

> A woman in a low-income household is more likely to be poorly nourished during pregnancy and to produce a low birth weight or premature baby. A child growing up in a low-income household is more likely to be disadvantaged in terms of diet, crowding, safe areas in which to play and opportunities for educational achievement. An adolescent from a low-income household is more likely to leave education at the minimum school-leaving age, with few qualifications and to experience unemployment before entering a low-paid, insecure and hazardous occupation, with no occupational pension scheme. An adult working in this sector of the labour market is more likely to experience periods of unemployment, to raise a family in financially difficult circumstances and to retire early because their prematurely expended health can no longer cope with the physical demands of their work. A retired person who does not have an occupational pension is more likely to experience financial deprivation in the years leading up to their death[17].

The earliest paper in the present volume (Chapter 12), written before (and cited by) the 1990 review article discussed above, concluded that the "differential prevalence rates of disease in these middle-aged men will reflect socioeconomic factors over their life courses". However, the main focus of that paper was on adulthood risk factors, and there was what I now consider an over-reliance on height as an indicator of childhood social circumstances when attempting to examine the contribution of early-life deprivation to later-life health inequalities. After having been briefly (but inadequately) flagged up in this paper, the ways in which health inequalities could have their origins in early life became an increasing focus of subsequent work.

Early life influences on later disease

Lifecourse approaches to health inequalities explicitly consider how exposures acting from before conception through to death could have important health consequences. The novel aspect of these approaches, however, was certainly the inclusion of early-life factors, since previous explanatory approaches to adult health inequalities had generally concentrated on influences acting in adulthood. Thus there was a considerable focus of lifecourse researchers on previously neglected early-life influences, as reflected in the limited coverage of conventional adult risk factors for chronic adulthood disease seen in the Kuh and Ben-Shlomo edited collection[9].

Many progenitors of lifecourse epidemiology could be resurrected to provide a historical lineage for work in this field. Chapter 33 discusses work from the first half of the 20th century, while the particular contribution of William Ogilvy Kermack is covered in detail elsewhere[21]. The contention of Antonio Ciocco in 1941 that many held the view that "disease in adulthood is often brought about by the cumulative effects over a long period of time of many pathological conditions, many incidents, some of which take place and are even perceived in infancy"[22] illustrates that this was not a minority viewpoint. However, after the Second World War, as epidemiology came to focus on adult 'lifestyles', there was little interest in the childhood origins of adult disease until late in the century. The exceptions were the few studies relating to the aetiology of particular diseases – such as Gutensohn and Cole's work on childhood social environment and Hodgkin's disease[23] – but such work was generally not referred to within the health inequalities field.

Interest in childhood social circumstances and adult health in the UK developed within the context of the national birth cohorts – in particular, the 1946 and 1958 cohorts – that had collected data from the time of birth onwards. Much of the initial focus was on how relating childhood social position and health to adulthood social position and health could address the question of health-related selection, a contentious issue in the mid-1980s. Mike Wadsworth[24], Chris Power[25] and their colleagues reported detailed analyses of these issues from the birth cohorts. The contribution of social circumstances in childhood to adult morbidity and mortality followed on from this, both in the birth cohorts[26,27,28] and elsewhere, including in several of the papers reprinted in this book (Chapters 15, 17, 19, 20, 21 and 32). My main interest in this regard was in the processes linking childhood disadvantage to particular health outcomes, such as cardiovascular disease mortality, which could not be examined in the national birth cohorts as they were too young to have experienced many such events.

Models of lifecourse influences on adult disease

Many analyses of how socially patterned exposures acting at different stages of the lifecourse affect health outcomes use unspecific measures such as all-cause mortality or overall subjective health ratings. These composite outcomes will be influenced by a wide range of exposures – for example, all the aetiological factors relating to the component causes of death will relate to all-cause mortality. Detailed models of how exposures acting at different stages of life come together to influence health outcomes cannot be clearly specified with respect to such summary measures.

The development of lifecourse epidemiology within particular health domains made it clear that different processes come into play with respect to different health outcomes. Yoav Ben-Shlomo and Diana Kuh have developed a helpful typology of models for lifecourse epidemiology[29] (see Table 1), some of which are illustrated by material in this book.

A simple model of lifecourse influences is that the *accumulation of risk* occurs, such that an adverse exposure early in life has an additive effect with later life adverse influences to increase disease risk. When examining all-cause mortality or a broad cause of death group like cardiovascular mortality, this appears to be true, as demonstrated in Chapter 15, where a cumulative exposure measure of lifecourse socioeconomic circumstances is created by simply adding up the instances of being in particular social locations across life. Similar analyses have been carried out for an overall measure of self-perceived health status in the 1958 birth cohort (Figure 4)[30]. Cumulative effects are also seen with respect to cardiovascular disease mortality when combining early and later life socioeconomic and behavioural factors (smoking and excess drinking), as shown in Chapter 19. In these cases, the adverse exposures could either be uncorrelated – for example,

Table 1: Conceptual lifecourse models[29]

Critical period model
      with or without later life risk factors
      with later life effect modifiers

Accumulation of risk
      with independent and uncorrelated insults
      with correlated insults
            'risk clustering'
            'chains of risk' with additive or trigger effects

Figure 4: Poor health at age 33 and cumulative socioeconomic circumstances (birth to age 33), Britain (1958-91)[30]

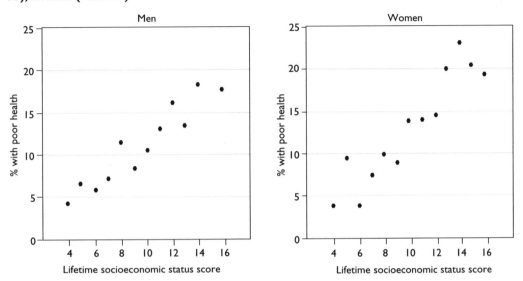

Note: 'Poor health' includes subjects who rated their health as 'fair'.

high alcohol consumption is not strongly related to childhood or adulthood social class – or they could cluster. Clustering could occur because poor social circumstances are related to a variety of other exposures, such as smoking, or clustering could reflect more direct causal links – as when poor childhood educational attainment leads to an unfavourable adulthood occupation and toxic exposures in the workplace.

An alternative set of models sees the time window of exposure as key. Negative consequences of exposures in a specific developmental time window are well established in a variety of situations, such as with pre-natal infections or drug exposure, where during a particular period of fetal development these can lead to devastating permanent developmental changes, whereas if they are experienced just a few days earlier or later they will have no long-term impact. Such *critical period* effects can be seen from before conception right through the growing period and beyond. Tables 2 and 3 list some infectious and environmental exposures for which critical periods seem to apply. The 'fetal origins of adult disease' hypothesis is, of course, one example of a critical period model of adult disease. Infections acquired early in life may have adverse consequences, consistent with a critical period model. In the present book the demonstration that stomach cancer appears to be particularly dependent on adverse social circumstances in childhood (see Chapter 17) presumably reflects this. Infection with *Helicobacter pylori* early in life is enhanced by social conditions that mitigate against good hygiene practices, and during a time when *H pylori* was unrecognised, or infection was not diagnosed and treated, this acquisition can lead, many decades later, to stomach cancer (a process not understood when Chapter 14 was written). More recently we have shown that the number of siblings a person has – which is also related to risk of *H pylori* infection in early life – is related to risk of stomach cancer[31]. The exact age of acquisition of *H pylori* seems to be related to the particular disease outcomes that result (*H pylori* also causes stomach and duodenal ulcers), as with other infections; for example, very early hepatitis B infection (which mainly occurs in 'developing' countries) appears to increase the risk many decades later of developing liver cancer. The age of acquisition of human papilloma virus through unprotected sexual intercourse may also influence the risk of subsequently developing cervical cancer, just as the particular age at which lead exposure occurs will influence its neurodevelopmental consequences. Of course the ultimate outcome of exposures experienced at critical periods can depend on later life influences. A simple illustration of this is that antibiotic treatment to eradicate *H pylori* dramatically reduces risk of developing stomach cancer[32], and low birthweight appears to have greater detrimental consequences if followed by obesity in later life[33].

The absence of infections or the experience of a particularly hygienic environment during a critical period may adversely influence later health, and it has been proposed that such a lack of exposure may increase the risk of asthma, hayfever, Hodgkin's disease, non-Hodgkin's lymphoma and type I diabetes, among other conditions. Some of the conditions show a positive socioeconomic gradient (that

Table 2: Infections with age dependency of acquisition and health consequences

Hepatitis B
TB
Polio
H Pylori
Epstein-Barr virus
Rheumatic heart disease
Chagas disease
Schistosomiasis
Congenital infections
Filariasis

Table 3: Environmental exposures with age-dependency

Lead
Iodine deficiency
Indoor air pollution
Protein-energy malnutrition
Birth trauma

is, more affluent people are at higher risk), which may reflect this exposure characteristic.

Disease occurring in later life clearly reflects the influence of factors acting at different stages, from before birth through to late adulthood. Therefore socioeconomic inequalities in these conditions will reflect the social patterning of the relevant exposures across the lifecourse. The interplay of the accumulation of risk and critical period exposures in generating health inequalities differs with respect to the particular health outcome under investigation[34].

Inequalities in health: general or specific explanations?

One issue within the health inequalities field that has, in my view, been illuminated by lifecourse approaches is the consideration of the degree to which such inequalities reflect the outcome of a general process – with the component health outcome composition of the overall pattern of inequality being, in some senses, a mere contingency – or whether a case-by-case analysis of each health outcome contributing to overall health inequality is required. This issue is not exclusive to the health inequality field, being of relevance to epidemiology more generally. An influential exponent of what has been termed a 'general susceptibility' view of health inequalities was the US epidemiologist John Cassel, whose classic paper 'The contribution of the social environment to host resistance'[35] is a touchstone for debates in this field. Cassel was largely concerned with what some consider to be stress-related morbidity and mortality. He concluded that it was more feasible to strengthen resistance to stressors than to reduce exposure, and thought that there was little aetiological specificity between breakdowns in host resistance and the health outcomes seen in particular settings. Cassel's ideas were widely adopted in social epidemiology, particularly with respect to socioeconomic differentials in health[36,37]. At the same time researchers in other branches of public health and epidemiology were focusing on susceptibility. For example, Thomas McKeown's influential thesis regarding the importance of improved nutrition in relation to mortality declines in Britain across the second half of the 19th and 20th centuries implied that inadequate nutrition is a factor underlying many diseases[38]. Height trends in Britain over the past two centuries have been cited as evidence that nutritional status, as reflected in height, has been a driving force behind mortality change[39,40].

We can examine the relevance of general susceptibility accounts of health inequalities by answering a series of simple questions: have health inequalities always existed? Do all current populations show general patterns of health inequality? Do all or most health outcomes show social patterning in the same direction, and with the same strength of association?

The first question is easy to answer: no, health inequalities have not always existed in the same way as they now do. In Britain, for example, before about 1750, the wealthiest groups – the major and minor aristocracy – experienced similar life expectancy and infant mortality to the overall population[40]. These aristocrats had, of course, enormously privileged existences, but this did not translate into longer life for them or their babies. Various aspects of aristocratic living could have been detrimental to health – in particular, servants and trades people coming into the home, more travel and more time spent in large congregations of people, would increase the risk of exposure to infectious agents. Notions of what was the best food encouraged early weaning and the introduction of meat among infants, possibly helped by pre-chewing of solid food by a nurse maid. Wet-nursing of aristocratic children by poor women in their own homes was common. In terms of nutrition and subjective social status the aristocracy were highly privileged, but this failed to prevent them developing disease as frequently – or more frequently – than those in considerably less favourable social positions. As Sheila Ryan Johansson has suggested[40], knowledge and power were required to convert wealth into health. Once the modes of existence that were salubrious became obvious, the better-off could afford to practice them, and began to live longer. A straightforward – but dramatic – example of how knowledge, wealth and power together could benefit the health of

Figure 5: Deaths in Genoa attributed to the plague (1656-57)[41]

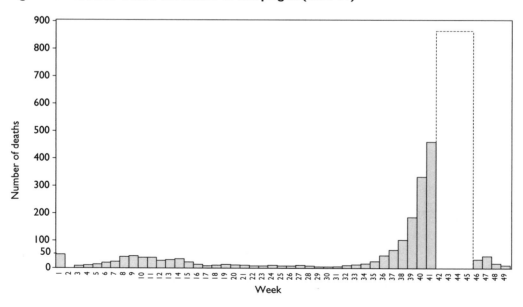

the rich relates to deaths from the plague in the middle of the 17th century in Italy[41]. Figure 5 shows the number of deaths occurring in Genoa on a week-to-week basis in 1656 and 1657. The data come from searchers – often widows who were paid to inspect the corpses of the dead and report cases of apparent plague. The period of missing data during the epidemic reflects the fact that the wealthy – who paid for this data collection – left the city, and thus they avoided the plague during epidemics. The less well-off could not afford to leave. Once knowledge could be translated into action to avoid disease through the use of material resources, the better-off began to dramatically improve their health compared to (and sometimes at the expense of) the poor.

The second question – whether health inequalities exist in the same way in all contemporary populations – also gets a negative answer. While in fully industrialised societies there is generally a strong association between, for example, income and overall mortality, at the aggregate level exceptions exist. Within a country such as Japan, areas of higher average incomes had worse life expectancy profiles until the middle of the 20th century[42]. In countries that are not yet fully industrialised the lack of any area-level association between socioeconomic circumstances and health outcomes has on occasion been noted[43]. At an individual level there are a few good data from 'developing' countries, but a recent study from Tanzania, for example, demonstrated no socioeconomic gradient in the incidence of diarrhoeal disease among children, but a strong gradient in terms of the treatments the ill children received[44]. For specific causes of ill-health rather than overall measures, the situation – as discussed below – is of considerable heterogeneity in the directions of association across different societies. Thus, while in the great majority of cases social circumstances do go along with worse poor health, and across the world today poverty is a very major determinant of sickness, exceptions to this situation exist.

Many of the exceptions to the usual pattern of worse overall health among those who are less well off probably reflect the adverse consequences of urbanisation and industrialisation, at least during their early stages[45]. The British aristocracy in the 17th and 18th centuries managed to create a pseudo-urban environment in their own homes, and suffered the 'urban penalty' even without experiencing the slums and cesspools of developing cities. Similarly, in countries that are currently industrialising people in urban areas may have higher incomes, and own more assets (such as televisions), compared with the people remaining in rural areas, but they often experience worse health. Thus across the whole population higher income may be associated with worse health, because of the link between urbanisation and access to economic resources. The health consequences of urbanisation are largely due to the exposure patterns that concentrated living conditions bring with them, providing a demonstration of the importance of differential exposure patterns.

The third question relates to the socioeconomic distribution of different causes of ill-health. The specific factors contributing to the socioeconomic distribution of particular diseases have been investigated in less detail than have the determinants of more general outcomes, such as overall mortality or self-rated poor health. This partly reflects the availability of data: most of the data sources used for documenting health inequalities do not contain detailed information regarding underlying social factors, potential mediators and specific health outcomes, in large enough populations to allow such analytical approaches[46]. However, the lack of attention to cause-specific analyses may also reflect investigators holding to a 'general susceptibility 'model' discussed above[35,36,37,47,48].

Several processes have been postulated which could lead to increased susceptibility to disease in general among the less economically favoured, including psychosocial stress, poor diet, inadequate coping resources and genetic differences[49,50,51]. A wide range of physiological measures have been advanced as potential mechanisms for the increased susceptibility, largely within the stress paradigm[52,53,54]. Data from several sources suggest that the general susceptibility argument is inconsistent with the true complexity of socioeconomic differentials in health. When particular causes of death are examined there is a considerable degree of heterogeneity in their association with socioeconomic position. Figure 6 summarises data from Chapter 14, relating to cancer mortality in the Whitehall Study of London civil servants, in which there was a marked gradient in the association between employment grade and all-cause mortality[37] (see Chapter 12). For overall cancer mortality the lower grade civil servants (clerical and manual) had a 48% higher risk than the higher grades (administrators, professionals and executives). However, for the 13 specific cancer

Figure 6: Relative risks of cancer by employment grade in the Whitehall Study (relative rate for low versus high grade civil servants)

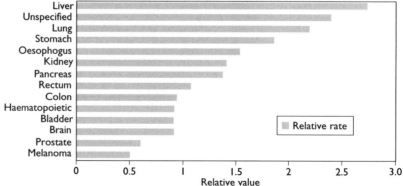

sites examined grade-related risk varied by site. The low grade civil servants had a greater mortality risk for seven of the cancer sites, the higher grades had a greater risk for six. Similar findings with respect to the heterogeneity of site-specific cancer risk with socioeconomic position have come from other studies[55,56].

In Table 4, data for a wider range of causes of death are presented from the mortality follow-up of a third of a million men in the US MRFIT study (from Chapter 5). Relative risks are given for mortality associated with $10,000 lower median income of the area of residence (zip code areas being used for this purpose). For some causes of death – including AIDS, homicide, respiratory disease, diabetes and rheumatic heart disease – there are large differentials, with relative risks greater than 1.5 per $10,000 lower zip code income. For other causes of death – including such major contributors to all-cause mortality as CHD, lung cancer and stroke – the relative risks associated with $10,000 lower income were in the range 1.21-1.50. For a large number of causes of death – many of them relatively minor contributors to all-cause mortality – there were weak or reversed gradients between income and risk.

For some conditions that show a gradient of increasing risk with better-off social circumstances the reason seems straightforward. Melanoma risk is increased by exposure to sunlight, and the higher grade civil servants in the 1960s and 1970s would have been more likely to be able to afford summer holidays in places where intense sunlight exposure occurs more often than in Britain. Thus the better-off civil servants had twice the risk of dying of melanoma. In the MRFIT study it is not surprising that people from higher income areas are more likely to die in flying accidents – airline tickets (and private planes) are relatively expensive. For a large number of cancers that show either a reverse of the usual gradient, or no gradient, such as prostate cancer, breast cancer and lymphoma, there is evidence that better nutrition and growth in childhood are associated with increased risk – taller people are also at greater risk of these conditions (see Chapter 22)[57]. People in better social circumstances across their lives are, on average, taller, and this is reflected in their cancer risk. The marked heterogeneity in the strength and even direction of the associations between socioeconomic position and cause-specific mortality draws attention to the need for explanatory models which account both for the overall and specific health effects of socioeconomic position.

Lifecourse approaches to inequalities in health make some contribution to considerations of general or specific susceptibility through identifying the particular times during life when socially patterned exposures act to generate inequalities in health outcomes. The evidence in this regard suggests that for different health outcomes these aetiologically relevant periods differ. For example, stomach

Table 4: Proportional increase in cause-specific mortality (relative risk) per $10,000 decrease in median income of area of residence (zip code) in US men screened in the MRFIT study

RR >1.50	RR 1.21-1.50	RR 1.00-1.20	RR <1.00
AIDS	Infection	Aortic aneurysm	Blood disease
Diabetes	CHD	Suicide	Motor neurone disease
Rheumatic heart disease	Stroke	Nervous system disease	Flying accidents
Heart failure	Cirrhosis	Oesophageal cancer	Lymphoma
COPD	Genitourinary disease	Stomach cancer	Hodgkin's disease
Pneumonia/ influenza	Symptoms/signs	Pancreatic cancer	Melanoma
Homicide	Accidents	Prostate cancer	Bone/connective tissue cancer
	Lung cancer	Bladder cancer	
	Liver cancer	Kidney cancer	
	Colorectal cancer	Brain cancer	
		Myeloma	
		Leukaemia	

cancer reflects adverse social conditions, leading to *H pylori* infection, in childhood; haemorrhagic stroke similarly appears to be particularly dependent on deprivation in early life[31]; some non-smoking related cancers, such as prostate cancer, appear to be influenced by calorie intake and growth rates in childhood, as discussed above, while others, such as Hodgkin's disease, may be influenced by an absence of infections in childhood; and for others – such as lung cancer – exposures during adult life, in this case smoking, is key. For CHD and breast cancer exposures acting right the way across the lifecourse appear to be of importance, yet even in these cases some periods are more sensitive to exposures than others. For CHD, for example, the intra-uterine environment may be a key period, while for breast cancer the period between puberty and first birth may be of particular importance.

It is clear that when examining the aetiology of particular conditions the lifecourse periods during which the particular exposures act differ considerably[34]. This leads to differences in the direction and strength of gradients between social position and various health outcomes. This, however, is against a background in which most environmental exposures that are known to be – or in a common-sense way appear to be – noxious, are more concentrated on people in adverse social circumstances. A recent review, for example, demonstrated how hazardous wastes, outdoor and indoor air pollution, water quality, ambient noise, household over-crowding and quality, safety at schools, childcare provider–child interactions, work environments and neighbourhood quality show strong social gradients in such a way as to generate inequalities in health outcomes[58]. In this sense there will be a reasonably general association between adverse social position and health, but one that works through social processes leading to the exploited, excluded and oppressed receiving the worst of what life has to offer with regard to those resources that can be appropriated by groups of people with the economic or social power to do so.

The embodiment of social advantage and disadvantage across the lifecourse

In the early decades of the 19th century it was evident that disease and death were concentrated on the poorest urban residents[59,60,61], and the abject physical condition of the poor was widely discussed. Frederich Engels[59] quoted a Dr Hawkins as saying that visitors to Manchester were struck "by the lowness of stature, the leanness and the paleness which present themselves so commonly to the eye". In London Engels had seen "pale, lank, narrow-chested, hollow-eyed ghosts" with "languid, flabby faces, incapable of the slightest energetic expression". The physical effects of the living conditions of the poor started early; the female factory operatives worked when pregnant until the hour of delivery (because otherwise they lost their wages) and their offspring were said to be feeble. As children they shared the poor diets of their parents, and "the food of the labourer, indigestible enough in itself, is utterly unfit for young children, and he has neither means nor time to get his children more suitable food. Moreover the custom of giving children spirits, and even opium, is very general; and these two influences, with the rest of the conditions of life prejudicial to bodily development, give rise to the most diverse affections of the digestive organs, leaving life-long traces behind them"[59].

These characteristics – reflected in the short, scrawny, pale and physically degenerate factory worker – were considered to be produced by long working hours, hot, damp, dusty and overcrowded working environments, repetitive arduous work, physical abuse from overseers, poor food, lack of sleep and inadequate exposure to sunlight[59,60,61]. The resultant poor constitution increased susceptibility to disease and death and, in the words of a Leeds surgeon, "never a year passes, but I see several instances where children are in the act of being worn to death by thus working in factories"[61].

With some improvement in social conditions and standards of living from the mid-19th century[62] the focus on the inadequate physical condition of the poor may have decreased, although echoes of previous viewpoints continued to be heard. At the beginning of the next century the Interdepartmental Committee on Physical Deterioration – discussed in Chapter 33 – was established in 1903 in response to the high proportion of men found unfit for military service in the Boer War. The Committee reported that while (despite its title) there was no evidence of actual deterioration, the physical condition of the British worker was poor.

With the economic depression of the 1930s there was a resurgence of popular and academic interest in the effects of poverty on health. Again a particular focus was on physical condition. In their well-known book *Poverty and public health*, M'Gonigle and Kirby[63] detailed the shorter stature, lower weight, greater dental decay, greater prevalence of rickets and other bone diseases, worse posture and greater prevalence of squint among the inadequately nourished children from poor households. According to these authors, "Children ... cannot survive unscathed prolonged deprivations or deficiencies of certain essentials for normal nutrition". The social medicine movement of the period became much concerned with social physiology; John Ryle, one of its leading figures, stated: "The comparison of social class with social class in respect of height, weight, the routine clinical examination of systems, radiographic appearances, the common disabilities, and of mental and physical function tests ... should have much to teach us"[64]. It is not for nothing that the initiators of the celebrated Peckham Health Centre – a pioneering project in integrated healthcare, much lauded today as a model that should be recreated – called their first book *Biologists in search of material*[65].

It is clear that discussions of poverty and health over the 19th and first half of the 20th century were much concerned with the effects of social disadvantage on the physique and constitution of the poor. However, the explosion of research into inequalities in health which followed the 1980 publication of the Black Report[11,15,66] has largely been disinterested in differences in macroscopic physiology. A major concern has been the extent to which socioeconomic differentials in major causes of death, such as CHD, are explicable in terms of differences in behavioural patterns, such as smoking, drinking and exercise, and of conventional risk factors, such as blood pressure and cholesterol levels[11] (see Chapter 12). Much explanatory research has focused on psychological and psychosocial factors, such as lack of job control, hostility, depression, and lack of social support among individuals[67], and social anxiety within populations[68]. If biological factors are invoked these tend to revolve around over- or under-activation of the conventional stress system, the hypothalamic-pituitary-adrenal axis, and the consequences of this[54].

Why has the inequalities in health literature either not been interested in biology or had a particularly constrained view of the biological factors of interest? An answer to this question may come from inspecting the limited literature which has taken a macro-biological approach. This literature tends to focus on genetic explanations, an example being Lee Ellis' work which postulates a fundamental genetic determination of socioeconomic differences in height, birth weight, brain size, intelligence, parental investment, work motivation, drug use and altruism, and thus of health[69]. This is, of course, playing a very old tune indeed: in the 1840s the short stature and poor constitution of children working in mines was blamed on heredity[70]. The uncomfortable reaction produced by such hereditarian thinking – which Ellis anticipates – is surely conditioned by its resonance with the biologism that underlay eugenic theories, and thus the consequences of eugenics.

There has been a convergence of several lines of thought that have constrained consideration of the role of biology in generating health inequalities. First, there is the common-sense view that if something is biological it is resistant to change. Second, that the appropriate focus of inequalities in health research should be on the ways in which inequalities can be reduced and the health of the poor improved. Third, there are linguistic similarities and sometimes conceptual confusion between social selection views of the origins of health inequalities and Darwinian natural selection. The confluence of these ideas has been combined with an understandable distaste for genetic approaches to social problems to limit consideration of the biological basis of health inequalities to a discussion of the unseen – and comfortably metaphorical – workings of the stress systems.

The dismissal of what are seen as overly-biological approaches to health inequalities may have unfortunate consequences if it focuses attention on areas that actually contribute little to the generation (and thus potential amelioration) of health inequalities, while simultaneously neglecting the more important socially produced (but biologically embodied) aspects of life which generate inequalities. In *Lifelines* the biologist Steven Rose lays out the multilevel, historically contingent and highly mutable nature of biological processes[71]. Taking a similar approach to the production of health inequalities may help us out of this impasse.

A key step is to consider time as a crucial dimension. Health is fundamentally shaped by time: at a given level of absolute standard of living, mortality rates are considerably lower today than they were in the 1930s. The conditions of life a particular society (and individuals within that society) experiences depends crucially on historical circumstances. The individual lifecourse (even if artificially abstracted from its social location) unfolds over time, with each step being partially dependent on what has happened before and partially shaped by existing conditions, which are integrated into the nature of the individual who faces (and reacts to) succeeding events.

Lifecourse approaches are clearly consistent with models that see social inequality as being literally incorporated, as being written onto (and into) the body. For example, maternal social environment is related to fetal growth and development, which appears to have long-term influence on disease risk in adulthood. Following birth, nutrition and infections are related to growth in early infancy, which in turn helps determine adult height. Both fetal development and environmental exposures in infancy and childhood influence the development of lung function, and thus respiratory health. Later life exposures, such as occupational dusts and smoking, also permanently influence lung capacity. Infections acquired in childhood can become permanent – people may retain the infectious agents right the way through their lives, as with *H pylori* infection during early childhood and later risk of peptic ulcer and stomach cancer. In this collection height receives particular attention (Chapter 22); the components of height – leg length and trunk length – also receive attention (Chapter 23), because evidence suggests that socially patterned exposures in childhood are particularly related to leg length, both in childhood and adulthood[72,73].

Epidemiological implications of lifecourse approaches

There has been considerable recent debate regarding the individualistic focus of much epidemiology on the lifestyles or physiological profiles of people abstracted from their social context[74,75,76,77]. These authors point out that there are broader social determinants of the risks to health that people suffer, and that attempts to reduce these risks should recognise this fundamental social determination. Others have taken issue with this view[78].

The many weaknesses of epidemiological approaches which fail to locate exposure-disease associations within their historical, political and social context have been convincingly elaborated on[76,79,80]. Perhaps less widely acknowledged is that the abstraction of such associations from their particular context can lead to severely misleading conclusions. Take, for example, the extensive research on vitamin C consumption and the risk of cardiovascular disease. A strong observational inverse association between plasma vitamin C levels and CHD risk[81] was rendered implausible by a subsequent large randomised controlled trial (RCT) of a vitamin supplement that raised plasma vitamin C levels substantially, but left five-year CHD mortality unchanged[82]. In this case the range of plasma vitamin C levels in the observational study and the change introduced by supplementation were similar, yet the outcomes of observation and experiment were very different (see Figure 7)[81,82]. There are now a series of similar examples, including hormone replacement therapy, vitamin E and beta carotene intake in relation to cardiovascular disease. What these examples have in common is that the groups of people who were apparently receiving protection from these substances in the observational studies were very different from the groups not using them, on a whole host of characteristics of their lives. In a

Figure 7: Estimates of the effects of an increase of 15.7micromol/l plasma vitamin C on CHD five-year mortality estimated from the observational epidemiological EPIC study and the randomised controlled Heart Protection Study (relative risks and 95% confidence interval)

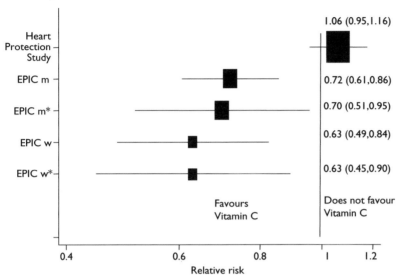

Notes: EPIC m = men, age-adjusted; EPIC m* = men, adjusted for systolic blood pressure, cholesterol, BMI, smoking, diabetes and vitamin supplement use; EPIC w = women, age-adjusted; EPIC w* = women, adjusted for systolic blood pressure, cholesterol, BMI, smoking, diabetes and vitamin supplement use.

cross-sectional study of late middle-aged women, blood vitamin C levels were measured and it was found that women with higher vitamin C levels were less likely to have had a father in a manual social class job, less likely to have had no bathroom and no hot water in their homes as a child, less likely to have come from a family with no car, less likely to have only completed minimal education, less likely to be in a manual social class in adulthood, less likely to have no car as an adult, less likely to be a smoker, more likely to have moderate daily alcohol intake, more likely to exercise in their leisure time, more likely to eat a low fat diet, less likely to be obese, more likely to be tall, and more likely to have longer legs[83]. It is clear that a large range of confounding factors acting right across the lifecourse would generate an apparent protective effect of vitamin C levels on CHD, even when no causal association exists.

Believing that these differences could be summed up in measures of a few 'potential confounders' and adequately adjusted for in statistical analyses fails to recognise the complexity of the reasons why people differ with regard to particular and general characteristics of their lives. It also fails to recognise the limited ability of statistical models to adjust for confounding factors, given the inherent problems of measurement error and unmeasured confounding factors[84]. It would be gratifying if the refutation of observational studies by RCT evidence in these areas led to a critical evaluation of approaches which abstract single elements – which are almost always behavioural, psychological or therapeutic – from the complexity of the life and times of people, and relate these to single health outcomes. It is likely, however, that as in many decaying research programmes auxiliary hypotheses will be mobilised to explain each apparent 'mistake', on a case-by-case basis.

Stress, psychosocial factors and health inequalities

Much current research into health inequalities is concerned with the potential aetiological contribution of stress, negative emotions and other psychosocial factors (such as low levels of social support or control at work). I started work in the health inequalities field much concerned with such factors; indeed in an article I wrote some years before the first paper reprinted in this collection I included a polemic against approaches that failed to take into account the contribution of stress[85]. However, the current research evidence falls short of convincingly demonstrating that such psychosocial factors make an independent *direct* aetiological contribution to disease. Such factors do, of course, influence the patterns of exposure that people receive to known noxious agents, and in this way they are clearly causes of health inequalities. This is not what is implied in much of the literature in the field, in which psychosocial factors are viewed as direct aetiological agents (acting through the stress systems in the body).

In a recent comprehensive review article[86] Linda Gallo and Karen Matthews discuss the conditions that must be met for psychosocial factors to be accepted as mediators between social circumstances and health outcomes. Research must show that:

- social position relates to health;
- social position relates to psychosocial factors;
- psychosocial factors relate to health;
- when all factors are examined within a single framework the relationship between social position and health is attenuated if the effects of psychosocial factors are taken into account.

What does a lifecourse approach add to this? The first condition is, of course, easily met, and lifecourse approaches merely add that social position across the lifecourse relates to health outcomes. The second condition is also met, with additional evidence that social circumstances in early life (as well as during later life) relate to some (but not all) psychosocial factors[87]. The third condition is problematic:

for those psychosocial factors that meet the second condition – that is, are related to social position – it is unlikely that they would not be related to health, even if they had no causal role. Confounding by social circumstances and by socially patterned causes of disease would guarantee that such psychosocial factors were associated with disease outcomes. Indeed, associations of psychosocial factors with social circumstances across the lifecourse would render this confounding more pervasive. Lack of convincing evidence of a causal association between some psychosocial factors and health outcomes makes the interpretation of the fourth condition problematic – statistical adjustment for psychosocial factors that are correlates of social position may attenuate the association between social position and health even if these correlates are not causes of disease, depending on the particular measurement characteristics of the variables included in the statistical model[88].

In the West of Scotland Collaborative study (the source of data in Chapters 15, 16, 17, 18 and 19 in this volume) we examined a measure of the stress of daily (including working) life[89,90]. We found no convincing evidence that this was causally related to CHD or various other health outcomes (although it was related to admission to psychiatric hospital, suggesting that it did actually measure stress)[89]. We also demonstrated empirically that confounding could distort the association between psychosocial factors and health outcomes[89], and that reporting bias could generate spurious associations between psychosocial factors and health outcomes in situations where reports of both could be influenced by a tendency to accentuate the negative aspects of life[90].

John Macleod and I have recently reviewed the evidence on the contribution of psychosocial factors to health inequalities[91]. We considered the current evidence to be inconclusive. We also reasoned that a focus on such factors might lead to the well-established material causes of health inequalities remaining unaddressed. Although many (but by no means all) of the researchers in the psychosocial field emphasise the structural determinants of stress, the interventions that have been developed and tested so far have generally had a highly individualistic focus. Further research within a lifecourse framework could help illuminate this area, with the consequences of psychosocial stress in early life being investigated along with later life stress, and full consideration given to confounding by socially patterned exposures acting across the lifecourse.

A lifecourse approach would, for example, focus attention on the long-term consequences of sexual and non-sexual abuse in infancy and childhood for health outcomes. Research in this tradition suggests that such mistreatment in early life is associated with worse health in adulthood[92]. This reflects, at least in part, an influence of abuse in early life on a wide range of health-damaging behaviours that develop from childhood, through adolescence, into adulthood[92]. The chains of causation that run from early-life experiences through later life dispositions and that ultimately lead to major adverse health outcomes can be importantly illuminated by consideration of life trajectories.

Although not possible in many cases, experimental or quasi-experimental studies are preferable to observational studies, as the problems of confounding are reduced. This study design has produced suggestive preliminary evidence that job insecurity may have detrimental health effects[93], and further research utilising this methodology would be valuable.

One particular issue that may be illuminated by the lifecourse perspective is the suggestion that as the gradient in health outcomes is continuous across the socioeconomic spectrum it cannot be due to absolute material standards. Thus, with respect to the Whitehall Study of British civil servants (see Chapters 12, 13 and 14) it has been argued that the "gradient in mortality among civil servants who are not poor argues for the importance of psychosocial factors linked to the position in the hierarchy"[94]. However, this argument ignores the earlier life experience of these civil servants. The top-grade civil servants will almost all have come from privileged backgrounds, while the lower-grade (but still middle-class) civil servants will in many cases have come from poorer backgrounds. Indeed, the top-grade civil servants are considerably taller (Chapter 12) and have a considerably lower risk of mortality due to stomach cancer (Chapter 14) than the lower-grade (but middle-class) civil servants, suggesting that their childhood circumstances were more favourable[87]. A comprehensive survey of the social origins of civil servants was conducted around the time the Whitehall Study was established[95]. This demonstrated that around three quarters of administrative grade civil servants had fathers in social class I and II occupations, as opposed to 34% of executive grade and 23% of clerical grade civil servants. Conversely, virtually no administrative grade civil servants had fathers who were semi-skilled or unskilled manual workers, whereas 15% of executive grade and 22% of clerical grade employees did so. Only around 1 in 10 administrative grade civil servants had skilled manual fathers, whereas a third of executive grade and nearly 40% of clerical grade civil servants had fathers in these occupations. It is clear that the social origins – and therefore the social circumstances in early life – of the administrative grade and other grades of civil servants differ considerably. Whereas very few administrative grade civil servants would have experienced deprivation in childhood, a higher proportion of executive and clerical grade civil servants would have done so. Many studies have demonstrated that deprived circumstances in childhood increase the risk of poor health outcomes in adulthood, independent of later-life social circumstances[96,97] (and Chapters 17, 20 and 21). When lifetime social circumstances are taken into consideration, the gradient is not mysterious and need not be attributed to psychosocial influences.

Income inequality, social capital and population health

Much recent research in the health inequalities field has considered the potential contribution of general social inequality – and income inequality in particular – to overall levels of population health. Richard Wilkinson and others have argued that higher levels of income inequality within a country or region lead to worse overall health[98]. Other investigators have suggested that 'social capital' mediates between income inequality and population health. The term 'social capital' has been used in a variety of ways[99,100], but one definition given by a group of prominent investigators within the social epidemiology tradition is "the features of social organization, such as civic participation, norms of reciprocity, and trust in others, that facilitate cooperation for mutual benefit"[101]. Researchers in this tradition tend to see psychosocial factors as mediating between income inequality and health outcomes.

The evidence on income inequality and population health has come from cross-national studies and also from within-country investigations, in particular from studies carried out across the states of the USA[102]. Chapter 34 is an editorial written to mark the publication of the initial studies from within the US. It pointed out that given the known latency periods with respect to some chronic adulthood diseases – with aetiological processes set in train many decades before the development of illness or death – income inequality must be working as a marker for long-term underinvestment in human resources if it is related to adult mortality. Recent evidence showing that adjustment for education – in part a measure of childhood socioeconomic circumstances (as discussed in Chapter 16) – abolishes the association between income inequality and mortality across the states of the US supports this interpretation[103].

Turning to the cross-national data the same caveats may apply. The original finding by Richard Wilkinson[98] is not robust to the inclusion of data from additional countries[104] (Figure 8). This may reflect changes within and between countries, such that income inequality does not remain a stable indicator of investment in human and social resources across the lifecourse. Similarly, our recent investigation of associations between income inequality, markers of social capital and various health outcomes across countries[104] did not provide support for the notion that markers of social capital and the psychosocial environment account for health differences between countries. Indeed, where associations were found, they tended to be

Figure 8: Income inequality and life expectancy[104]

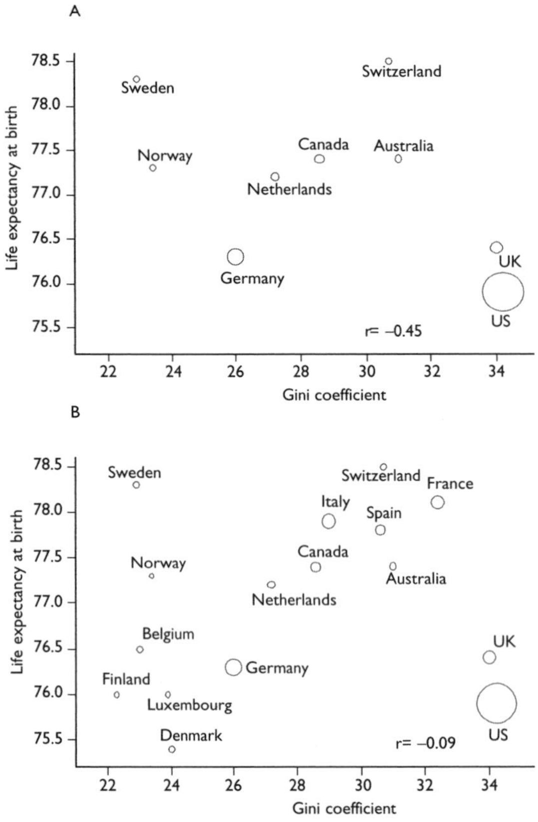

A

B

Notes: Circles represent country population size.

A For the same nine countries reported by Wilkinson et al[98], but with information updated to 1989-91.

B After adding the other seven countries for which income inequality data are now available in the Luxembourg Income Study, for the period 1989-91.

in the opposite direction to those expected. For example, countries where people reported high levels of control over their lives – which would be expected to protect against CHD[105] – actually had *higher* rates of CHD mortality (correlation between control and CHD mortality 0.63, p=0.02; also see Chapter 8). Higher income inequality was associated with higher infant mortality – which might be expected, since the lag period for factors influencing infant mortality will be shorter than for adult mortality. Higher income inequality was associated with *lower* rates of late adulthood mortality, demonstrating that an acute mortality-increasing effect of income inequality is not observed in this case.

Time trend data also fail consistently to support the notion that income inequality and social capital influence adult mortality in the short term. Figure 9 demonstrates that during a period when income inequality increased dramatically in the US, mortality rates for both

Figure 9: Income inequality (gini) and sex-specific age-adjusted all-cause mortality, US (1968-98)[106]

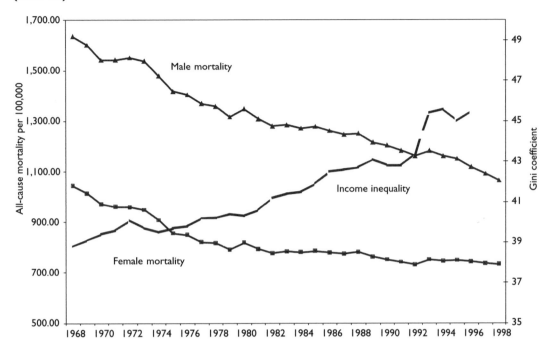

men and women continued to fall dramatically[106]. Equivalent data have been reported from the UK[107]. Similarly, the percentage of the population voting – which has been taken by the leading social capital theorist Robert Putnam as an important indicator of social capital[108] – has declined substantially over the past two decades in the US, a period during which mortality has also fallen (Figure 10). In Chapter 9 we show that the proportion of people not voting in British parliamentary elections – an indicator of low levels of social capital – is less strongly related to mortality rates across parliamentary constituencies than is the proportion voting Labour. Labour voting is perhaps a more direct marker of the material circumstances within areas.

Despite considerable popularity psychosocial interpretations of the effects of social organisation on population health receive little support from empirical data. In Chapter 35 we suggested that unitary accounts of the determinants of population health – whether focused on psychosocial factors, lifestyle issues or genetic influences – appear inadequate. A lifecourse approach, that considers the social and economic factors that have acted across the lifecourses of people currently developing disease and dying, may be a more successful way of explaining population health differences. While currently few data exist, the available evidence is encouraging. For example,

Figure 10: Ethnic-group specific voting participation in presidential elections and age-adjusted, all-cause mortality, US (1968-98)[106]

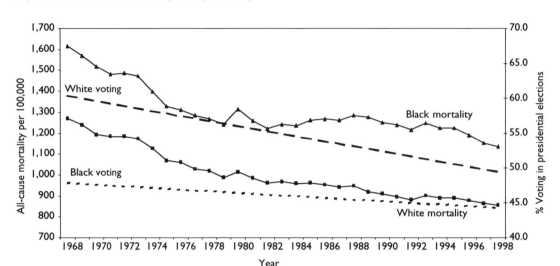

lung cancer mortality rates across time fit well with the lifetime smoking patterns of successive birth cohorts[109]. Similarly, when David Leon and I examined cross-national rates of late adulthood mortality in relation to infant mortality rates around the time these older adults were born, we found strong correlations with conditions known to be influenced by early-life circumstances – stomach cancer, stroke and tuberculosis (see Figure 11)[110]. This suggests that for some causes of death early-life circumstances determine population differences in death rates 70 years after the populations experienced these exposures. With respect to the data presented in Figure 11 this perspective may make sense of why Russia, Japan and Chile currently have high rates of stomach cancer mortality. It is difficult to think of similarities between these countries in current levels of particular exposures that could lead them to be grouped in this way, but they are all countries that experienced high rates of infant mortality (and thus, presumably, of childhood diarrhoea and *H pylori* infection) in the early decades of the 20th century. It is this that is reflected in the high rates of stomach cancer mortality towards the end of the 20th century.

The lifecourse approach to population health, examining the degree to which determinants of socioeconomic differentials in health within countries relate coherently to population health differences between countries and to time trends in disease rates – as a form of triangulation – is an area which merits further research. Factors which could coherently account for all three of these important demographic health patterns are more plausible aetiological candidates than are factors that could explain only one or two of them. As discussed in detail

Figure 11: Infant mortality (1921-23) against stomach cancer mortality (1991-93) for men aged 65-74 in 27 countries[110]

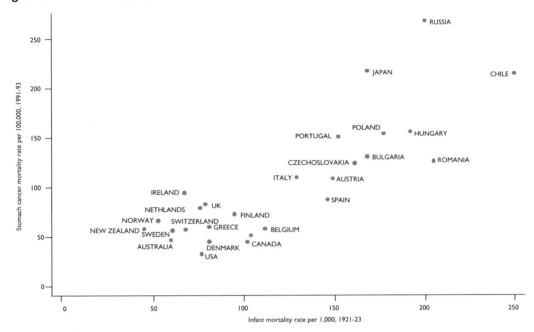

elsewhere[87,91,100,104,111] psychosocial factors, stress and social capital fail to meet this requirement in my view.

What is in, and what is not, in this book

This collection contains work with which I have been involved over the last 14 years. It therefore cannot claim to be a comprehensive treatment of lifecourse approaches within the health inequalities field, since it reflects my main interests and the data sources available to me.

The first section, *Patterns of health inequality*, reprints several largely descriptive papers demonstrating the extent of health inequalities, trends over time, the importance of area-based as well as individual socioeconomic characteristics, the specificity of associations between different indices of social circumstances and different causes of death, and the heterogeneity in the magnitude and direction of the associations between socioeconomic circumstances and particular causes of death. The continuing increase in socioeconomic differentials in mortality in Britain until the end of the 20th century (Chapter 1), against a background of overall declining mortality, makes sense when viewed from a lifecourse perspective. The overall accumulation of adverse exposures across the lifecourse will have improved for successive birth cohorts, but the degree to which these are socially differentiated will have increased. The improvement is reflected in declining overall mortality rates, while the increasing socioeconomic disparity relates to the increasing socioeconomic gradient in mortality. In my view models that see psychosocial factors as the key influence on health inequalities do not sit coherently with the improvements in overall population health. This issue was recognised in a different context by Jerry Morris in his seminal text book *Uses of epidemiology*[112,113] with respect to the then popular theory that stress caused peptic ulcer. Jerry noted the striking declines in peptic ulcer that were evident by 1975, when the 3rd edition of his book was published[114], and pointed out that if psychosomatic factors were the major determinants of peptic ulcer then the social environment must have become considerably less stressful, which, as he pointed out, was "scarcely conceivable"[114]. Of course in retrospect we recognise the decline in peptic ulcer as reflecting falling levels of *H pylori* infection[115,116], an infection acquired in childhood. Perhaps the major consequence of the continuing increases in social inequalities – including income inequality – in Britain will only be seen when the long-term effects of this concentration of poverty on families with children becomes apparent.

The second section, *Voting and mortality*, starts with a paper that was written for the Christmas issue of the *British Medical Journal*. This seasonal issue traditionally contains papers intended to entertain as well as inform, and several other papers in this collection were originally published in this forum (Chapters 27, 28, 29, 31, 32, 35). The title of the paper, "I'm all right, John", referred to the British Conservative Prime Minister, John Major; we had to fight hard to stop the copy-editor changing John to the 'Jack' of the common British saying.

Our paper infuriated the Conservative government then in power, and the *British Medical Journal* was denounced as having published "outrageous propaganda", despite the fact that we showed that constituencies that elected Conservative Members of Parliament had lower death rates. The reaction was presumably because of our conclusion that people "living in better circumstances and who have better health, who are at least likely to require unemployment benefit and free school meals or to rely on a state pension in old age, and who are most able to opt out of state subsidised provision of transport, education, and the National Health Service, vote for the party that is most likely to dismantle the welfare state". It is unfortunate that, as our later papers on this issue point out, the incoming Labour government after the 1997 election showed little more enthusiasm for redistributing wealth and equalising life chances than the government that preceded them.

The third section, *The Whitehall Study*, reprints three papers concerning a study that had, earlier, produced one of the most influential papers of recent times in the health inequality field, authored by Michael Marmot and colleagues[37]. The study had little data on lifecourse influences, although Michael had presciently interpreted the inverse association between height and CHD mortality as probably reflecting height serving as a marker of those factors operating in early life that influence CHD risk[37]. The second Whitehall Study, established in 1985[117], has gathered exquisitely detailed data on factors determining inequalities in health[93,105,118] and will certainly continue to substantially influence thinking in the health inequalities field.

Section IV, *Health and lifetime social circumstances: the Collaborative Study*, reprints papers concerning a study instigated in the west of Scotland in the early 1970s by Victor Hawthorne and Charles Gillis. Unusually for epidemiological studies established at this time Victor and Charles included questions about lifetime social circumstances, education, family formation, employment history and day-to-day stress. These have served as a basis for a large number of reports in addition to those reprinted here (see Box), including a paper showing that adverse social circumstances in childhood are related to high adulthood body mass index (a marker of obesity), independent of later life social position[119]. We have recently replicated this finding in the Glasgow Students cohort[120]. Carole Hart has also demonstrated the small contribution of health-related social mobility to inequalities in mortality by adulthood social position using data from this study[121].

Section V, *Further lifecourse influences on health*, reports additional data on the influence of childhood circumstances on mortality using data from various studies. These papers suggest that the pattern of mortality by childhood deprivation is similar to that seen with height, reflecting that, to an extent, height serves as an indicator of childhood social circumstances. We also demonstrate that this observation could be taken forward through examining components of height, with leg length being the component that best indexes early life factors[72,73]. Debbie Lawlor has since replicated the inverse association between leg length and insulin resistance reported in Chapter 23[122] and has also shown that among women leg length is the component of height most strongly related to the birth weight of their offspring[123]. The latter finding demonstrates how factors acting early in the life of one generation may influence the health, in late adulthood, of a subsequent generation.

Section VI, *Ethnicity and health inequalities*, contains two review articles that propose the importance of considering lifecourse factors when attempting to explain ethnic group differences in health. The third article presents data suggesting that the pattern of differences in mortality between African Americans and Americans of European origin indicate a possible major contribution of early-life factors.

Collaborative study: additional papers on social factors and health

Stress

MacLeod, J., Davey Smith, G., Heslop, P., Metcalfe, C., Carroll, D. and Hart, C. (2001) 'Are the effects of psychosocial exposures attributable to confounding? Evidence from a prospective observational study on psychological stress and mortality', *Journal of Epidemiology and Community Health*, vol 55, pp 878-84.

Heslop, P., Davey Smith, G., Carroll, D., Macleod, J., Hyland, F. and Hart, C. (2001) 'Perceived stress and coronary heart disease risk factors: the contribution of socio-economic position', *British Journal of Health Psychology*, vol 6, pp 167-78.

Macleod, J., Davey Smith, G., Heslop, P., Metcalfe, C., Carroll, D. and Hart, C. (2002) 'Psychological stress and cardiovascular disease: empirical demonstration of bias in a prospective observational study on Scottish men', *BMJ*, vol 324, pp 1247-51.

Heslop, P., Davey Smith, G., Metcalfe, C., Macleod, J. and Hart, C. (2002) 'Change in job satisfaction, and its association with self-reported stress, cardiovascular risk factors and mortality', *Social Science and Medicine*, vol 54, pp 1589-99.

Metcalfe, C., Davey Smith, G., Macleod, J., Heslop, P. and Hart, C. (2003) 'Self-reported stress and subsequent hospital admissions as a result of hypertension, varicose veins and haemorrhoids', *Journal of Public Health Medicine*, vol 25, pp 62-8.

Lifetime social circumstances

Blane, D., Hart, C.L., Davey Smith, G., Gillis, C.R., Hole, D.J. and Hawthorne, V.M. (1996) 'Association of cardiovascular disease risk factors with socioeconomic position during childhood and during adulthood', *BMJ*, vol 313, pp 1434-8

Hart, C.L., Davey Smith, G. and Blane, D. (1998) 'Inequalities in mortality by social class measured at 3 stages of the lifecourse', *American Journal of Public Health*, vol 88, pp 471-4.

Hart, C.L., Hole, D.J., Davey Smith, G. (2000) 'Influence of socioeconomic circumstances in early and later life on stroke risk among men in a Scottish cohort study', *Stroke*, vol 31, pp 2093-7.

Heslop, P., Davey Smith, G., Macleod, J. and Hart, C. (2001) 'The socioeconomic position of employed women, risk factors and mortality', *Social Science and Medicine*, vol 53, pp 477-85.

Social mobility

Hart, C.L., Davey Smith, G. and Blane, D. (1998) 'Social mobility and 21 year mortality in a cohort of Scottish men', *Social Science and Medicine*, vol 47, pp 1121-30.

Blane. D., Davey Smith, G. and Hart, C. (1999) 'Some social and physical correlates of intergenerational social mobility: evidence from the West of Scotland Collaborative Study', *Sociology*, vol 33, pp 169-83.

Employment history

Metcalfe, C., Davey Smith, G., Sterne, J.A.C., Heslop, P., Macleod, J. and Hart, C. (2003) 'Frequent job change and associated health', *Social Science and Medicine*, vol 56, pp 1-15.

Metcalfe, C., Davey Smith, G., Sterne, J.A.C., Heslop, P., Macleod, J. and Hart, C. (2001) 'Individual employment histories and subsequent cause specific hospital admissions and mortality: a prospective study of a cohort of male and female workers with 21 years follow up', *Journal of Epidemiology and Community Health*, vol 55, pp 503-4.

Sleep

Heslop, P., Davey Smith, G., Metcalfe, C., Macleod, J. and Hart, C. (2002) 'Sleep duration and mortality: the effect of short or long sleep duration on cardiovascular and all-cause mortality in working men and women', *Sleep Medicine*, vol 3, pp 305-14.

Family structure

Hart, C.L. and Davey Smith, G. (2003) 'Relation between number of siblings and adult mortality and stroke risk: 25 year follow up of men in the Collaborative study', *Journal of Epidemiology and Community Health*, vol 57, pp 385-91.

Intelligence

Hart. C.L., Deary, I.J., Taylor, M.D., MacKinnon, P.L., Davey Smith, G., Whalley, L.J., Wilson, V., Hole, D.J. and Starr, J.M. (2003) 'The Scottish Mental Survey 1932 linked to the Midspan studies: a prospective investigation of childhood intelligence and future health', *Public Health*, vol 117, pp 187-95.

Taylor, M.D., Hart, C.L., Davey Smith, G., Starr, J.M., Hole, D.J., Whalley, L.J., Wilson, V. and Deary, I.J. (2003) 'Childhood mental ability and smoking cessation in adulthood: prospective observational study linking the Scottish Mental Survey 1932 and the Midspan studies', *Journal of Epidemiology and Community Health*, vol 57, pp 464-5.

However, the study in question had no data to directly test this hypothesis and this is one area that certainly merits the considerable ongoing research that is attempting to address it.

Section VII, *Diversions*, and Section VIII, *Health inequalities – past and present*, mainly consist of papers from the Christmas *British Medical Journal*, which shows an interest in history not seen in the usual weekly issues. These papers generally illustrate, in different ways, issues raised by earlier papers in the collection. Mary Shaw, Danny Dorling and I recently edited a volume of material illustrating the trajectory of interest in inequalities in health in Britain from 1800 to 2000[124], which substantially elaborates on the historical papers in these sections.

Section IX, *Social inequality and population health*, briefly raises issues discussed earlier in this introduction regarding the degree to which factors underlying health inequalities may relate to differences in health between populations and over time. Combining the individual lifecourse and population health perspectives remains, in my view, one of the most important agendas for research in this field.

Finally, Section X, *Reducing health inequalities, now and in the future*, discusses some policy approaches to health inequalities that are cognisant of the lifecourse approach. In common with many areas of research, the health inequalities field is peopled by researchers interested in influencing policy. However, it is arguable that rather little real influence from research has been seen. There is, of course, no direct translation of research evidence into policy making, indeed policy makers may cherry-pick the evidence that fits with the decisions they have already made. This is a somewhat depressing – although probably realistic – conclusion.

This collection suffers from many deficiencies, but two particular ones stand out. First, there is no detailed consideration of gender issues. This partly reflects the datasets that were available to me – these were generally studies set up to investigate cardiovascular disease at a time when this was perceived to be a particular problem for men, and consequently only men were recruited into the studies. Other datasets available for long-term follow-up – such as the Glasgow Students Cohort (Chapter 20) – contain some women, but have a large gender imbalance that, coupled with the lower death rates among women, did not allow robust examination of influences of early life factors on adult mortality. The Renfrew and Paisley study (Chapter 7) contained approximately equal numbers of men and women and demonstrated – as do national data – that overall health inequalities are of similar magnitude in the two genders. The major weakness, however, remains that the data required to allow for detailed consideration of how gender and social position interact were not available in these studies, and the focus on mortality in my work has compounded this problem. Luckily several recent books provide excellent introductions to this field[125,126,127]. Secondly, this collection contains no material on health inequalities outside wealthy industrialised countries. This ignores the vast burden of poverty-produced ill-health in the world. Unfortunately few data on lifecourse influences on health inequalities in non-industrialised countries exist, although a useful start in this regard is made by a recent review of how the effects of poverty are transmitted within and between generations[128].

Conclusions

When we recently reviewed lifecourse influences on inequalities in selected specific health problems it became clear that socioeconomic position at different stages of the lifecourse influenced particular conditions in particular ways[34]. Two conditions – haemorrhagic stroke and stomach cancer – appear to be particularly responsive to early-life influences while others – CHD, chronic obstructive respiratory disease, breast cancer and suicide – appear to be influenced by socially patterned exposure acting right across life. Some conditions – for example most forms of accidental and violent death and lung cancer – appear to be mostly determined by socially patterned factors acting in adulthood. Thus there is no single answer to the question that Yoav Ben-Shlomo and I posed rhetorically on whether deprivation in childhood or adulthood is a more important determinant of adult mortality risk[10]. Not only is there a difference between particular health conditions at one point in time with respect to early or later life determination of risk, but the relative importance of factors can change over time. For example, tuberculosis (TB) morbidity and mortality in adulthood has long been considered to reflect infection acquired in childhood[21,129,130] (with social conditions in early life therefore being of key importance in determining adulthood TB risk). However, with the advent of HIV infection, in many places the major driving force for resurgent adulthood TB rates will for many be an adulthood phenomenon – acquisition of HIV.

The changing importance of early and later life determinants of adulthood mortality risk can be seen in the long-term trends in mortality in Britain over the last 160 years. In 1934 Kermack and colleagues[21,131] (and see Chapter 33) demonstrated that all-cause mortality began to decline after about 1850 in a cohort-specific manner, with falls being seen first in young children, then young adults and then older adults. The mortality rates behaved as if people who were children after around 1850 took with them, as they aged, better health potential that had been established in early life. Interestingly Kermack and colleagues pointed out that as infant mortality did not decline until the turn of the century it was unlikely that this improvement reflected intra-uterine development; they therefore interpreted their data as suggesting that nutrition and health in childhood determined later health. Thus, over the period 1850–1930 mortality risk in adulthood appeared to be importantly influenced by childhood environment. After 1930, however, serious disruption to the cohort-specific mortality trends occurred[21,132] (and see Chapter 33), with age-specific mortality rates changing together, rather than in the earlier age-related way. This suggests that environmental factors acting in adulthood became of greater importance. The rise of smoking in the British population is one obvious candidate here. Another is the introduction of medical therapies which influenced mortality risk and a change in the balance of causes of death, such that diseases with predominantly early life determination (including TB, stomach cancer, rheumatic heart disease and haemorrhagic stroke) decreased in importance, while those with adulthood determination (including lung cancer and accidental/violent death) or determination over the lifecourse (including CHD, ischaemic stroke and breast cancer) became of relatively greater importance. After 1930, therefore, the dominance of the early-life determination of mortality risk seems to have been replaced by a greater contribution of adulthood influences.

Specific patterns of lifecourse exposure are related to specific diseases[34] and, as discussed earlier, there is little support for a simple model of general susceptibility entrained by psychosocial stress, nutritional status or other such factors. Inequalities in overall health status result from the tendency for the important causes of ill-health – for example, CHD, stroke, lung cancer and respiratory disease – to show large socioeconomic differentials. The social processes which concentrate the exposures that increase the risk of these diseases on particular disadvantaged groups therefore underlie inequalities in overall health status.

The social structure leads to the clustering – over time and cross-sectionally – of a multitude of adverse or beneficial factors within the lives of the same individuals. Furthermore, the coexistence of a series of exposures within one person's life may generate greater health problems than would be anticipated from the known effect of single exposures. For example, the combination of an occupational exposure (arsenic or asbestos) and smoking generates a greater risk of lung cancer than would be expected from the simple addition of the known effects of the exposures experienced on their own[133,134]. This synergistic effect of combined exposures would contribute to the poor health outcomes of people who experience disadvantage in several aspects of their lives.

A striking phenomenon, mentioned above, is the tendency for the most common causes of death to demonstrate the most marked socioeconomic gradients. Indeed, as particular causes of death have become more important health problems over the course of the 20th century, the tendency for them to be concentrated among the most deprived greatly increases. Table 5 presents data on male lung cancer from 1931-91. In 1931, when lung cancer caused 1% of deaths, it showed no social class gradient; by 1991 there was a marked gradient – with the mortality rate in social class V men 4.6 times that of social class I men. A similar picture could be seen with respect to social class differences in CHD during the period of rapid increase in this condition as a cause of death. This partially results from more favourable social circumstances providing people with the ability to

Table 5: Lung cancer mortality, 1931-91: social class differences and contribution to total mortality among men of working age (relative rates)

			Social class				% all
	I	II	IIIN	IIIM	IV	V	deaths
1931	1.07	0.96	1.01		0.91	1.12	1.0
1951	0.81	0.82	1.07		0.91	1.18	7.8
1971	0.53	0.68	0.84	1.18	1.23	1.43	11.7
1991	0.45	0.61	0.87	1.38	1.32	2.06	9.9

avoid identified noxious exposures. The influence of these exposures is experienced against the background of less avoidable exposures (for example, poor growth, health and development in infancy and childhood) to determine the overall pattern of disease. It should be remembered in this regard that even lung cancer – a disease for which a particularly important adult risk factor can be identified – shows sociodemographic differentials over and above those created in any simple way by smoking[135].

While 'general susceptibility' as a unitary biological phenomenon does not appear to underlie health inequalities it is certainly possible to identify social processes which lead to unfavourable exposures being concentrated on those in less privileged social circumstances, from birth to death. Human bodies in different social locations become crystallised reflections of the social experiences within which they have developed. The socially patterned nutritional, health and environmental experiences of the parents and of the individuals concerned influence birthweight, height, weight and lung function, for example, which are in turn important indicators of future health prospects. These biological aspects of bodies (and the histories of bodies) should be viewed as frozen social relations, rather than as asocial explanations of health inequalities which, once accepted, exclude the social from consideration[136]. The lifecourse approach to health inequalities views the physical and the social as being mutually constitutive, since aspects of bodily form can influence social trajectory in the same way as social experiences become embodied. Comprehending the ways in which the social becomes biological – and the biological in turn becomes part of the social world – must be a central aspect of an agenda aimed at improved understanding of how health inequalities arise and how they can be reduced.

Notes

[1] Barker, D.J.P. and Osmond, C. (1986) 'Infant mortality, childhood nutrition and Ischaemic heart disease in England and Wales', *Lancet*, vol i, pp 1077-81.

[2] Forsdahl, A. (1973) 'Momenter til belysning ar den høye dødelighet; Finnmark Fylke', *Tidsskr Nor Lægeforen*, vol 93, pp 661-7. (Translated as A. Forsdahl [2002] 'Observations throwing light on the high mortality in the county of Finnmark. Is the high mortality today a late effect of very poor living conditions in childhood and adolescence?', *International Journal of Epidemiology*, vol 31, pp 302-8.)

[3] Forsdahl, A. (1977) 'Are poor living conditions in childhood and adolescence an important risk factor for arteriosclerotic heart disease?', *British Journal of Preventive and Social Medicine*, vol 31, pp 91-5.

[4] Forsdahl, A., Salmi, H. and Forsdahl, F. (1974) 'Finskættede i Sør-Varanger kommune II', *Tidsskrift for den Norske Lægeforening*, vol 94, pp 1565-72.

[5] Forsdahl, A. (1978) 'Living conditions in childhood and subsequent development of risk factors for arteriosclerotic heart disease', *Journal of Epidemiology and Community Health*, vol 32, pp 34-7.

[6] Barker, D.J.P., Osmond, C., Winter, P.D., Margetts, B. and Simmonds, S.J. (1989) 'Weight in infancy and death from Ischaemic heart disease', *Lancet*, vol ii, pp 577-80.

[7] Forsen, T., Eriksson, J., Tuomilehto, J., Reunanen, A., Osmond, C. and Barker, D. (2000) 'The fetal and childhood growth of persons who develop type 2 diabetes', *Annals of Internal Medicine*, vol 133, pp 176-82.

[8] Barker, D.J.P., Forsen, T., Uutela, A., Osmond, C. and Eriksson, J.G. (2001) 'Size at birth and resilience to the effects of poor living conditions in adult life: longitudinal study', *BMJ*, vol 323, p 1273.

[9] Kuh, D. and Ben-Shlomo, Y. (1997) (eds) *A life course approach to chronic disease epidemiology*, Oxford: Oxford University Press.

[10] Ben-Shlomo, Y. and Davey Smith, G. (1991) 'Deprivation in infancy or in adult life: which is more important for mortality risk?', *Lancet*, vol 337, pp 530-4.

[11] DHSS (Department of Health and Social Security) (1980) *Inequalities in health: Report of a research working group*, London: DHSS.

[12] Berridge, V. (2002) 'The Black Report and the health divide', *Contemporary British History*, vol 16, pp 131-72.

[13] Morris, J.N. and Heady, J.A. (1955) 'Social and biological factors in infant mortality', *Lancet*, vol i, pp 343-9.

[14] Blane, D. (1985) 'An assessment of the Black report's "explanations of health inequalities"', *Sociology of Health and Illness*, vol 7, pp 423-45.

[15] Davey Smith, G., Bartley, M. and Blane, D. (1990) 'The Black report on socio-economic inequalities in health 10 years on', *BMJ*, vol 301, pp 373-7.

[16] Blane, D., Davey Smith, G. and Bartley, M. (1993) 'Social selection: what does it contribute to social class differences in health?', *Sociology of Health Illness*, vol 15, pp 1-15.

[17] Davey Smith, G., Blane, D. and Bartley, M. (1994) 'Explanations for socio-economic differentials in mortality: evidence from Britain and elsewhere', *European Journal of Public Health*, vol 4, pp 131-44.

[18] Bartley, M., Blane, D. and Davey Smith, G. (1996) 'Poverty, inequality and health', *Benefits*, vol 17, pp 2-4.

[19] Blane, D., Bartley, M. and Davey Smith, G. (1997) 'Disease aetiology and materialist explanations of socio-economic mortality differentials', *European Journal of Public Health*, vol 7, pp 385-91.

[20] Blane, D. (1987) 'The meaning of social class differences in health: people's experiences of risk factors', *Radical Community Medicine*, vol 29, pp 31-7.

[21] Davey Smith, G. and Kuh, D. (2001) 'William Ogilvy Kermack and the childhood origins of adult health and disease', *International Journal of Epidemiology*, vol 30, pp 696-703.

[22] Ciocco, A., Klein, H. and Palmer, C.E. (1941) 'Child health and the selective service physical standards', *Public Health Reports*, vol 56, pp 2365-75.

[23] Gutensohn, N. and Cole, P. (1981) 'Childhood social environment and Hodgkin's Disease', *New England Journal of Medicine*, vol 394, no 3, pp 135-40.

[24] Wadsworth, M. (1986) 'Serious illness in childhood and its association with later-life achievement', in R.G. Wilkinson (ed) *Class and health*, London: Tavistock.

[25] Power, C., Manor, O. and Fox, A.J. (1991) *Health and class: The early years*, London: Chapman Hall.

[26] Power, C., Matthews, S. and Manor, O. (1998) 'Inequalities in self-rated health: explanations from different stages of life', *Lancet*, vol 351, pp 1009-14.

[27] Power, C. and Matthews, S. (1997) 'Origins of health inequalities in a national population sample', *Lancet*, vol 350, pp 1584-9.

[28] Kuh, D., Hardy, R., Langenberg, C., Richards, M. and Wadsworth, M.E.J. (2002) 'Mortality in adults aged 26-54 years related to socioeconomic conditions in childhood and adulthood: post war birth cohort study', *BMJ*, vol 325, pp 1076-80.

[29] Ben-Shlomo, Y. and Kuh, D. (2002) 'A lifecourse approach to chronic disease epidemiology: conceptual models, empirical challenges and interdisciplinary perspectives', *International Journal of Epidemiology*, vol 31, pp 285-93.

[30] Power, C., Manor, O. and Matthews, S. (1999) 'The duration and timing of exposure: effects of socioeconomic environment on adult health', *American Journal of Public Health*, vol 89, pp 1059-65.

[31] Hart, C.L. and Davey Smith, G. (2003) 'Relation between number of siblings and adult mortality and stroke risk: 25 year follow up of men in the Collaborative study', *Journal of Epidemiology and Community Health*, vol 57, pp 385-91.

[32] Uemura, N., Okamoto, S., Yamamoto, S., Matsumura, N., Yamaguchi, S., Yamakido, M., Taniyama, K., Sasaki, N. and Schlemper, R.J. (2001) '*Helicobacter Pylori* infection and the development of gastric cancer', *New England Journal of Medicine*, vol 345, pp 784-9.

[33] Frankel, S., Elwood, P., Sweetnam, P., Yarnell, J. and Davey Smith, G. (1996) 'Birthweight, body-mass index in middle age, and incident coronary heart disease', *Lancet*, vol 348, pp 1478-80.

[34] Davey Smith, G., Gunnell, D. and Ben-Shlomo, Y. (2000) 'Life-course approaches to socio-economic differentials in cause-specific adult mortality', in D. Leon and G. Walt, *Poverty, inequality and health*, Oxford: Oxford University Press, pp 88-124.

[35] Cassel, J. (1976) 'The contribution of the social environment to host resistance', *American Journal of Epidemiology*, vol 104, pp 107-23.

[36] Berkman, L.F. and Syme, S.L. (1979) 'Social networks, host resistance and mortality: a nine-year follow-up study of Alameda County residents', *American Journal of Epidemiology*, vol 109, pp 186-204.

[37] Marmot, M.G., Shipley, M.J. and Rose, G. (1984) 'Inequalities in death – specific explanations of a general pattern?', *Lancet*, vol i, pp 1003-6.

[38] McKeown, T. (1979) *The role of medicine*, Oxford: Blackwell.

[39] Floud, R., Wachter, K. and Gregory, A. (1990) *Height, health and history: Nutritional status in the United Kingdom 1750-1980*, Cambridge: Cambridge University Press.

[40] Johansson, S.R. (1999) *Death and the doctors: Medicine and elite mortality in Britain from 1500 to 1800*, Cambridge Group for the History of Population and Social Structure Working Paper Series No 7, Cambridge: Cambridge University Press.

[41] Del Panta, L. (1980) *Le epidemie nella storia demografica italiana (secoli xiv-xix)*, Torino: Loescher Editore.

[42] Mosk, C. and Johansson, S. (1986) 'Income and mortality', *Population and Development Review*, pp 414-40.

[43] Asthana, S. (1995) 'Variations in poverty and health between slum settlements: contradictory findings from Visakhapatnam, India', *Social Science and Medicine*, vol 40, pp 177-88.

[44] Schellenberg, J.A., Victora, C.G., Mushi, A., de Savigny, D., Schellenberg, D., Mshinda, H. and Bryce, J. (2003) 'Inequities among the very poor: health care for children in rural southern Tanzania', *Lancet*, vol 361, pp 561-6.

[45] Szreter, S. (1997) 'Economic growth, disruption, deprivation, disease and death: on the importance of the politics of public health for development', *Population and Development Review*, vol 23, pp 693-728.

[46] Hummer, R.A., Rogers, R.G. and Eberstein, I.W. (1998) 'Sociodemographic differentials in adult mortality: a review of analytical approaches', *Population and Development Review*, vol 24, pp 553-78.

[47] Najman, J.M. and Congalton, A.A. (1979) 'Australian occupational mortality, 1965-1967: cause specific or general susceptibility?', *Sociology of Health and Illness*, vol 1, pp 158-76.

[48] Pearce, N.E., Davis, P.B., Smith, A.H. and Foster, F.H. (1983) 'Mortality and social class in New Zealand II: male mortality by major disease groupings', *New Zealand Medical Journal*, vol 96, pp 711-16.

[49] Valkonen, T. (1987) 'Social inequality in the face of death', in European Population Conference, Helsinki: Central Statistical Office of Finland, pp 201-61.

[50] Thurlow, H.J. (1967) 'General susceptibility to illness: a selective review', *Canadian Medical Association Journal*, vol 97, pp 1397-404.

[51] Najman, J.M. (1980) 'Theories of disease causation and the concept of general susceptibility: a review', *Social Science and Medicine*, vol 14A, pp 231-7.

[52] Sterling, P. and Eyer, J. (1981) 'Biological basis of stress-related mortality', *Social Science and Medicine*, vol 15E, pp 3-42.

[53] Totman, R. (1987) *Social causes of illness*, London: Souvenir Press.

[54] Brunner, E. (1997) 'Stress and the biology of inequality', *BMJ*, vol 314, pp 1472-6.

[55] Faggiano, F., Partanen, T., Kogevinas, M. and Boffetta, P. (1997) 'Socioeconomic differences in cancer incidence and mortality', in M. Kogevinas, N. Pearce, M. Susser and P. Boffeta (eds) *Social inequalities in cancer*, IARC Scientific Publications No 138, Lyon: IARC, pp 65-176.

[56] Fernandez, E. and Borrell, C. (1999) 'Cancer mortality by educational level in the city of Barcelona', *British Journal of Cancer*, vol 79, pp 684-9.

[57] Gunnell, D., Okasha, M., Davey Smith, G., Oliver, S.E., Sandhu, J. and Holly, J.M.P. (2001) 'Height, leg length and cancer risk: a systematic review', *Epidemiologic Reviews*, vol 23, pp 313-42.

[58] Evans, G.W. and Kantrowitz, E. (2002) 'Socioeconomic status and health: the potential role of environmental risk exposure', *Annual Review of Public Health*, vol 23, pp 303-31.

[59] Engels, F. (1845) *The condition of the working class in England in 1844*, Harmondsworth: Penguin.

[60] Thackray, C.T. (1832) *The effects of the arts, trade, and professions, and of the civic states and habits of living, on health and longevity*, Leeds: Baines and Newsome.

[61] Wing, C. (1837) *Evils of the factory system demonstrated by parliamentary evidence*, London: Saunders and Otley.

[62] Feinstein, C.H. (1998) 'Pessimism perpetuated: real wages and the standard of living in Britain during and after the Industrial Revolution', *Journal of Economic History*, vol 58, pp 625-58.

[63] M'Gonigle, G.C.M. and Kirby, J. (1936) *Poverty and public health*, London: Victor Gollancz.

[64] Ryle, J. (1947) 'The meaning of the normal', *Lancet*, vol i, pp 1-5.

[65] Williamson, G.S. and Pearse, I.H. (1938) *Biologists in search of material*, London: Faber and Faber.

[66] Graham, H. (1998) 'Observations on the UK experience of promoting research on inequality in health', in B. Arve-Pares, *Promoting research on inequality in health*, Stockholm: Swedish Council for Social Research.

[67] Hemingway, H. and Marmot, M.G. (1999) 'Psychosocial factors in the aetiology and prognosis of coronary heart disease: systematic review of prospective cohort studies', *BMJ*, vol 318, pp 1460-7.

[68] Wilkinson, R.G. (1999) 'Health, hierarchy, and social anxiety', *Annals of the New York Academy of Sciences*, vol 896, pp 48-63.

[69] Ellis, L. (1994) 'Relationships between height, health and social status (plus birth weight, mental health, intelligence, brain size, and fertility): a broad theoretical integration', in L. Ellis (ed) *Social stratification and socioeconomic inequality volume 2: Reproductive and interpersonal aspects of dominance and status*, Westport, CT: Praeger.

[70] Kirby, P. (1995) 'Causes of short stature among coal-mining children 1823-1850', *Economic Historical Review*, vol 48, pp 687-99.

[71] Rose, S. (1997) *Lifelines*, Harmondsworth: Penguin.

[72] Gunnell, D.J., Davey Smith, G., Frankel, S.J., Kemp, M. and Peters, T.J. (1998) 'Socio-economic and dietary influences on leg length and trunk length in childhood: a reanalysis of the Carnegie (Boyd Orr) survey of diet and health in prewar Britain (1937-39)', *Paediatric and Perinatal Epidemiology*, vol 12, Suppl 1, pp 96-113.

[73] Wadsworth, M.E.J., Hardy, R.J., Paul, A.A., Marshall, S.F. and Cole, T.J. (2002) 'Leg and trunk length at 43 years in relation to childhood health, diet and family circumstances; evidence from the 1946 national birth cohort', *International Journal of Epidemiology*, vol 31, pp 383-90.

[74] Diez-Roux, A.V. (1998) 'Bringing context back into epidemiology: variables and fallacies in multilevel analysis', *American Journal of Public Health*, vol 88, pp 216-22.

[75] Koopman, J.S. and Lynch, J.W. (1999) 'Individual causal models and population system models in epidemiology', *American Journal of Public Health*, vol 89, pp 1170-4.

[76] Krieger, N. (1994) 'Epidemiology and the web of causation: has anyone seen the spider?', *Social Science and Medicine*, vol 39, pp 887-903.

[77] Davey Smith, G. (2001) 'Reflections on the limitations of epidemiology', *Journal of Clinical Epidemiology*, vol 54, pp 325-31.

[78] Rothman, K.J., Adami, H.O. and Trichopoulos, D. (1998) 'Should the mission of epidemiology include the eradication of poverty?', *Lancet*, vol 352, pp 810-13.

[79] Schwartz, S. and Carpenter, K.M. (1999) 'The right answer for the wrong question: consequences of type III error for public health research', *American Journal of Public Health*, vol 89, pp 1175-80.

[80] Pearce, N. (1996) 'Traditional epidemiology, modern epidemiology, and public health', *American Journal of Public Health*, vol 86, pp 678-83.

[81] Khaw, K.-T., Bingham, S., Welch, A., Luben, R., Wareham, N., Oakes, S. and Day, N. (2001) 'Relation between plasma ascorbic acid and mortality in men and women in EPIC-Norfolk prospective study: a prospective population study', *Lancet*, vol 357, pp 657-63.

[82] Heart Protection Study Collaborative Group (2002) 'MRC/BHF Heart Protection Study of antioxidant vitamin supplementation in 20,536 high-risk individuals: a randomised placebo-controlled trial', *Lancet*, vol 360, pp 23-33.

[83] Lawlor, D.A. (2003) personal communication.

[84] Davey Smith, G. and Phillips, A.W. (1992) 'Confounding epidemiological studies: why "independent" effects may not be all they seem', *BMJ*, vol 305, pp 757-9.

[85] Radical Statistics Health Group (1987) 'Health education; blaming the victim?', in *Facing the figures*, London: Radical Statistics Health Group, pp 155-64.

[86] Gallo, L.C. and Matthews, K.A. (2003) 'Understanding the association between socio-economic status and physical health: do negative emotions play a role?', *Psychological Bulletin*, vol 129, pp 10-51.

[87] Davey Smith, G., Ben-Shlomo, Y. and Lynch, J. (2002) 'Life course approaches to inequalities in coronary heart disease risk', in S.A. Stansfeld and M.G. Marmot, *Stress and the heart*, London: BMJ Books.

[88] Phillips, A. and Davey Smith, G. (1991) 'How independent are "independent" effects? Relative risk estimation when correlated exposures are measured imprecisely', *Journal of Clinical Epidemiology*, vol 44, pp 1223-31.

[89] MacLeod, J., Davey Smith, G., Heslop, P., Metcalfe, C., Carroll, D. and Hart, C. (2001) 'Are the effects of psychosocial exposures attributable to confounding? Evidence from a prospective observational study on psychological stress and mortality', *Journal of Epidemiology and Community Health*, vol 55, pp 878-84.

[90] Macleod, J., Davey Smith, G., Heslop, P., Metcalfe, C., Carroll, D. and Hart, C. (2002) 'Psychological stress and cardiovascular disease: empirical demonstration of bias in a prospective observational study of Scottish men', *BMJ*, vol 324, pp 1247-51.

[91] Macleod, J. and Davey Smith, G. (2003) 'Psychosocial factors and public health: a suitable case for treatment?', *Journal of Epidemiology and Community Health*, vol 57, pp 565-70.

[92] Felitti, V.J., Anda, R.F., Nordenberg, D., Williamson, D.F., Spitz, A.M., Edwards, Koss, M.P. and Marks, J.S. (1998) 'Relationship of childhood abuse and household dysfunction to many of the leading causes of death in adults', *American Journal of Preventive Medicine*, vol 14, pp 245-58.

[93] Ferrie, J.E., Shipley, M.J., Marmot, M.G., Stansfeld, S. and Davey Smith, G. (1995) 'Health effects of anticipation of job change and non-employment: longitudinal data from the Whitehall II study', *BMJ*, vol 311, pp 1264-9.

[94] Marmot, M. and Bobak, M. (2000) 'International comparators and poverty and health in Europe', *BMJ*, vol 321, pp 1124-8.

[95] Kelly, M.P. (1980) *White-collar proletariat: The industrial behaviour of British civil servants*, London: Routledge and Kegan Hall.

[96] Paulton, R., Caspi, A. and Milne, B.J. et al (2002) 'Association between children's experience of socioeconomic disadvantage and adult health: a lifecourse study', *Lancet*, vol 360, pp 1640-5.

[97] Claussen, B., Davey Smith, G. and Thelle, D. (2003) 'Impact of childhood and adulthood socioeconomic position on cause specific mortality: the Oslo Mortality Study', *Journal of Epidemiology and Community Health*, vol 57, pp 40-5.

[98] Wilkinson, R.G. (1996) *Unhealthy societies: The afflictions of inequality*, London: Routledge.

[99] Woolcock, M. and Narayan, D. (2000) 'Social capital: implications for development theory, research and policy', *World Bank Research Observer*, vol 15, pp 225-49.

[100] Muntaner, C., Lynch, J. and Davey Smith, G. (2001) 'Social capital, disorganised communities, and the third way: understanding the retreat from structural inequalities in epidemiology and public health', *International Journal of Health Services*, vol 31, pp 213-37.

[101] Kawachi, I., Kennedy, B.P., Lochner, K. and Prothrow-Stith, D. (1997) 'Social capital, income inequality, and mortality', *American Journal of Public Health*, vol 87, pp 1491-8.

[102] Kaplan, G.A., Pamuk, E.R. and Lynch, J.W. et al (1996) 'Inequality in income and mortality in the United States: analysis of mortality and potential pathways', *BMJ*, vol 312, pp 999-1003.

[103] Muller, A. (2002) 'Education, income inequality and mortality: a multiple regression analysis', *BMJ*, vol 324, pp 23-5.

[104] Lynch, J., Davey Smith, G., Hillemeier, M., Shaw, M., Raghunathan, T. and Kaplan, G. (2001) 'Income inequality, the psychosocial environment, and health: comparisons of wealthy nations', *Lancet*, vol 358, pp 194-200.

[105] Marmot, M.G., Bosma, H., Hemingway, H., Brunner, E. and Stansfeld, S. (1997) 'Contribution of job control and other risk factors to social variations in coronary heart disease incidence', *Lancet*, vol 350, pp 235-9.

[106] Lynch, J. and Davey Smith, G. (2003: in press) 'Rates and states: reflections on the health of nations', *International Journal of Epidemiology*.

[107] Lynch, J., Davey Smith, G., Kaplan, G. and House, J. (2000) 'Income inequality and mortality: importance to health of individual income, psychosocial environment, or material conditions', *BMJ*, vol 320, pp 1200-4.

[108] Putnam, R.D. (2000) *Bowling alone*, New York, NY: Simon and Schuster.

[109] Strachan, D.P. and Perry, I.J. (1997) 'Time trends', in D. Kuh and Y. Ben-Shlomo (eds) *A life course approach to chronic disease epidemiology*, Oxford: Oxford University Press.

[110] Leon, D. and Davey Smith, G. (2000) 'Infant mortality, stomach cancer, stroke, and coronary heart disease: ecological analysis', *BMJ*, vol 320, pp 1705-6.

[111] Pearce, N. and Davey Smith, G. (2003) 'Is social capital the key to inequalities in health?', *American Journal of Public Health*, vol 93, pp 122-9.

[112] Morris, J.N. (1957) *Uses of epidemiology*, Edinburgh: Livingstone.

[113] Davey Smith, G. (2001) 'The uses of "Uses of epidemiology"', *International Journal of Epidemiology*, vol 30, pp 1146-55.

[114] Morris, J.N. (1975) *Uses of epidemiology* (3rd edn), Edinburgh: Churchill Livingstone.

[115] Banatvala, N., Mayo, K., Megraud, F., Jennings, R., Deeks, J.J. and Feldman, R.A. (1993) 'The cohort effect and Helicobacter pylori', *Journal of Infectious Disease*, vol 168, pp 219-21.

[116] Marshall, B. (2002) 'Helicobacter as the "environmental factor" in Susser and Stein's cohort theory of peptic ulcer disease', *International Journal of Epidemiology*, vol 31, pp 21-2.

[117] Marmot, M.G., Davey Smith, G., Stansfeld, S., Patel, C., North, F., Head, J., White, I., Brunner, E. and Feeney, A. (1991) 'Health inequalities among British civil servants: the Whitehall II study', *Lancet*, vol 337, pp 1387-94.

[118] Marmot, M., Shipley, M., Brunner, E. and Hemingway, H. (2001) 'Relative contribution of early life and adult socioeconomic factors to adult morbidity in the Whitehall II study', *Journal of Epidemiology and Community Health*, vol 55, pp 301-7.

[119] Blane, D., Hart, C.L., Davey Smith, G., Gillis, C.R., Hole, D.J. and Hawthorne, V.M. (1996) 'Association of cardiovascular disease risk factors with socioeconomic position during childhood and during adulthood', *BMJ*, vol 313, pp 1434-8.

[120] Okasha, M., McCarron, P., McEwen, J., Durnin, J. and Davey Smith, G. (2003) 'Childhood social class and adulthood obesity: findings from the Glasgow Alumni Cohort', *Journal of Epidemiology and Community Health*, vol 57, pp 508-9.

[121] Hart, C.L., Davey Smith, G. and Blane, D. (1998) 'Social mobility and 21 year mortality in a cohort of Scottish men', *Social Science Medicine*, vol 47, pp 1121-30.

[122] Lawlor, D.A., Davey Smith, G. and Ebrahim, S. (2003) 'Life course influences on insulin resistance: findings from the British Women's heart and Health Study', *Diabetes Care*, vol 26, pp 97-103.

[123] Lawlor, D.A., Davey Smith, G. and Ebrahim, S. (2003) 'Association between leg length and offspring birthweight: partial explanation for the transgenerational association between birthweight and cardiovascular disease', *Paediatric and Perinatal Epidemiology*, vol 17, pp 148-55.

[124] Davey Smith, G., Dorling, D and Shaw, M. (2001) *Poverty, inequality and health in Britain, 1800-2000*, Bristol: The Policy Press.

[125] Wamala, S.P. and Lynch, J. (eds) (2002) *Gender and social inequities in health*, Stockholm: Studentlitteratur.

[126] Annandale, E. and Hunt, K. (2000) *Gender inequalities in health*, Buckingham: Open University Press.

[127] Kuh, D. and Hardy, R. (2002) *A lifecourse approach to women's health*, Oxford: Oxford University Press.

[128] Harper, C., Marcus, R. and Moore, K. (2003) 'Enduring poverty and the conditions of childhood: lifecourse and intergenerational poverty transmissions', *World Development*, vol 31, pp 535-54.

[129] Frost, W.H. (1939) 'The age selection of mortality from tuberculosis in successive decades', *American Journal of Hygiene*, vol 30, pp 91-6.

[130] Springet, V.H. (1952) 'An interpretation of statistical trends in tuberculosis', *Lancet*, vol i, pp 521-5, 575-80.

[131] Kermack, W.O., McKendrick, A.G. and McKinlay, P.L. (1934) 'Death rates in Great Britain and Sweden: some general regularities and their significance', *Lancet*, vol 226, pp 698-703. (Reprinted in the *International Journal of Epideiology*, 2001, vol 30, pp 678-83.)

[132] Kuh, D. and Davey Smith, G. (1993) 'When is mortality risk determined? Historical insights into a current debate', *Social History of Medicine*, vol 6, pp 101-23.

[133] Hertz-Picciotto, I., Smith, A.H., Holtzman, D., Lipsett, M. and Alexeeff, G. (1992) 'Synergism between occupational arsenic exposure and smoking in the induction of lung cancer', *Epidemiology*, vol 3, pp 23-31.

[134] Erren, T.C., Jacobsen, M. and Piekarski, C. (1999) 'Synergy between asbestos and smoking on lung cancer risks', *Epidemiology*, vol 10, pp 405-11.

[135] Hart, C.L., Hole, D.J., Gillis, C.R., Davey Smith, G. and Watt, G.C.H. (2001) 'Social class differences in lung cancer mortality: risk factor explanations using two Scottish cohort studies', *International Journal of Epidemiology*, vol 30, pp 268-74.

[136] Najman, J.M. and Davey Smith, G. (2000) 'The embodiment of social class and health inequalities policies in Australia', *Australian and New Zealand Journal of Public Health*, vol 24, pp 3-4.

Section I
Patterns of health inequality

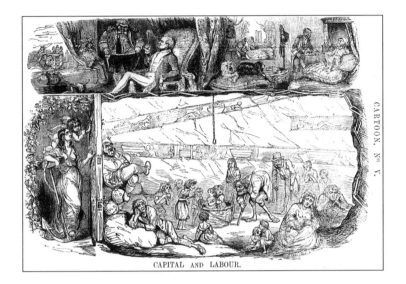

Working conditions in the mines: capital and labour.
The Wellcome Library, London. Reproduced with permission.

1

Health inequalities in Britain: continuing increases up to the end of the 20th century

George Davey Smith, Daniel Dorling, Richard Mitchell and Mary Shaw

Introduction

Socioeconomic inequalities in premature mortality in Britain increased over the second half of the 20th century, particularly from the early 1970s onwards.[1] The magnitude of mortality differentials reflects the trend in income inequality, which has also undergone a dramatic increase over the last quarter century.[1] The present British government has stressed their commitment to reducing health inequalities. For example the Minister for Health, Alan Milburn, has stated that, "Our ambition is to do something that no government – Tory or Labour – has ever done. Not only to improve the health of the nation, but also to improve the health of the worst off at a faster rate".[2] A set of targets for the reduction of health inequalities has been presented. To monitor progress in this regard we have produced updated analyses of premature mortality rates running through to the end of 1999.

Methods

The mortality data are the Office for National Statistics' (ONS) digital records of all deaths in England and Wales, and equivalent records from the General Register Office (Scotland). The full postcode of the usual residence of the deceased was used to assign each death to the parliamentary constituency in which the deceased usually lived. The death data were provided for single years since 1990 and have been grouped into two-year aggregates.

Journal of Epidemiology and Community Health,
2002, vol 56, pp 434-5

Poverty was indexed by a modified version of the Breadline Britain index, based on lack of basic amenities and car access, unskilled and semi-skilled manual occupations, unemployment, non-owner-occupier households and lone-parent households. This is a validated indicator of deprivation.[3] Parliamentary constituencies were ranked according to the poverty measure and divided into equal population size deciles on the basis of this ranking. The same deciles, based on 1991 Census data, are used for each of the time periods. Standardised mortality ratios (SMRs) were calculated separately for men and women for these deciles, using their overall age-specific mortality rates for England and Wales for the periods under consideration.

Population by age group and sex have to be estimated for parliamentary constituencies in the 1990s. The ONS and General Record Office (Scotland) produce mid-year population estimates for years up to 1999 at local authority district level. In order to maintain a geographical base consistent with previous studies of Britain's health gap, these district-level estimates were extrapolated to electoral ward level, and then aggregated to parliamentary constituencies. The interpolation was based on population estimates for 1996 which were available at electoral ward level, and was carried out such that $W_{ij} = (P_{ij} \times C_{ij}) + Y_{ij}$, where W_{ij} is the 1999 ward level population count for age group i and sex j, P_{ij} is the proportion of the 1996 district level population count for age/sex group ij resident in ward W, C_{ij} is the change in district level population count 1996-99 for age/sex group ij from ONS and General Register Office (Scotland) mid-year estimates, and Y_{ij} is the 1996 ward level population count for age/sex group ij.

Results

The age and sex standardised mortality ratios (SMRs) for premature mortality (death before 75) for the period 1990-99 are presented in Table 1, together with the relative index of inequality (RII),[4] which is the relative rate of mortality for the hypothetically poorest compared to the hypothetically richest person in the population, assuming an essentially linear association between poverty and mortality risk. As is apparent from Table 1, the assumption of linearity in this relationship is reasonable.

The RII for mortality increased steadily across the decade. In Table 2 the RII is shown according to age/sex groups.[5] The RIIs are generally greater for men than women and the increase has been more consistent in the former. The inequalities are greatest for older adult men (45-64) but show the greatest increase over time in the younger male age group (20-44). The inequalities are still evident in the age group 65-74, although diminished in magnitude. An increase in inequality over time is, however, seen in this older age group.

Income inequality data[5] are presented in Figure 1. Income inequality increased steadily from the mid–1970s to early 1990s, showed small reversals in the middle of the decade, but has steadily increased from 1997 until the middle of 2000.

Table 1: Age and sex-standardised SMRs (ages 0-74) according to decile of poverty, and the RII

SMR 0-74	1990-91	1992-93	1994-95	1996-97	1998-99
Decile 1	129	132	134	136	138
Decile 2	117	119	118	120	122
Decile 3	110	112	111	113	114
Decile 4	109	109	109	110	111
Decile 5	101	100	100	101	103
Decile 6	96	95	96	95	97
Decile 7	92	91	91	92	92
Decile 8	87	88	87	87	87
Decile 9	85	83	84	84	83
Decile 10	81	81	81	80	80
RII	1.68	1.74	1.75	1.80	1.85

Table 2: RIIs by age group and sex, 1990-99

	1990-91	1992-93	1994-95	1996-97	1998-99
Men					
0-19	1.47	1.62	1.55	1.47	1.62
20-44	1.66	2.04	2.10	1.98	2.20
45-64	2.02	2.09	2.17	2.26	2.39
65-74	1.54	1.57	1.58	1.67	1.69
0-74	1.71	1.78	1.80	1.87	1.95
Women					
0-19	1.47	1.59	1.55	1.46	1.56
20-44	1.48	1.58	1.58	1.62	1.67
45-64	1.76	1.77	1.77	1.86	1.80
65-74	1.57	1.64	1.63	1.63	1.69
0-74	1.63	1.68	1.67	1.70	1.72

Figure 1: Gini coefficients for the distribution of income (1981 to 1999-2000)[5]

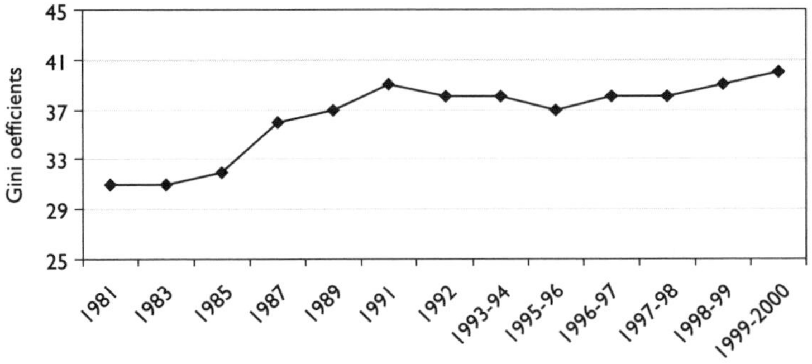

Note: From 1996-97 values are based on estimates for the sample grossed up to population totals.

Discussion

Inequalities in health according to area of residence increased from the 1970s after 20 years of little change,[1] in parallel to changes in income inequality in the population.[1] In this chapter we demonstrate that the increasing trend in mortality inequalities has accelerated from the mid-1990s. This parallels trends in income inequality, which was relatively stable from the early 1990s until 1997 and has now increased. The increase in income inequality since 1997 demonstrates that the underlying economic tendency to widening disparities in income – before tax, benefit and goods-in-kind exchanges have occurred – has a greater influence than the minor attempts at redistribution through fiscal policy which have been implemented.

The increases in inequalities in mortality have been particularly marked for young adults, dramatically so in the case of men. From a perspective which sees health (or inequalities in health) as being determined across the lifecourse,[1] this suggests that continuing increases in mortality differentials at older ages are currently being set in train. This will undermine attempts to reduce inequalities in health and meet the targets which the government has set. Similarly, income inequality increases have been concentrated on families with children,[5] which are generally the ones also containing younger adults. This will also feed into the reproduction across generations of inequalities in both material circumstances and health outcomes.

References

[1] Shaw, M., Dorling, D., Gordon, D. and Davey Smith, G. (1999) *The widening gap: Health inequalities and policy in Britain*, Bristol: The Policy Press.

[2] Milburn, A. (1999) 'Killer that shames Britain', *The Observer*, 12 December, p 13.

[3] Gordon, D. (1995) 'Census based deprivation indices: their weighting and validation', *Journal of Epidemiology and Community Health*, suppl 2, vol 49, pp S39-S44.

[4] **Davey Smith, G., Hart, C., Hole, D., MacKinnon, P., Gillis, C., Watt, G., Blane, D. and Hawthorne, V. (1998) 'Education and occupational social class: which is the more important indicator of mortality risk?', *Journal of Epidemiology and Community Health*, vol 52, pp 153–60.**

[5] Lakin, C. (2001) 'The effects of taxes and benefits on household income, 1999-2000', *Economic Trends*, vol 569, pp 35-74.

2

Shrinking areas and mortality

George Davey Smith, Daniel Dorling and Mary Shaw

Differences in mortality rates according to residential areas have been reported for many years in the UK. Such differences were believed by William Farr 150 years ago[1] to show the "comparative salubrity of every part of England and Wales". A wide range of socioenvironmental factors, including climate, altitude, water constituents, latitude, specific occupational factors, pollution, the long-term effects of development during early life, and deprivation, have been advanced as determinants of the differentials.

An important characteristic of residential areas that has not been investigated in relation to mortality is the change in population because of people moving in and out of them. Areas with unfavourable social and physical environments are the ones people will, if possible, leave to move to more attractive places.[2] We therefore investigated the association between population change and mortality across Britain between 1971 and 1991. We used a previously described database,[3] to calculate the population changes between 1971 and 1991 as percentage increases or decreases. These data include the gold standard population estimates, to protect against shrinking areas seeming to have raised standardised mortality ratios (SMRs) simply because of population under-numeration. We investigated the association between mortality in 1990-92 and population change in the two preceding decades across 292 areas (county boroughs and urban and rural remainders of counties) in Britain (Figure 1).

In places where the population has shrunk, the average mortality is high compared with places in which the population has grown. The correlation between population change and all-cause SMRs was -0.62 ($p<0.001$); for SMRs for the male population, the correlation was -0.68 ($p>0.001$); and for the female population it was -0.50 ($p<0.001$). All correlations were weighted by population size in 1991, but weighting made little difference to the findings. Analysis of male and female cause-specific mortality showed strong correlations between population change and most broad cause-of-death groups (accidental deaths excepted).

Lancet, 1998, vol 352, pp 1439-40

Figure1: Population change (aged under 65) between 1971 and 1991 and absolute change in SMR for deaths under 65 (1991-95 minus 1981-85) for British constituencies

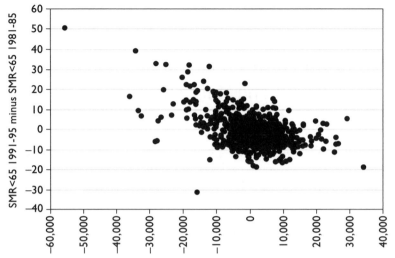

Population change 1971-91 (aged under 65)

To investigate whether the relation between population change and mortality merely reflects differences in degree of deprivation, we calculated partial correlations between all-cause SMRs in men and women together and population changes between 1971 and 1991. The correlation was weakened but remained substantial at −0.49 ($p<0.001$). Finally, we found the correlations between population change between 1971 and 1991 and change in SMRs during 1969-73 and 1990-92 to be −0.37 ($p<0.001$), which suggests that change in population size and change in mortality accompany each other.

Although most studies have tended to focus on economic factors (work and wages), people also move to improve their physical and social environment. The quality of life factors include issues such as cost of living, the image and ambience of a place, available amenities and services, notions of community, crime, pace of life, degrees of pollution, healthcare provision, and quality of housing.[2-4] These factors are thought to underlie differences in health statuses between areas, but they are not adequately indexed by conventional measures of deprivation. The people who remain in shrinking areas need environmental improvement and health services. At present, resources are allocated largely according to population size, and local and health authority budgets have therefore fallen most in these shrinking areas over time. New funding arrangements, such as health action zones,[5] will not reverse this trend.

References

[1]   Britton, M. (1990) 'Introduction', in M. Britton (ed) *Mortality and geography: A review in the mid-1980s*, London: HMSO, pp 1-3.

[2]   Findlay, A. and Rogerson, R. (1993) 'Migration, places and quality of life: voting with their feet?', in T. Champion (ed) *Population matters*, London: Paul Chapman Publishing, pp 33-49.

[3]   Dorling, D. and Atkins, D.J. (1995) *Population density, change and concentration in Great Britain 1971, 1981 and 1991*, Studies in Medical Population Subjects No 58, London: HMSO.

[4]   Boyle, P., Halfacree, K. and Robinson, V. (1998) *Exploring contemporary migration*, Harlow: Longman.

[5]   Jacobson, B. and Yen, L. (1998) 'Health action zones', *British Medical Journal*, vol 316, p 164.

3

Population change and mortality in men and women

George Davey Smith, Mary Shaw and Daniel Dorling

The association between population change and mortality has been investigated for over a century. In the *Supplement to the 35th Annual Report of the Registrar-General (1861-1870)* it was evident that rapidly urbanising areas, with increasing populations, experienced relatively adverse mortality trends, while districts with declining populations did rather better.[1] In 1930 Lewis-Faning[1] showed that between 1860 and 1910 more rapid population growth was associated with declining relative mortality, albeit weakly. These data were taken to suggest that rapid industrialisation and urbanisation had unfavourable health effects during a period when infectious diseases were the most important cause of morbidity and mortality. Conversely Hoffman[2] examined the trend in death rates in large US cities between 1871 and 1904 and demonstrated that the cities with the greater population growth had the lower mortality rate. Thus the influence of population change on mortality appears to be specific in time and place. In Chapter Two we demonstrated that population changed between 1971 and 1991 was inversely correlated with mortality around the 1991 Census across 292 county boroughs and urban and rural remainders of counties in Britain.[3] The correlations between population change and all-cause standardised mortality ratios (SMRs) were -0.68 ($p<0.001$) for men and -0.50 ($p<0.001$) for women. Adjusting for the proportion of the population in semi-skilled and unskilled manual jobs or with unclassified social class in 1991 attenuated the correlations, but they remained substantial. Furthermore the change in SMR between the early 1970s and the early 1990s correlated at -0.37 ($p<0.001$) with the change in population between these times demonstrating that change in population size and change in mortality accompany each other.

Molarius and Janson[4] studied 16 municipalities of the county of Värmland (Sweden) and found a similar correlation between

Journal of Epidemiology and Community Health,
2001, vol 55, p 9

population change and male all-cause mortality, but no correlation with all-cause mortality in women. This may reflect the very small sample size in this ecological study, with there being considerable sampling variation around the estimated correlation coefficients. They also report correlations with particular causes of death, but the problems here of sample size are even greater, and few of these correlations are robust. We have therefore repeated our analysis using population change between 1971 and 1991 and cause-specific mortality for two periods, 1981-89 and 1990-98. As can be seen in Table 1, the correlations with all-cause and cause-specific mortality

Table 1: Correlations between population change 1981-91 and SMRs, weighted by population size

SMR	1981-89	Adjusted[a]	1990-98	Adjusted[a]
Men				
All-cause	−0.70	−0.57	−0.72	−0.61
Stomach cancer	−0.50	−0.30	−0.46	−0.27
Lung cancer	−0.71	−0.59	−0.69	−0.56
Other cancer	−0.57	−0.39	−0.52	−0.30
Alcohol and drugs	−0.46	−0.38	−0.42	−0.29
Chronic heart disease	−0.61	−0.41	−0.69	−0.55
Stroke	−0.62	−0.44	−0.67	−0.53
Other cardiovascular	−0.63	−0.48	−0.58	−0.51
Respiratory	−0.70	−0.58	−0.68	−0.60
Cirrhosis	−0.61	−0.51	−0.68	−0.57
Suicide	−0.39	−0.23	−0.40	−0.16
Other accidents	0.10*	0.24	−0.07*	0.19
All others	−0.66	−0.52	−0.71	−0.59
Women				
All-cause	−0.68	−0.64	−0.66	−0.62
Stomach cancer	−0.37	−0.28	−0.42	−0.34
Lung cancer	−0.63	−0.58	−0.63	−0.58
Breast cancer	0.01*	0.01*	0.20	0.21
Other cancer	−0.32	−0.19	−0.29	−0.16
Alcohol and drugs	−0.39	−0.40	−0.36	−0.33
Chronic heart disease	−0.49	−0.39	−0.60	−0.54
Stroke	−0.52	−0.43	−0.53	−0.44
Other cardiovascular	−0.60	−0.54	−0.58	−0.53
Respiratory	−0.60	−0.54	−0.62	−0.56
Cirrhosis	−0.51	−0.48	−0.57	−0.52
Suicide	−0.49	−0.50	−0.50	−0.44
Other accidents	−0.07*	−0.05*	−0.09*	−0.00*
All others	−0.60	−0.53	−0.61	−0.55

[a] Partial correlations controlling for percentage of the population in social classes IV, V or of unclassified social class.

Note: All correlations are significant at *p* < 0.01 except those marked*.

are similar for the two time periods and show a clear pattern for all-cause, lung cancer, coronary heart disease, stroke, respiratory disease and cirrhosis mortality – which show strong negative correlations only partly attenuated by adjustment for social class composition of areas. For breast cancer, we have failed to confirm the positive correlation of 0.39 (but p = 0.14) found by Molarius and Janson,[4] instead finding a negligible correlation for mortality between 1981 to 1989 and a weak positive correlation for mortality between 1990 and 1998. We hypothesised that mortality from causes related to social fragmentation – in particular due to alcohol and drugs or suicide – would be strongly associated with population change, but these correlations were, if anything, weaker than the correlations with the major causes of death such as cardiovascular disease and lung cancer.

We think that the conclusion of our original study – that the broad range of factors which underlie differences in health status between areas, such as cost of living, the image and ambience of the place, available amenities and services, notions of community, pace of life, degree of pollution, healthcare provision, type of jobs available, quality of housing and safety of traffic – are ones which people clearly recognise as noxious, but that are not automatically incorporated into conventional measures of deprivation. People leave areas with a high prevalence of these factors when they can, so that relative population shrinkage occurs, while at the same time the areas have high mortality rates. The need for resources to be allocated to the most disadvantaged areas both in terms of conventional deprivation measures and the wider aspects of the local environment should be considered.

References

[1] Lewis-Faning, E. (1930) 'A survey of the mortality in Dr Farr's 63 healthy districts of England and Wales during the period 1851-1925', *Journal of Hygiene*, vol 30, pp 121-53.

[2] Hoffman, F.L. (1906) 'The general death-rate of large American cities, 1871-1904', *American Statistical Association*, vol 73, pp 1-69.

[3] **Davey Smith, G., Shaw, M. and Dorling, D. (1998) 'Shrinking areas and mortality', *Lancet*, vol 352, pp 1439-40.**

[4] Molarius, A. and Janson, S. (2000) 'Population change and mortality in men and women', *Journal of Epidemiology and Community Health*, vol 54, p 772.

4

Area-based measures of social and economic circumstances: cause-specific mortality patterns depend on the choice of index

George Davey Smith, Elise Whitley, Daniel Dorling and David Gunnell

Introduction

Indices of deprivation based on the characteristics of areas of residence are widely used in epidemiology and public health, and have a number of possible applications. First, they may be used when data describing an individual's socioeconomic circumstances have not been, or cannot be, collected directly.[1] Second, they may inform the distribution of health service resources, for primary care, community health services and hospital services.[2] Third, in ecological studies examining the effects of local environmental conditions on health they allow investigators to control for possible socioeconomic confounding.[3] Lastly, they can be used when the main analytic interest lies in the effects of characteristics of place of residence on health.[3,5]

Methods and results

Since the particular socioeconomic and demographic characteristics of areas which are related to ill health could differ for different diseases, we have compared how two indices – the Townsend deprivation index and a measure developed by Congdon which has been referred to as an anomie index[4,5] – relate to cause-specific mortality. The first

Journal of Epidemiology and Community Health,
2001, vol 55, pp 149-50

of these indices was developed as a measure of deprivation; the second as a measure of social fragmentation, based on Durkheim's theoretical concept of social integration. Since Durkheim's concept of social integration differs from his notion of anomie, we refer to the Congdon measure as an index of social fragmentation.[7] Mortality data from 1981-92 for 633 parliamentary consistencies of Britain (as defined in 1991) were used. The Townsend deprivation score was based on 1981 and 1991 Census data regarding unemployment, car ownership, overcrowded housing and housing tenure. The social fragmentation index was derived from 1981 and 1991 Census data on private renting, single-person households (aged <65), unmarried persons, and mobility in the previous year. Averages of these scores in 1981 and 1991 were used. The Townsend and social fragmentation index were reasonably strongly correlated; r=0.7. Table 1 presents correlations between the two indices and death from several illustrative causes, with simple correlations and partial correlations – with each index controlled for the other index – being presented.

While both Townsend and anomie indices are associated with all-cause mortality, the association of the former is of considerably greater magnitude. Partial correlation analysis leaves the association between all-cause mortality and Townsend deprivation unchanged, whereas the direction of association with anomie is actually reversed. For three causes of death strongly related to Townsend deprivation – coronary

Table 1: Correlation between indices and SMRs

	Simple correlations		Partial correlations	
	Townsend	Social fragmentation	Townsend	Social fragmentation
Men				
All-cause	0.87	0.46	0.86	−0.40
CHD	0.67	0.13	0.80	−0.60
Stroke	0.67	0.24	0.71	−0.40
Lung cancer	0.84	0.44	0.82	−0.34
Stomach cancer	0.60	0.15	0.69	−0.45
Suicide	0.58	0.71	0.18	0.53
Cirrhosis	0.70	0.67	0.45	0.36
Women				
All-cause	0.82	0.35	0.85	−0.50
CHD	0.66	0.12	0.81	−0.62
Stroke	0.58	0.12	0.68	−0.46
Lung cancer	0.81	0.51	0.73	−0.12
Stomach cancer	0.60	0.15	0.69	−0.45
Suicide	0.38	0.58	−0.04	0.48
Cirrhosis	0.63	0.56	0.40	0.23

heart disease (CHD), stroke and stomach cancer – the associations with social fragmentation are small to moderate and these reverse after controlling for the Townsend deprivation score. For suicide, on the other hand, the association with social fragmentation is of greater magnitude than with Townsend deprivation, a finding amplified in the partial correlation analysis. Cirrhosis mortality is equally related to social fragmentation and Townsend deprivation.

Comment

These findings suggest that socioeconomic and demographic characteristics of areas have specific associations with particular forms of ill health and death. Socioeconomic deprivation is related to overall mortality rates and to cardiovascular disease, lung and stomach cancer mortality – causes of death known to be strongly related to low socioeconomic position. Controlling for social fragmentation has little effect on these associations. Social fragmentation, on the other hand, shows inverse associations with these causes of death once deprivation is controlled for. Suicide – the cause of death most plausibly linked to social disintegration – is more strongly associated with the fragmentation score than with general levels of deprivation. Social fragmentation could be expected to be related to use of legal and prescribed drugs and in these data this appears to be the case for alcohol consumption, as reflected in cirrhosis mortality.

There has been relatively little development of different area-based indices of social circumstances which are hypothesised to have differential influences on particular health outcomes. An exception is the use of historical and current measures of social circumstances, where it has been shown that stroke, stomach cancer and respiratory disease mortality seem to be related to early-life socioeconomic conditions in within-country and cross-national ecological studies,[6,7,8] in agreement with findings from prospective studies of individuals.[9] This correspondence in findings between ecological and individual level studies is suggestive that they reflect underlying causal processes which can be indexed through specific area-based measures (in this case indices relating to social circumstances during early life) or through collecting the relevant information on individuals. The notion that specific social factors are related to particular causes of death has also been examined in time-series analyses, which show plausible differential associations, for example the divorce rate being strongly positively related to suicide and cirrhosis mortality and negatively related to stomach cancer mortality.[10]

Socioeconomic data have been used to provide evidence on a wide variety of human experiences ranking from levels of misery to scales of isolation, the effects of racism, feelings of contentment, freedom, opportunity and general happiness. To continue to simply use socioeconomic data to produce measures of deprivation as a unidimensional and purely cross-sectional phenomenon is to ignore the wealth of other aspects of people's lives that affect their health and are of great potential importance for particular conditions.

References

[1] Danesh, J., Gault, S., Semmence, J. et al (1999) 'Postcodes as useful markers of social class: population based study in 26,000 British households', *British Medical Journal*, vol 318, pp 843-4.

[2] Sheldon, T.A. (1997) 'Formula fever: allocating resources in the NHS', *British Medical Journal*, vol 315, p 964.

[3] MacIntyre, S., MacIver, S. and Sooman, A. (1993) 'Area, class and health: should we be focusing on places or people?', *Journal of Social Policy*, vol 22, pp 213-34.

[4] Congdon, P. (1996) 'Suicide and parasuicide in London: a small-area study', *Urban Studies*, vol 33, pp 137-58.

[5] Whitley, E., Gunnell, D.J., Dorling, D. and Davey Smith, G. (1999) 'Ecological study of social fragmentation, poverty and suicide', *British Medical Journal*, vol 319, pp 1034-7.

[6] Ben-Shlomo, Y. and Davey Smith, G. (1991) 'Deprivation in infancy and in adult life: which is more important for mortality risk?', *Lancet*, vol 337, pp 530-4.

[7] Guallar-Castillon, P., Artalejo, F.R., Banegas, J.R.B. et al (1999) 'Factores ambientales en la vida temprana y nivel socioeconomico en la actualidad', *Medicina Clinica (Barc)*, vol 113, pp 444-6.

[8] Leon, D.A. and Davey Smith, G. (2000) 'Infant mortality, stomach cancer, stroke and coronary heart disease: ecological analysis', *British Medical Journal*, vol 320, pp 1705-6.

[9] **Davey Smith, G., Hart, C., Blane, D. and Hole, D. (1998) 'Adverse socioeconomic conditions in childhood and cause specific adult mortality: prospective observational study', *British Medical Journal*, vol 316, pp 1631-5.**

[10] Leenaaars, A.A. and Lester, D. (1998) 'Social factors and mortality from NASH in Canada', *Crisis*, vol 19, no 2, pp 73-7.

5

Socioeconomic differentials in mortality risk among men screened for the Multiple Risk Factor Intervention Trial: Part I – results for 300,685 white men

George Davey Smith, James D. Neaton,
Deborah Wentworth, Rose Stamler
and Jeremiah Stamler

Abstract

Objectives: This study examined socioeconomic differentials in risk of death from a number of specific causes in a large cohort of white men in the US.

Methods: For 300,685 white men screened for the Multiple Risk Factor Intervention Trial between 1973 and 1975, data were collected on median income of white households in the zipcode of residence, age, cigarette smoking, blood pressure, serum cholesterol, previous myocardial infarction and receipt of drug treatment for diabetes. The 31,737 deaths that occurred over the 16-year follow-up period were grouped into specific causes and related to median white family income.

Results: There was an inverse association between age-adjusted all-cause mortality and median family income. There was no attenuation of this association over the follow-up period and the association was similar for the 22 clinical centres carrying out the screening. The gradient was seen for many – but not all – of the specific causes of death. Other risk factors accounted for some of the association between income and coronary heart disease and smoking-related cancers.

American Journal of Public Health, 1996, vol 86, pp 486-96

Conclusions: Socioeconomic position, as measured by median family income of area of residence, is an important determinant of mortality risk.

Introduction

In 1865 in Providence, Rhode Island, less than one quarter of the population were taxpayers. These individuals constituted the affluent section of Providence society, and, for most age groups, their mortality rates were less than half of those of the less affluent non-taxpayers.[1] Data reported over the following 125 years indicate that socioeconomic position has remained an important predictor of mortality risk in the US[2-13] in a period in which the relative importance of different causes of death has changed dramatically.[14]

The magnitude of the socioeconomic mortality differentials has changed over time in the US, the disparities having increased over the last three decades.[10,11,15,16] While mortality differentials are seen in essentially all of the industrialised countries in which they have been sought,[17,18] their magnitude differs between countries.[19,20] In formal comparisons of the size of mortality differences associated with education level,[20] it appears that larger differentials exist in the US than in several European countries. The geographical and temporal variations in socioeconomic differentials in mortality indicate that their reduction could be achievable, with important gains for the overall health profile of the US.

Previous studies of socioeconomic position and mortality have often originated from government data, in which case no information was generally available regarding characteristics other than age, gender, 'race'/ethnicity and, occasionally, socioeconomic position.[2,4,6,9,12,13] Studies with additional information have tended to deal with relatively small groups of individuals,[8] in which case there were limitations in the ability to examine socioeconomic differentials in risk of mortality from particular causes and/or the shape of the relationship between socioeconomic position and mortality risk. Data for men screened in the early 1970s for the Multiple Risk Factor Intervention Trial (MRFIT), which included a 16-year mortality follow-up, allow for detailed examination of the socioeconomic gradient in mortality risk. Mortality differentials from a wide range of causes can be studied, providing evidence as to the possible etiologic roles of socioeconomic differences in susceptibility to disease in general and of distributions of socially determined adverse exposures.[21]

The contribution of key specific mortality risk factors, including smoking, blood pressure and serum cholesterol, to the mortality differentials can also be investigated. Since income levels varied significantly for white and black men screened,[22] the relationship of income with mortality was investigated separately among black and white men. This report gives the results for white men; a companion report gives findings for black men (see Chapter Six in this volume).[22]

Methods

Methods used to recruit participants and collect baseline data on the men screened have been reported.[23,24] In brief, from November 1973 to November 1975, 361,662 men aged 35 to 57 years were screened at 20 MRFIT centres in 18 cities. Centres used a variety of recruitment methods, including house-to-house canvassing and screening government or industrial employee populations, civic groups, unions and churches.

Name, address, date of birth, self-reported race, social security number and number of cigarettes smoked per day were recorded. Serum cholesterol levels were determined at one of 14 local laboratories with an Auto Analyser II and with standardisation by the Lipid Standardisation Program, Centres for Disease Control in Atlanta.[25] Three blood pressure measurements were taken with a standard mercury sphygmomanometer. Averages of the second and third readings are used in this chapter. Participants also reported whether they had been hospitalised for heart attack, or were taking medication for diabetes. Vital status was determined in December 1990, an average of 16 years of follow-up (range = 15 to 17 years) by matching identifying information obtained from participants at the time of screening with the National Death Index (1979 to 1990) and data files obtained from the Social Security Administration (1973 to 1979). Vital status ascertainment was estimated to be 95% complete.[26] For decedents, death certificates were obtained and coded by a trained nosologist using the ninth revision of the International Classification of Diseases.[27]

The socioeconomic position of each participant, although not recorded at screening, was indexed by matching the participant's postal zipcode with data from the 1980 US Census,[28] this information coming from a period around five to seven years after the screening examinations had been carried out. Median income for families headed by a white householder in the zipcode area of residence is used as an ecologic marker of socioeconomic position. Baseline characteristics and mortality rates for men with known and unknown income data (Table 1) show that the latter had a less favourable risk factor profile and a slightly higher mortality rate than the former. The age-adjusted relative risk of mortality for the group without income data was 1.06 (95% confidence interval [CI]: 1.02-1.11). Adjustment for smoking, diastolic blood pressure, serum cholesterol, prior heart attack and medication for diabetes reversed this association, producing a relative risk of 0.90 (95% CI: 0.86-0.93).

Table 1: Baseline data on white men screened between 1973 and 1975, by availability of income data for zipcode area: MRFIT

	Income data available	Income data not available
Number of men	300,685	24,699
Mean age (years)	46.0	46.2
Cigarette smokers (%)	35.2	45.2
Mean systolic blood pressure (mm Hg)	129.8	131.2
Mean diastolic blood pressure (mm Hg)	83.5	86.6
Mean serum cholesterol (mg/dl)	214.5	220.0
Prior hospitalisation for heart attack (%)	1.5	1.7
Medication for diabetes (%)	1.4	1.3
Age-adjusted death rate (per 10,000 person years)	69.4	74.4

Mortality rates were age-standardised by the direct method, based on the age distribution for the entire study population, and are presented as rates per 10,000 person-years of follow-up. Proportional hazards regression analyses,[29] stratified by the 22 clinical centres (one MRFIT centre had three separate clinics), were performed to compute relative risks. These models included either age alone or age, diastolic blood pressure, serum cholesterol, number of cigarettes smoked per day, history of hospitalisation for heart attack, and medication for diabetes as covariates in examinations of the relationship between income and mortality. In the latter case, essentially all of the available explanatory variables were included. Separate regression models were fit for each clinical centre to examine the consistency of the relationship of income with mortality after adjustment for age among the 22 clinical centres.

For an analysis of risk of total mortality, median income of families headed by white householders was categorised into fifteen $2,000 interval groups ranging from $10,000 to $36,000. For other analyses and analyses of particular causes, median family income was divided into six groups, based on the bottom and top deciles of income, together with quartiles of the men from zipcode areas with median family incomes lying between these levels. These cut-offs were chosen to allow examination of differentials in cause-specific mortality, with manageable tables. For these analyses, the group of men from zipcode areas with the highest median family income were assigned a relative risk of unity.

Regression coefficients are also presented from proportional hazards models in which zipcode area median census tract income was treated as a continuous variable. The negative values of these coefficients were exponentiated to estimate change in risk associated with a $10,000 lower income.

Results

Characteristics of the 300,685 white men for whom zipcodes were available are presented in Table 2 according to income. For the six income groups considered, there were weak trends of lower age and blood pressure with greater income and a very weak trend of higher cholesterol concentration with higher income. Lower prevalence rates of current cigarette smoking, previous heart attack and diabetes with higher income were more pronounced findings. There was a strong correlation between income and other socioeconomic measures available to characterise zipcode areas. In lower income zipcode areas unemployment was higher, the education level and the percentage of individuals in managerial or professional occupations were lower, and more people were below the poverty line.

Table 2: Characteristics of white men screened, by level of median family income for zipcode of residence and characteristics of zipcode areas of residence

	Income ($)[a]					
	<18,571 (n=29,701)	18,571-21,585 (n=58,832)	21,586-24,057 (n=60,932)	24,058-27,372 (n=60,834)	27,373-31,952 (n=59,993)	≥31,953 (n=30,393)
Characteristics of men screened						
Mean age (years)	46.8	46.3	46.0	45.9	45.6	45.9
Mean systolic blood pressure (mm Hg)	131.1	131.2	130.2	129.1	128.8	127.9
Mean diastolic blood pressure (mm Hg)	84.2	84.0	83.6	83.1	83.1	82.7
Mean serum cholesterol (mg/dl)	214.0	213.9	214.8	214.2	214.9	215.4
Cigarette smokers (%)	40.6	38.7	37.1	34.6	31.0	28.5
Cigarettes per day for smokers (mean)	27.2	26.8	26.9	26.8	26.1	26.2
Prior hospitalisation for heart attack (%)	1.8	1.8	1.5	1.5	1.3	1.0
Medication for diabetes (%)	1.9	1.7	1.4	1.3	1.2	1.0
Population characteristics of zipcode areas[a]						
Unemployment (%)	4.6	3.7	3.4	2.8	2.3	2.0
Average years of schooling	13.1	13.6	14.0	14.4	14.8	15.4
Managerial or professional occupations (%)	6.4	8.9	11.3	14.1	17.4	22.7
Below the poverty line (%)	12.2	6.3	4.4	3.1	2.2	1.9

[a] Based on data from the 1980 US Census.

All-cause mortality

Over the 16 years of follow-up, 31,737 deaths were identified among the 300,685 men in the cohort. Mortality rates and relative risk estimates, according to median zipcode area family income (henceforth 'income') categorised into 14 groups, are presented in Table 3.

The relationship between income and mortality is similar among smokers and non-smokers – the change in risk associated with a $10,000 lower income were 1.22 (95% CI: 1.19-1.26) for smokers and 1.18 (95% CI: 1.15-1.22) for non-smokers. The graded association between income and mortality was also similar by age; relative risks associated with a $10,000 lower income were 1.17 (95% CI: 1.12-1.23) for men 35 to 44 years old at screening, 1.20 (95% CI: 1.16-1.23) for men 45 to 54 years old at screening, and 1.16 (95% CI: 1.11-1.21) for those 55 to 57 years old at screening.

Cumulative mortality over the follow-up period for six income groups, presented in Figure 1, demonstrates that the differentials persisted over time. Cumulative mortality at 15 years for men in the six income groups (lowest to highest) was 12.7%, 10.9%, 9.8%, 8.9%, 7.9% and 7.4%.

There was a considerable range in income both within and between clinical centres among the white men screened. This permitted an

Table 3: All-cause mortality among white men screened, by level of median family income for zipcode of residence

Income ($)	Number of men	Number of deaths	Age-adjusted rate[a]	Age-adjusted relative risk (95% CI)	Age- and risk factor-adjusted relative risk (95% CI)
≤10,000	3,541	525	91.8	1.75 (1.56-1.96)	1.55 (1.38-1.74)
10,000-11,999	6,312	882	87.6	1.67 (1.51-1.85)	1.47 (1.33-1.62)
12,000-13,999	16,545	2,258	86.5	1.62 (1.49-1.77)	1.44 (1.32-1.56)
14,000-15,999	28,136	3,501	78.9	1.50 (1.39-1.63)	1.35 (1.24-1.47)
16,000-17,999	37,931	4,595	78.2	1.49 (1.37-1.61)	1.36 (1.25-1.47)
18,000-19,999	42,430	4,564	70.1	1.33 (1.23-1.44)	1.23 (1.14-1.33)
20,000-21,999	50,644	5,174	68.1	1.31 (1.21-1.42)	1.22 (1.13-1.32)
22,000-23,999	39,704	3,901	64.5	1.25 (1.15-1.35)	1.18 (1.09-1.28)
24,000-25,999	24,921	2,226	61.9	1.19 (1.09-1.30)	1.13 (1.04-1.23)
26,000-27,999	19,681	1,702	59.0	1.15 (1.06-1.26)	1.13 (1.03-1.23)
28,000-29,999	13,631	1,093	56.5	1.10 (1.00-1.21)	1.07 (0.97-1.20)
30,000-31,999	7,971	680	58.2	1.10 (0.99-1.23)	1.08 (0.97-1.20)
32,000-33,999	4,709	357	51.9	1.01 (0.89-1.15)	1.00 (0.88-1.13)
34,000+	8,943	709	51.4	1.00 (Reference)	1.00 (Reference)

[a] Per 10,000 person years.

Note: Family income levels were based on data from the 1980 US Census. Risk factors were diastolic blood pressure, serum cholesterol level, cigarettes per day, prior hospitalisation for heart attack, and medication for diabetes.

Figure 1: Cumulative morality among white men screened, for six income categories

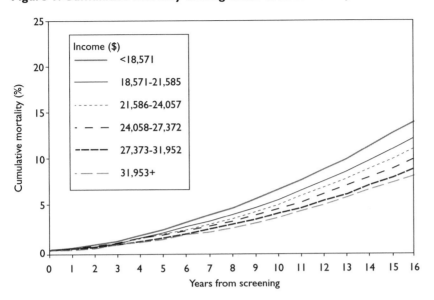

estimate of the relationship between income and mortality to be obtained for each centre. Figure 2 plots adjusted relative risk estimates and 95% confidence intervals for all-cause mortality corresponding to a $10,000 lower income. These estimates were all greater than one (range 1.12-1.55), and the association was significant at $p<0.05$ in 21 of 22 centres.

Cause-specific mortality

Mortality data for specific causes of death are presented in Tables 4 through 6. For each cause the tables show age-adjusted and risk-factor adjusted relative risks. While risks of most causes of death increased with decreasing income, there was considerable heterogeneity in the strength of these relationships. Table 7 summarises this, by presenting relative risks of mortality adjusted for age and for both age and risk factors, associated with a $10,000 lower income for both broad cause of death groups and individual causes.

The degree to which adjustment for risk factors attenuated the income–mortality associations was greatest for cardiovascular causes of death and smoking-related cancers, reflecting that the limited set of risk factors measured was most applicable to the aetiology of these conditions. For example, the relative risks associated with a $10,000 lower income was reduced from 1.25 to 1.16 for coronary heart disease after adjustment for other risk factors. For non-haemorrhagic stroke, this relative risk declined from 1.43 to 1.31. For lung cancer, the relative risk declined from 1.40 to 1.27 as a consequence of the larger percentage of men who reported using cigarettes in the lower income as compared to higher income groups.

Figure 2: Relative risk of death associated with a $10,000 lower income among white men screened in each of 22 clinical centres

Clinical centre	Number of white men	Number of deaths
Baltimore	11,963	1,407
New York	15,973	1,587
Minneapolis	29,680	3,072
San Fransisco	13,098	1,272
St Louis	16,290	1,574
Boston (Harvard)	11,960	1,145
Davis	16,537	1,792
Chicago (Northwestern)	5,237	521
Chicago (St Joseph's)	4,501	514
Chicago (University)	2,513	297
Portland	12,550	1,303
Boston (University)	11,550	1,130
Dayton	17,474	1,907
Newark	18,834	2,012
Philadelphia	15,085	1,409
Birmingham	18,424	2,016
Pittsburgh	18,463	2,581
Chicago (Rush)	13,155	1,166
Piscataway (Rutgers)	16,685	1,695
Columbia	10,063	1,189
Los Angeles	12,989	1,207
Miami	7,661	941
All centres	300,685	31,737

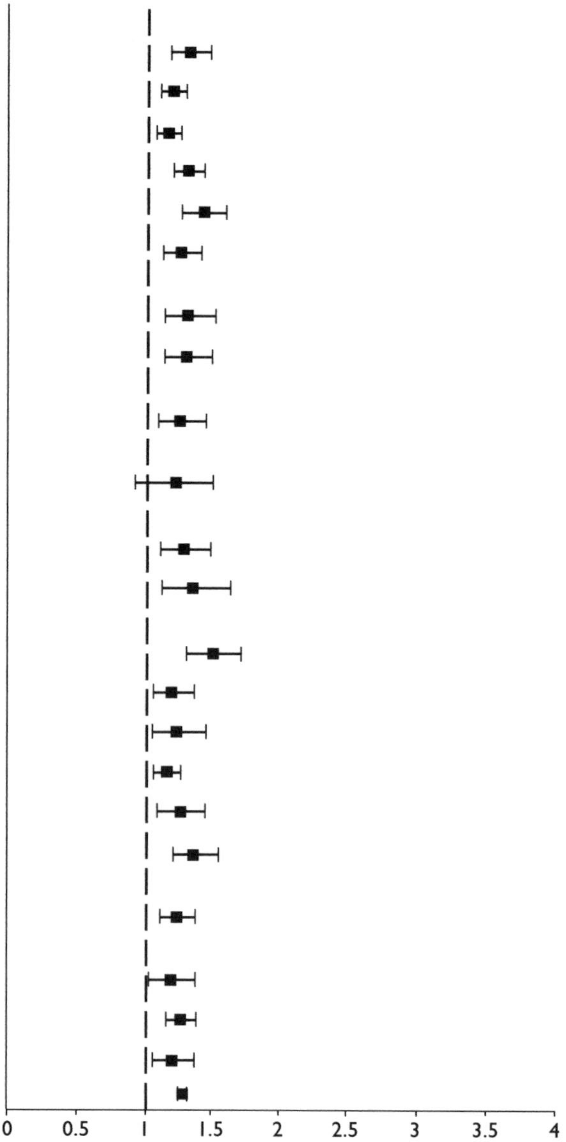

Table 4: Relative risk estimates, adjusted for age and all risk factors, of all-cause and cardiovascular disease mortality among white men screened, by level of median family income for zipcode of residence

Cause of death (Number of deaths)	<18,571	Income ($) 18,571- 21,585	21,586- 24,057	24,058- 27,372	27,373- 31,952	≥ 31,953
All causes (31,737)						
Age	1.59**	1.41**	1.32**	1.22**	1.10**	1.00
Risk factors	1.41**	1.28**	1.22**	1.15**	1.07**	1.00
Coronary heart disease (10,579)						
Age	1.62**	1.47**	1.37**	1.25**	1.16**	1.00
Risk factors	1.39**	1.30**	1.24**	1.16**	1.11*	1.00
Stroke (986)						
Age	1.63**	1.26	1.08	1.01	0.85	1.00
Risk factors	1.39**	1.11	0.98	0.94	0.82	1.00
Intracranial haemorrhage (265)						
Age	1.04	1.24	0.69	0.83	0.70	1.00
Risk factors	0.91	1.11	0.63	0.78	0.68	1.00
Nonhaemorrhagic stroke (560)						
Age	2.39**	1.54*	1.47*	1.31	0.98	1.00
Risk factors	2.01**	1.35	1.33	1.22	0.94	1.00
Other cardiovascular disease (2,537)						
Age	1.65**	1.35**	1.25*	1.24*	1.09	1.00
Risk factors	1.45**	1.22*	1.15	1.17	1.06	1.00
All cardiovascular disease (14,102)						
Age	1.63**	1.43**	1.33**	1.23**	1.12**	1.00
Risk factors	1.40**	1.27**	1.21**	1.15**	1.08*	1.00

Note: Family income levels were based on data from the 1980 US Census. Risk factors were diastolic blood pressure, serum cholesterol level, cigarettes per day, prior hospitalisation for heart attack, and medication for diabetes, as well as age; these were included in the regression model as covariates.

*p<0.05; **p<0.01.

Table 5: Relative risk estimates, adjusted for age and all risk factors, of cancer mortality among white men screened, by level of median family income for zipcode of residence

Cause of death (number of deaths)	<18,571	Income ($) 18,571- 21,585	21,586- 24,057	24,058- 27,372	27,373- 31,952	≥ 31,953
Oesophagus (309)						
Age	1.64	1.32	1.47	1.56	1.26	1.00
Risk factors	1.50	1.23	1.39	1.49	1.23	1.00
Stomach (437)						
Age	1.31	1.05	1.02	0.99	1.02	1.00
Risk factors	1.23	0.99	0.98	0.96	1.00	1.00
Colon (1,192)						
Age	1.50**	1.27	1.21	1.25	1.01	1.00
Risk factors	1.50**	1.26	1.20	1.25	1.00	1.00
Rectum (204)						
Age	1.98*	1.30	1.63	1.37	0.94	1.00
Risk factors	1.98*	1.30	1.63	1.37	0.94	1.00
Pancreas (658)						
Age	1.14	1.19	1.12	1.13	0.96	1.00
Risk factors	1.06	1.13	1.07	1.09	0.95	1.00
Lung (3,729)						
Age	1.76**	1.79**	1.66**	1.41**	1.12	1.00
Risk factors	1.49**	1.57**	1.48**	1.30**	1.12	1.00
Melanoma (293)						
Age	0.53*	0.81	0.79	1.00	0.89	1.00
Risk factors	0.52*	0.80	0.79	0.99	0.88	1.00
Prostate (658)						
Age	1.23	1.34	1.10	1.16	1.20	1.00
Risk factors	1.19	1.31	1.08	1.15	1.19	1.00
Brain (485)						
Age	1.03	0.87	1.06	0.82	0.82	1.00
Risk factors	1.03	0.87	1.06	0.82	0.82	1.00
Lymphatic (529)						
Age	0.91	0.91	0.87	0.76	0.97	1.00
Risk factors	0.89	0.89	0.86	0.75	0.97	1.00
Haematopoietic (583)						
Age	1.38	1.22	1.23	1.16	1.10	1.00
Risk factors	1.34	1.19	1.21	1.14	1.09	1.00
All cancer (11,111)						
Age	1.38**	1.32**	1.26**	1.17**	1.03	1.00
Risk factors	1.26**	1.23**	1.18**	1.12**	1.02	1.00

Note: Family income levels were based on data from the 1980 US Census. Risk factors were diastolic blood pressure, serum cholesterol level, cigarettes per day, prior hospitalisation for heart attack, and medication for diabetes, as well as age; these were included in the regression model as covariates.

*p<0.05; **p<0.01.

Table 6: Relative risk estimates, adjusted for age and all risk factors, of noncardiovascular, noncancer causes of death among white men screened, by level of median family income for zipcode of residence

Cause of death (Number of deaths)	<18,571	18,571- 21,585	21,586- 24,057	24,058- 27,372	27,373- 31,952	≥ 31,953
			Income ($)			
Infection (351)						
Age	1.73*	1.37	1.53*	0.79	0.77	1.00
Risk factors	1.65*	1.32	1.48*	0.77	0.76	1.00
AIDS (178)						
Age	2.13 **	1.56	2.15**	0.67	0.49	1.00
Risk factors	2.02 *	1.54	2.10**	0.68	0.50	1.00
Diabetes (402)						
Age	5.22**	3.72**	2.54**	2.16**	2.07*	1.00
Risk factors	3.66**	2.86**	2.00*	1.81*	1.86*	1.00
Respiratory (1,270)						
Age	2.47**	1.94**	1.78**	1.36*	1.36	1.00
Risk factors	2.13**	1.73**	1.62**	1.27	1.35*	1.00
Chronic obstructive pulmonary disease (677)						
Age	2.70**	2.24**	1.95**	1.40	1.45	1.00
Risk factors	2.30**	1.98**	1.76**	1.30	1.46	1.00
Pneumonia and influenza (345)						
Age	2.46**	1.83*	1.35	1.25	1.14	1.00
Risk factors	2.15**	1.65*	1.23	1.17	1.11	1.00
Other respiratory (248)						
Age	2.06*	1.48	2.07*	1.52	1.55	1.00
Risk factors	1.89	1.38	1.96*	1.47	1.54	1.00
Digestive (1,047)						
Age	2.21**	1.71**	1.83**	1.47**	1.37*	1.00
Risk factors	1.89**	1.51**	1.66**	1.37*	1.33*	1.00
Cirrhosis (603)						
Age	2.25**	1.84**	1.94**	1.61*	1.59*	1.00
Risk factors	1.91**	1.62*	1.76**	1.50*	1.55*	1.00
Other digestive (444)						
Age	2.16**	1.56*	1.70*	1.31	1.10	1.00
Risk factors	1.85**	1.38	1.54*	1.21	1.08	1.00
Symptoms, signs and ill-defined conditions (227)						
Age	2.08*	1.82*	1.32	1.27	0.92	1.00
Risk factors	1.85*	1.65	1.22	1.19	0.90	1.00
Violent causes (1,933)						
Age	1.73**	1.39**	1.22*	1.23*	1.14	1.00
Risk factors	1.61**	1.31**	1.16	1.18	1.13	1.00
Accidents (1,073)						
Age	1.63**	1.29	1.15	1.13	1.04	1.00
Risk factors	1.53*	1.23	1.10	1.09	1.03	1.00
Suicide (705)						
Age	1.61**	1.40*	1.29	1.40*	1.35	1.00
Risk factors	1.47*	1.30	1.21	1.34	1.33	1.00
Homicide (153)						
Age	3.15**	2.22*	1.38	1.24	0.91	1.00
Risk factors	2.90**	2.09*	1.32	1.19	0.90	1.00
All noncancer, noncardiovascular disease (6,168)						
Age	1.96**	1.58**	1.47**	1.28**	1.20**	1.00
Risk factors	1.74**	1.44**	1.36**	1.21**	1.17**	1.00

Note: Family income levels were based on data from the 1980 US Census. Risk factors were diastolic blood pressure, serum cholesterol level, cigarettes per day, prior hospitalisation for heart attack, and medication for diabetes, as well as age; these were included in the regression model as covariates. *p<0.05; **p<0.01.

Table 7: Relative risks of mortality associated with a $10,000 lower median income of zipcode of residence for white men screened

Cause (ICD-9 Code or Codes)	Age-adjusted relative risk (95% CI)	Age- and risk factor-adjusted relative risk (95% CI)
Broad cause groups		
All-causes	1.26 (1.23, 1.28)	1.18 (1.16, 1.21)
Cancer	1.21 (1.16, 1.25)	1.15 (1.11, 1.19)
Cardiovascular disease	1.26 (1.22, 1.30)	1.17 (1.13, 1.21)
Noncancer, noncardiovascular disease	1.36 (1.29, 1.43)	1.28 (1.22, 1.34)
Specific causes		
Infection (1-139)	1.35 (1.12, 1.62)	1.31 (1.09, 1.58)
AIDS (42-4)	1.57 (1.22, 2.01)	1.52 (1.19, 1.95)
Oesophageal cancer (150)	1.20 (0.96, 1.48)	1.15 (0.93, 1.42)
Stomach cancer (151)	1.13 (0.94, 1.35)	1.09 (0.91, 1.31)
Colon cancer (153)	1.23 (1.10, 1.37)	1.22 (1.10, 1.37)
Rectal cancer (154)	1.25 (0.96, 1.64)	1.25 (0.96, 1.64)
Liver cancer (155)	1.35 (1.00, 1.83)	1.27 (0.94, 1.72)
Pancreatic cancer (157)	1.17 (1.01, 1.35)	1.13 (0.98, 1.30)
Lung cancer (162)	1.40 (1.31, 1.50)	1.27 (1.19, 1.36)
Bone cancer, connective tissue (170, 171)	0.95 (0.66, 1.37)	0.93 (0.65, 1.34)
Melanoma (172)	0.86 (0.71, 1.05)	0.86 (0.70, 1.04)
Prostate cancer (185)	1.11 (0.96, 1.27)	1.09 (0.95, 1.26)
Bladder cancer (191)	1.13 (0.85, 1.50)	1.08 (0.82, 1.43)
Kidney cancer (189)	1.01 (0.84, 1.22)	0.97 (0.80, 1.16)
Brain cancer (191)	1.04 (0.88, 1.23)	1.04 (0.88, 1.23)
Unspecified cancer (195-9)	1.13 (0.99, 1.29)	1.07 (0.94, 1.23)
Lymphatic cancer (200-2)	0.95 (0.81, 1.11)	0.94 (0.80, 1.10)
Hodgkin's disease (201)	0.91 (0.53, 1.57)	0.88 (0.51, 1.52)
Hematopoietic cancer (203-8)	1.16 (1.00, 1.26)	1.15 (0.98, 1.34)
Myeloma (203)	1.19 (0.89, 1.59)	1.17 (0.88, 1.55)
Leukemia (204-8)	1.15 (0.96, 1.38)	1.14 (0.95, 1.37)
Diabetes (250)	1.94 (1.57, 2.39)	1.62 (1.31, 1.99)
Diseases of the blood (280-9)	0.92 (0.66, 1.29)	0.89 (0.63, 1.24)
Diseases of the nervous system (320-89)	1.16 (0.95, 1.42)	1.14 (0.94, 1.39)
Motor neuron disease (335.2)	0.97 (0.68, 1.37)	0.95 (0.67, 1.34)
Rheumatic heart disease (390-8)	1.52 (0.98, 2.38)	1.52 (0.98, 2.37)
Coronary heart disease (410-14, 429.2)	1.25 (1.21, 1.30)	1.16 (1.12, 1.21)
Heart failure (428)	1.71 (1.24, 2.37)	1.57 (1.14, 2.18)
Stroke (430-8)	1.26 (1.12, 1.43)	1.17 (1.10, 1.23)
Intracranial haemorrhage (431-2)	1.14 (0.91, 1.42)	1.06 (0.85, 1.33)
Nonhaemorrhagic stroke (433-8)	1.43 (1.21, 1.69)	1.31 (1.11, 1.55)
Aortic aneurysm (441)	1.10 (0.90, 1.34)	1.01 (0.83, 1.24)
Respiratory (460-519)	1.56 (1.39, 1.75)	1.44 (1.28, 1.61)
Chronic obstructive pulmonary disease (460-96)	1.62 (1.38, 1.91)	1.47 (1.25, 1.72)
Pneumonia and influenza (480-7)	1.70 (1.37, 2.11)	1.59 (1.28, 1.97)
Digestive (520-79)	1.40 (1.24, 1.57)	1.28 (1.14, 1.45)
Cirrhosis (571)	1.36 (1.16, 1.58)	1.25 (1.07, 1.46)

cont.../

Table 7: contd.../

Cause (ICD-9 Code or Codes)	Age-adjusted relative risk (95% CI)	Age- and risk factor-adjusted relative risk (95% CI)
Genitourinary (580-629)	1.50 (1.11, 2.03)	1.39 (1.03, 1.88)
Symptoms, signs, etc (780-99)	1.48 (1.14, 1.92)	1.40 (1.08, 1.81)
Violent causes (800-999)	1.27 (1.17, 1.39)	1.23 (1.12, 1.34)
Accidents (800-919)	1.28 (1.14, 1.43)	1.24 (1.10, 1.39)
Flying accidents (840-3)	0.50 (0.31,0.79)	0.50 (0.31, 0.80)
Suicide (950-9, 980-9)	1.17 (1.01, 1.34)	1.11 (0.97, 1.28)
Homicide (960-9)	2.10 (1.51, 2.91)	2.00 (1.44, 2.78)

Note: Income levels were based on data from the 1980 US Census. Risk factors were diastolic blood pressure, serum cholesterol level, cigarettes per day, prior hospitalisation for heart attach, and medication for diabetes, as well as age. ICD-9 = International Classification of Diseases, Ninth Revision. CI = confidence interval.

Discussion

The cohort of men screened for the MRFIT provides a powerful database for study of the magnitude and causes of socioeconomic differentials in mortality. The differentials were of large magnitude and were seen for many – but not all – causes of death. There are, however, two major concerns regarding the data. The first relates to the degree to which the associations between socioeconomic position and mortality risk in the sample can be considered representative of the associations in the white population of the US at large. While, for some centres, it is possible to calculate response rates from employment group surveys,[30] this cannot be done generally, nor can participants recruited through different mechanisms be analysed separately. However, the consistency of the association of income with all-cause mortality for each of the 22 screening clinical centres provides evidence against the possibility that recruitment of men with both different average incomes and different mortality risks at the various screening centres underlies the observed relationships, and indicates that the results may be widely generalisable among US white men.

An external check on how representative the associations between income and mortality found in the MRFIT comes from a comparison with the equivalent associations seen in the National Longitudinal Mortality Study (NLMS).[12] The latter provides five-year follow-up data relating family income – applicable to the individuals themselves, not to their area of residence – to mortality for a representative sample of 155,346 white males aged 35-64 years at study entry.

There were 6,842 deaths among these men during follow-up, and standardised mortality ratios (SMRs) for that study are presented together with MRFIT data in Table 8. The trial cohort was divided into groups of equivalent size to those in the NLMS for comparison.

Table 8: Comparison of income–mortality associations in the MRFIT and the NLMS

Income group ($)	% population	SMRs[a] in NLMS	Age-adjusted relative risk in MRFIT (95% CI)
≤18,950	12.2	167	1.56 (1.48, 1.65)
18,951-21,062	12.3	122	1.44 (1.37, 1.52)
21,063-22,612	13.9	97	1.33 (1.26, 1.40)
22,613-24,827	16.2	87	1.29 (1.23, 1.36)
24,828-32,804	36.9	80	1.14 (1.09, 1.20)
32,805+	8.4	66	1.00

[a] SMR = 100 for total NLMS population.

Note: In the MRFIT, participants were 35 to 57 years of age at baseline; in the NLMS, participants were 35 to 64 years of age at baseline.

When analysed by equivalent group size, the mortality differentials between income groups are somewhat wider in the NLMS than in the MRFIT study.

However, when the range of mortality differentials in the MRFIT study presented in Table 3 are compared to those in the NLMS, they are similar. This suggests that the MRFIT data provide a good model for socioeconomic differentials in mortality in the general population in relative terms, but underestimate the absolute effect of these differentials because of under-representation of low income men.

A second concern relates to the use of an ecological index of socioeconomic position, median family income for zipcode area of residence. The fact that the income data relate to 1980 rather than the time of the survey (five to seven years earlier) is probably a minor concern; while changes occur in the characteristics of neighbourhoods, this is unlikely to seriously influence their ranking in terms of income of resident families in the period. If the actual family income of the participant is considered to be the underlying socioeconomic variable of interest, then the use of the ecological indicator could be seen as a source of misclassification. The relatively large populations of the zipcode areas – as compared with the census tracts or blocks often used in US studies – may lead to some attenuation of the underlying mortality differentials, due to the heterogeneity of socioeconomic level within individual zipcode areas. However, the similarity of the income–mortality gradients in the MRFIT study and studies in which income has been categorised at the level of the individual participant,[12,31] suggests that personal family income and median family income of the zipcode area of residence function in a similar manner as discriminators of mortality risk. Census-based data have been compared directly to individual socioeconomic indicators as predictors of health and health-related behaviours in US[32] and British[33] studies, the findings of which attest to the robustness of the area-based methodology.

The use of ecological indices of socioeconomic position has a long tradition in both the US[3,7,34,35] and the UK.[36-38] As well as median income, these indicators have included factors such as level of education, tenure and quality of housing, car ownership and the unemployment rate of areas. Ecological measures may, in some circumstances, provide more stable information regarding socioeconomic position than individual-based socioeconomic data. First, consider the situation of temporary loss of earnings of a family member around the time individual-level data were collected. This would lead to reduced family income, but not to a change of the ecological measure, the median family income of zipcode area of residence. In this case the ecological measure would be a better indicator of the usual socioeconomic circumstances of the study participant than individual-based data.

Second, family incomes in studies such as the NLMS are not adjusted for size of the family; therefore the same level of family income would have a different relationship to the actual economic circumstances of the individuals involved, depending on the size of the family and number of dependants. For a given level of family income, large families will generally be in worse economic circumstances than small families. This will be reflected in the area of residence in which the family can afford to live. Again, in this respect the ecological measure may be a better index of actual economic circumstances than the individual-based measure.

Third, even at a given level of personal family income there are many factors related to the physical and sociocultural environment of the area of residence, and thus to the median family income of the zipcode area, which could influence health.[39] In the Alameda County study, for example, it was shown that residents of 'poverty areas' experienced elevated mortality rates even after statistical adjustment for income, education, ethnicity, health status at study entry, availability of healthcare and a host of behavioural factors considered detrimental to health.[8]

In broad terms, the income differentials in mortality due to specific causes are similar in the MRFIT cohort and in the representative sample in the NLMS.[12] However, the smaller number of deaths in the NLMS in the equivalent age bands to the MRFIT cohort gives lower power for detailed examination of these associations. Furthermore, data on behavioural and physiological risk factors for mortality, available in the MRFIT screening study, are unavailable in the NLMS.

A striking finding from both this investigation and from the NLMS[12] is the graded and continuous nature of the association between income and mortality, with the differentials persisting into relatively privileged groups. This fine stratification of mortality risk has also been demonstrated in studies carried out in the UK and Canada.[18,31,40-43] The fact that socioeconomic differentials in mortality are not confined to groups which are, in any straightforward sense, materially deprived, presents a serious challenge to any simple interpretations couched in terms of absolute poverty.

The degree to which socioeconomic differentials in health are in some ways artefactual – that is, produced by the ways in which data are collected and analysed – has been debated.[44-47] In particular, the manner in which causes of death are coded could be related to the socioeconomic position of the deceased. This is likely to occur with respect to the category of symptoms, signs and ill-defined conditions (International Classification of Diseases, codes 780-99), which displays a marked gradient with income in the present study. Similarly, this category is used more frequently for deaths occurring among minority populations than among white people in the US.[48] However, such an excess of poorly categorised deaths among lower-income men is unlikely to greatly dilute the income–mortality associations for other causes, since a very small proportion of deaths end up with unspecified attribution.

In the UK an empirical study of cause of death coding in relation to social class demonstrated that, with regard to broad cause groups, social class differentials in mortality are not greatly affected by bias in cause of death coding.[49,50] In a large study of the accuracy of death certificate data for cancer mortality, carried out in the US,[51] the degree of misclassification between cancer sites is such that it is unlikely to account for differences in associations between income and particular cancers reported here. It could be, however, that in certain cases – such as with AIDS – differences in access to health services according to income level influence the manner in which cause of death is classified.

Socioeconomic differentials in mortality could be produced by health-related social mobility, if ill health leads to a worsening of socioeconomic position. The role of such health-related social selection in producing socioeconomic health differentials has been widely discussed,[45,46,52-54] but current evidence suggests that, at least acting in a direct manner, it has a relatively small influence on the magnitude of the differentials.[55]

Two aspects of the present study have a bearing on this. First, as discussed above, the area-based measure of socioeconomic position, median family income of place of residence, is less affected by loss of earnings due to poor health than an individually based measure. Therefore the socioeconomic indicator used in this study is protected, to an extent, from the influence of health-related social selection. Second, mortality differentials generated by health-related social selection would be expected to be greatest early in the follow-up period. This is because sick men who suffer downward social mobility have an elevated mortality risk. Their high rate of death removes them from the study population, so at each successive follow-up period they have less influence on mortality differentials.[56] In a mortality follow-up of a 1% sample from the 1971 Census in England and Wales it was demonstrated that socioeconomic differentials in mortality did not decrease with follow-up time, a finding which was interpreted as demonstrating that the role of health-related social mobility in producing socioeconomic differentials in mortality was small.[56] In this investigation, mortality differentials by income group also show no tendency to decrease as the time from screening increases (Figure 1).

The present study could not examine the influence on mortality risk of socioeconomic position in early life, or changes in social position from early childhood to adulthood. In the National Longitudinal Survey of Labor Market Experience of Mature Men, data are available on socioeconomic position at various stages of the life cycle.[57] Within the constraints of this small study (around 1,500 deaths occurring in a cohort of 5,000 men), the extent of family assets during middle-age are inversely associated with mortality risk, in line with the findings of the present study. However, level of education and first occupation on entry into the labour market have an influence on mortality which is apparently distinct from that of family assets. This highlights the need to consider socioeconomic careers, rather than socioeconomic position at one point in time, in future studies.

The degree to which known risk factors account for income differentials in mortality was examined through stratification and through statistical adjustment. Smoking is an important behavioural risk factor for mortality from a variety of causes and men in lower income groups were more likely to report smoking cigarettes. The stratification into smokers and non-smokers demonstrates that income–mortality risk gradients are similar for smokers and non-smokers. Similarly, even after adjustment for smoking and other risk factors, a $10,000 lower income was associated with a 18% higher mortality. While lack of data on lifetime smoking patterns does not permit separation of non-smokers into never and ex-smoking groups, other studies in which such data are available attest to the robustness of this finding.[40,47,58]

For some causes of death – notably coronary heart disease and lung cancer – adjustment for risk factors led to quite substantial attenuation of the excess mortality among lower income groups. This is not surprising since the risk factors measured at screening related to these diseases in particular. It is probable that the residual associations, seen after risk factor adjustment, are at least partially due to inaccuracy inherent in using single measurements of the risk factors that were measured.[59-62] Thus more detailed information on smoking behaviour and blood pressure would allow for better statistical adjustment for these risk factors, with the degree of attribution of income differentials in mortality to these factors consequently becoming more evident.

However, in the case of serum cholesterol, the lower cholesterol levels in the lower income groups should produce a gradient in coronary heart disease risk in the opposite direction to that actually seen. If the lower serum cholesterol in the lower income men were a lifelong phenomenon, rather than just a property of middle-age, better measurement of serum cholesterol and improved statistical adjustment would actually lead to magnification, rather than attenuation, of the inverse relationship between income and coronary heart disease risk.

It is also the case that the socioeconomic differentials in mortality could be more marked if better indicators of socioeconomic position than median family income of zipcode areas of residence were available. In a study of civil servants in London it was shown that improved characterisation of socioeconomic position, through the use of multiple indicators, led to the demonstration of mortality differentials which were considerably wider than those seen when less precise measures were used.[40] In this study, the large socioeconomic differentials in coronary heart disease mortality could only partly be accounted for by differences in smoking, blood pressure, cholesterol, glucose intolerance, physical activity, height and prevalent disease.[40,63] More detailed information on both known risk factors (including alcohol consumption, obesity, physical inactivity and diet) and socioeconomic position is required if the degree to which the former account for coronary heart disease and lung cancer mortality differentials is to be elucidated further.

The degree to which known risk factors 'explain' socioeconomic differentials in mortality should not be taken as a measure of reduced intrinsic importance of the differentials. The fact that smoking accounts for some of the difference in mortality rates between the income groups does not mean that social causes are themselves less important. Smoking – like alcohol use, exercise and diet – does not occur in a social vacuum. The reason why smoking breaks the rule that households with low incomes cope by decreasing the personal expenditure of adults cannot be reduced to personal failure. In constrained economic circumstances smoking can be one of the few activities undertaken for personal pleasure and one that provides some respite from the strain of coping with the consequences of material deprivation.[64] Similarly, in poorer areas less healthy food is available and is often more expensive.[65] The determination of socially patterned behaviours should be seen as part of the process generating socioeconomic differentials in health, not as a reason for considering social interventions unnecessary.[66,67]

In this investigation, for most causes of death, risk factor adjustment had little effect on the mortality differentials according to income group. This reflects lack of measurement of etiological factors – either because they were not included in the study or, more commonly, because they were not known – for most of these conditions.

It has been argued that unfavourable socioeconomic environments increase the susceptibility to disease in general[68-72] and the potential biological mechanisms of stress-related immune suppression and neuroendocrine activation have been advanced to account for this phenomenon.[73,74] Within the general pattern of increased mortality risk with lower income, however, there was a marked heterogeneity of the strength – or even existence and direction – of the associations in the present study. This has been remarked on by other researchers[3] and examined in relation to site-specific cancer mortality in some detail.[21] It demonstrates the need to move beyond simple notions of increased general susceptibility to disease in less favoured socioeconomic groups, presenting both a challenge and an opportunity to etiological investigations of particular diseases.

The extensive – and widening[10,15,16] – socioeconomic differentials in mortality indicate the depth of the social stratification which exists in the US. Recent increases in inequalities in mortality have also been seen in the UK,[75,76] and in both the US and UK these trends parallel widening inequalities in income.[75,77] In the public health tradition, mortality differentials should be taken to be an indicator of what could be achieved, since reducing mortality rates of all socioeconomic groups to those of the highest income stratum would constitute an important health gain. There is, however, no sign that a reversal of the recent upward redistribution of income, which is required to achieve this goal, is likely to occur in the short term.[75,77]

The findings present a challenge of a different nature to epidemiologists. Socioeconomic mortality differentials are continuous across the social hierarchy and do not appear to be explicable in terms of absolute deprivation during adult life. Investigating the degree to which the socioeconomic careers of moderately affluent people differ from those of people who are even better-off, together with the ways in which this can lead to different patterns of accumulation of exposures detrimental to health over the entire lifecourse, is necessary if further elucidation of the underlying factors is to occur.[38,57]

Acknowledgements

The principal investigators and senior staff of the clinical, coordinating and support centres, the National Heart, Lung, and Blood Institute project office, and members of the MRFIT Policy Advisory Board and Mortality Review Committee are listed in a previous report (*Journal of the American Medical Association*, 1982, vol 248, pp 1465-77). The mortality follow-up of the men screened for the MRFIT and data analysis for this report were supported by an NIH research grant, R01 HL28715.

References

[1] Chapin, C.V. (1924) 'Deaths among taxpayers and non-taxpayers: income tax, Providence, 1865', *American Journal of Public Health*, vol 14, pp 647-51.

[2] Britten, R.H. (1934) 'Mortality rates by occupational class in the US', *Public Health Reports*, vol 49, pp 1101-11.

[3] Coombs, L.C. (1941) 'Economic differentials in causes of death', *Medical Care*, vol 1, pp 246-54.

[4] Guralnick, G. (1963) 'Mortality by occupation and cause of death among men 20 to 64 years of age: US, 1950', *Vital Statistics Special Reports*, vol 53, no 3, DHEW.

[5] Antonovsky, A. (1967) 'Social class, life expectancy and overall mortality', *Milbank Memorial Fund Quarterly*, vol 45, pp 31-73.

[6] Kitagawa, E.M. and Hauser, P.M. (1973) *Differential mortality in the US: A study in socioeconomic epidemiology*, Cambridge, MA: Harvard University Press.

[7] Nagi, M.H. and Stockwell, E.G. (1973) 'Socioeconomic differentials in mortality by cause of death', *Health Service Reports*, vol 88, pp 449-56.

[8] Haan, M., Kaplan, G.A. and Camacho, T. (1987) 'Poverty and health: prospective evidence from the Alameda County study', *American Journal of Epidemiology*, vol 125, pp 989-98.

[9] Rogot, E., Sorlie, P.D., Johnson, N.J. et al (1988) *A mortality study of one million persons by demographic, social and economic factors: 1979-81 follow-up*, NIH Publication no 88-2896, Washington, DC: National Institute of Health.

[10] Feldman, J.J., Makuc, D.M., Kleinman, J.C. and Cornoni-Huntley, J. (1989) 'National trends in educational differences in mortality', *American Journal of Epidemiology*, vol 129, pp 919-33.

[11] Tyroler, H.A., Wing, S. and Knowles, M.G. (1993) 'Increasing inequality in coronary heart disease mortality in relation to educational achievement profiles of places of residence: US, 1962 to 1987', *Annals of Epidemiology*, vol 3, suppl, pp S51-4.

[12] Rogot, E., Sorlie, P.D., Johnson, N.J. and Schmitt, C. (1993) *A mortality study of 1.3 million persons by demographic, social, and economic factors: 1979-1985 follow-up*, US National Longitudinal Mortality Study, Washington, DC: National Institute of Health.

[13] Sorlie, P.D., Backlund, E. and Keller, J.B. (1995) 'US mortality by economic, demographic, and social characteristics: the National Longitudinal Mortality Study', *American Journal of Public Health*, vol 85, pp 949-56.

[14] Omran, A.R. (1977) 'A century of epidemiologic transition in the US', *Preventive Medicine*, vol 6, pp 30-51.

[15] Duleep, H.O. (1989) 'Measuring socioeconomic differentials over time', *Demography*, vol 26, pp 345-51.

[16] Pappas, G., Queen, S., Hadden, W. and Fisher, G. (1993) 'The increasing disparity in mortality between socioeconomic groups in the US, 1960-1986', *New England Journal of Medicine*, vol 329, pp 103-9.

[17] Fox, J. (1989) *Health inequalities in European countries*, Aldershot: Gower.

[18] Davey Smith, G., Bartley, M. and Blane, D. (1990) 'The Black Report on socioeconomic inequalities in health 10 years on', *British Medical Journal*, vol 301, pp 373-7.

[19] Lahelma, E. and Valkonen, T. (1990) 'Health and social inequities in Finland and elsewhere', *Social Science and Medicine*, vol 31, pp 257-65.

[20] Kunst, A.E. and Mackenbach, J.P. (1994) 'The size of mortality differences associated with educational level in nine industrialized countries', *American Journal of Public Health*, vol 84, pp 932-7.

[21] **Davey Smith, G., Leon, D., Shipley, M.J. and Rose, G. (1991) 'Socioeconomic differentials in cancer among men', *International Journal of Epidemiology*, vol 20, pp 339-45.**

[22] **Davey Smith, G., Wentworth, D., Neaton, J.D., Stamler, R. and Stamler, J. (1996) 'Socioeconomic differentials in mortality risk among men screened for the Multiple Risk Factor Intervention Trial: Part II – results for 20,224 black men', *American Journal of Public Health*, vol 86, pp 497-504.**

[23] Neaton, J.D., Kuller, L.H., Wentworth, D. and Borhani, N.O. (1984) 'Total and cardiovascular mortality in relation to cigarette smoking, serum cholesterol concentration, and diastolic blood pressure among black and white males followed for up to five years', *American Heart Journal*, vol 108, pp 759-69.

[24] Neaton, J.D., Grimm, R.H. and Cutler, J.A. (1987) 'Recruitment of participants for the Multiple Risk Factor Intervention Trial (MRFIT)', *Controlled Clinical Trials*, vol 8, pp 415-535.

[25] Lipid Research Clinics Program (1974) *Manual of operations, vol 1: Lipid and lipoprotein analysis*, Washington, DC: US Department of Health, Education and Welfare.

[26] Wentworth, D.N., Neaton, J.D. and Rasmussen, W.L. (1983) 'Evaluation of SSA master beneficiary files and the National Death Index in ascertainment of vital status', *American Journal of Public Health*, vol 73, pp 1270-4.

[27] International Classification of Diseases Ninth Revision (1981) *Clinical modification*, Ann Arbor, MI: Edwards Bros.

[28] US Department of Commerce, Bureau of the Census Population and Housing (1980) Summary Tape File 3, Washington, DC: US Department of Commerce.

[29] Cox, D.R. (1972) 'Regression models and life tables', *Journal of the Royal Statistical Society Series B – Statistical Methodology*, vol 34, pp 187-220.

[30] Kraus, J.F., Borhani, N.O. and Franti, C.E. (1980) 'Socioeconomic status, ethnicity, and risk of coronary heart disease', *American Journal of Epidemiology*, vol 111, pp 407-14.

[31] Wolfson, M., Rowe, G., Gentleman, J.F. and Tomiak, M. (1993) 'Career earnings and death: a longitudinal analysis of older Canadian men', *Journal of Gerontology: Social Sciences*, vol 48, pp S167-79.

[32] Krieger, N. (1992) 'Overcoming the absence of socioeconomic data in medical records: validation of a Census-based methodology', *American Journal of Public Health*, vol 82, pp 703-10.

[33] Sloggett, A. and Joshi, H. (1994) 'Higher mortality in deprived areas: community or personal disadvantage', *British Medical Journal*, vol 309, pp 1470-4.

[34] Sheps, C. and Watkins, J.H. (1947) 'Mortality in the socioeconomic districts of New Haven', *Yale Journal of Biology and Medicine*, vol 20, pp 51-80.

[35] Wing, S., Casper, M., Hayes, C.G., Dargent-Molina, P., Riggan, W. and Tyroler, H.A. (1987) 'Changing association between community occupational structure and ischaemic heart disease mortality in the US', *Lancet*, vol 2, pp 1067-70.

[36] Gardner, M.J. (1973) 'Using the environment to explain and predict mortality', *Journal of the Royal Statistical Society A – General*, vol 136, pp 421-40.

[37] Carstairs, V. and Morris, R. (1989) 'Deprivation: explaining differences in mortality between Scotland and England and Wales', *British Medical Journal*, vol 299, pp 886-9.

[38] Ben-Shlomo, Y. and Davey Smith, G. (1991) 'Deprivation in infancy or adult life: which is more important for mortality risk', *Lancet*, vol 337, pp 530-4.

[39] MacIntyre, S., MacIver, S. and Sooman, A. (1993) 'Area, class and health: should we be focusing on places or people?', *Journal of Social Policy*, vol 22, pp 213-34.

[40] **Davey Smith, G., Shipley, M.J. and Rose, G. (1990) 'The magnitude and causes of socioeconomic differentials in mortality: further evidence from the Whitehall Study', *Journal of Epidemiology and Community Health*, vol 44, pp 265-70.**

[41] Goldblatt, P. (1990) 'Mortality and alternative social classifications', in P. Goldblatt (ed) *Longitudinal study: Mortality and social organisation*, London: HMSO, pp 163-92.

[42] Moser, K., Pugh, H. and Goldblatt, P. (1990) 'Mortality and the social classification of women', in P. Goldblatt (ed) *Longitudinal study: Mortality and social organisation*, London: HMSO, pp 145-62.

[43] **Davey Smith, G., Carroll, D., Rankin, S. and Rowan, D. (1992) 'Socioeconomic differentials in mortality: evidence from Glasgow graveyards', *British Medical Journal*, vol 305, pp 1554-7.**

[44] Bloor, M., Samphier, M. and Prior, L. (1987) 'Artefact explanations of inequalities in health: an assessment of the evidence', *Sociology of Health and Illness*, vol 9, pp 231-64.

[45] Strong, P.M. (1990) 'Black on class and mortality: theory, method and history', *Journal of Public Health Medicine*, vol 12, pp 168-80.

[46] Davey Smith, G., Bartley, M. and Blane, D. (1991) 'Black on class and health: a reply to Strong', *Journal of Public Health Medicine*, vol 13, pp 350-7.

[47] Davey Smith, G., Blane, D. and Bartley, M. (1994) 'Explanations for socioeconomic differentials in mortality: evidence from Britain and elsewhere', *European Journal of Public Health*, vol 4, pp 131-44.

[48] Becker, T.M., Wiggins, C.L., Key, C.R. and Samet, J.M. (1990) 'Symptoms, signs and ill-defined conditions: a leading cause of death among minorities', *American Journal of Epidemiology*, vol 131, pp 664-8.

[49] Samphier, M.L., Robertson, C. and Bloor, M.J. (1988) 'A possible artefactual component in specific cause mortality gradients', *Journal of Epidemiology and Community Health*, vol 42, pp 138-43.

[50] Bloor, M.J., Robertson, C., Samphier, M.L. (1989) 'Occupational status variations in disagreements on the diagnosis of cause of death', *Human Pathology*, vol 20, pp 144-8.

[51] Percy, C., Stanek, E. and Gloeckler, L. (1981) 'Accuracy of cancer death certificates and its effect on cancer mortality statistics', *American Journal of Public Health*, vol 71, pp 242-50.

[52] Stern, J. (1983) 'Social mobility and the interpretation of social class mortality differentials', *Journal of Social Policy*, vol 12, pp 27-49.

[53] Illsley, R. (1986) 'Occupational class, selection and the production of inequalities in health', *Quarterly Journal of Social Affairs*, vol 2, pp 151-65.

[54] Wilkinson, R.G. (1986) 'Occupational class, selection and inequalities in health: a reply to Raymond Illsley', *Quarterly Journal of Social Affairs*, vol 2, pp 415-22.

55 Blane, D., Davey Smith, G. and Bartley, M. (1993) 'Social selection: what does it contribute to social class differences in health?', *Sociology of Health and Illness*, vol 15, pp 1-15.

56 Fox, A.J., Goldblatt, P.O. and Jones, D.R. (1985) 'Social class mortality differentials: artefact, selection or life circumstances?', *Journal of Epidemiology and Community Health*, vol 39, pp 1-8.

57 Mare, R.D. (1990) 'Socioeconomic careers and differential mortality among older men in the US', in J. Vallin, S. D'Souza and A. Palloni (eds) *Measurement and analysis of mortality: New approaches*, Oxford: Clarendon Press, pp 362-87.

58 Pekkanen, J., Tuomilehto, J., Uutela, A., Vartiainen, E. and Nissinen, A. (1995) 'Social class, health behaviour, and mortality among men and women in eastern Finland', *British Medical Journal*, vol 311, pp 589-93.

59 Spearman, C. (1904) 'The proof and measurement of association between two things', *American Journal of Psychology*, vol 15, pp 72-101.

60 Davey Smith, G. and Phillips, A.N. (1990) 'Declaring independence: why we should be cautious', *Journal of Epidemiology and Community Health*, vol 44, pp 257-8.

61 MacMahon, S., Peto, R., Cutler, J. et al (1990) 'Blood pressure, stroke and coronary heart disease. Part 1: prolonged differences in blood pressure: prospective observational studies corrected for the regression dilution bias', *Lancet*, vol 335, pp 765-74.

62 Phillips, A.N. and Davey Smith, G. (1991) 'How independent are "independent" effects? Relative risk estimation when correlated exposures are measured imprecisely', *Journal of Clinical Epidemiology*, vol 44, pp 1223-31.

63 Rose, G. and Marmot, M.G. (1981) 'Social class and coronary heart disease', *British Heart Journal*, vol 45, pp 13-19.

64 Graham, H. (1988) 'Women and smoking in the UK: the implications for health promotion', *Health Promotion*, vol 3, pp 371-82.

65 Sooman, A., MacIntyre, S. and Anderson, A. (1993) 'Scotland's health – a more difficult challenge for some? The price and availability of healthy foods in socially contrasting localities in the West of Scotland', *Health Bulletin*, vol 51, pp 276-84.

[66] Radical Statistics Health Group (1987) 'Health education: blaming the victim?', in *Facing the figures: What really is happening to the National Health Service?*, London: Radical Statistics.

[67] Link, B.G. and Phelan, J. (1995) 'Social conditions as fundamental causes of disease', *Journal of Health and Social Behavior*, extra issue, pp 80-94.

[68] Buell, P., Dunn, J.E. and Breslow, L. (1960) 'The occupational–social class risk of cancer mortality in men', *Journal of Chronic Diseases*, vol 12, pp 600-21.

[69] Thurlow, H.J. (1967) 'General susceptibility to illness: a selective review', *Canadian Medical Association Journal*, vol 97, pp 1397-404.

[70] Najman, J.M. (1980) 'Theories of disease causation and the concept of general susceptibility: a review', *Social Science and Medicine*, vol 14a, pp 231-7.

[71] Syme, S.L. and Berkman, L.F. (1976) 'Social class, susceptibility and sickness', *American Journal of Epidemiology*, vol 104, pp 1-8.

[72] Marmot, M.G., Shipley, M.J. and Rose, G. (1984) 'Inequalities in death – specific explanations of a general pattern?', *Lancet*, vol 1, pp 1003-6.

[73] Sterling, P. and Eyer, J. (1981) 'Biological basis of stress–related mortality', *Social Science and Medicine*, vol 15e, pp 3-42.

[74] Totman, R. (1987) *Social causes of illness*, London: Souvenir Press.

[75] Davey Smith, G. and Egger, M. (1993) 'Socioeconomic differentials in wealth and health: widening inequalities in health – the legacy of the Thatcher years', *British Medical Journal*, vol 307, pp 1085-6.

[76] McCarron, P.G., Davey Smith, G. and Womersley, J. (1994) 'Deprivation and mortality in Glasgow: increasing differentials from 1980 to 1992', *British Medical Journal*, vol 309, pp 1481-2.

[77] Plotnick, R.D. (1993) 'Changes in poverty, income inequality, and the standard of living in the US during the Reagan years', *International Journal of Health Services*, vol 23, pp 347-58.

6

Socioeconomic differentials in mortality risk among men screened for the Multiple Risk Factor Intervention Trial: Part II – results for 20,224 black men

George Davey Smith, Deborah Wentworth, James D. Neaton, Rose Stamler and Jeremiah Stamler

Abstract

Objectives: This study examined socioeconomic differentials in risk of death from a number of causes in a large cohort of black men in the US.

Methods: For 20,224 black men screened for the Multiple Risk Factor Intervention Trial between 1973 and 1975, data were collected on median family income of black households in zipcode of residence, age, cigarette smoking, blood pressure, serum cholesterol, previous heart attack, and drug treatment for diabetes. The 2,937 deaths that occurred over the 16-year follow-up period were grouped into specific causes and related to median black family income.

Results: There was an inverse association between age-adjusted all-cause mortality and median family income. There was no attenuation of this association over the follow-up period, and the association was similar for the 22 clinical centres carrying out the screening. The gradient was seen for most of the specific causes of death, although the strength of the association varied. Median income was markedly lower for the black men

American Journal of Public Health, 1996, vol 86, pp 497-504

screened than for the white men, but the relationship between income and all-cause mortality was similar.

Conclusions: Socioeconomic position is an important determinant of mortality risk for black men. Even though black men lived in areas with substantially lower median family income than white men, the association of income with mortality was similar for black and white men.

Introduction

In the US health differences between black and white citizens have been extensively discussed.[1-6] The intended interpretation of racial/ ethnic identity as an explanatory variable has sometimes been unclear. Black–white health differentials are often taken to be proxies for variations in health status related to socioeconomic position, a tendency that receives encouragement from the paucity of routine data regarding socioeconomic differentials in morbidity and mortality in the US.[7] This has meant that socioeconomic patterning of health status among African Americans has, to a degree, been neglected.[6,8]

The 1979 to 1985 follow-up of the National Longitudinal Mortality Study (NLMS)[9] demonstrated substantial differentials in mortality for black men and women according to family income. Only 965 deaths occurred among the 13,701 black men with known family income who were aged 35 to 64 years at study entry, however. Because of this, mortality differentials for particular causes of death could not be examined in detail. In this paper, data are presented on the mortality experience, over a 16-year follow-up period, of the large cohort of black men who were screened for the Multiple Risk Factor Intervention Trial (MRFIT).[10,11] Analyses of the gradients of total and cause-specific mortality risk by median income of zipcode area of residence have been carried out. Availability of data regarding smoking behaviour, blood pressure, cholesterol level and pre-existing disease allow for assessment of the influence of these key risk factors on observed income-mortality gradients. A companion report gives findings for white men (see Chapter Five in this volume).[12]

Methods

Methods used to recruit participants and a description of the men screened have been reported previously;[10,11] full details of the specific procedures related to the analysis of income differentials are being presented in the accompanying paper.[12] Of the men screened for the MRFIT, 23,490 indicated that they were black; income data regarding families with black heads of households (henceforth 'income') were available for 20,224 (86.1%) of these men living in 1,376 zipcode areas.

Fewer causes of death could be investigated for black than for white men because the cohort was substantially smaller. For analysing risk of total mortality, median zipcode area family income was categorised into ten groups, with $2,500 intervals, ranging from $7,500 to $27,500. For analyses of particular causes, median zipcode area family income was divided into three groups, based on tertiles of income. The group of men from the zipcode areas with the highest median family income was used as the reference group for calculation of relative risk estimates. Regression coefficients from proportional hazards models were used to estimate the relative risk associated with a $10,000 lower zipcode area median census tract income. Proportional hazards regression models with and without an interaction term between income and being black or white were compared to determine the magnitude and significance of any differences in the regression coefficients associated with income for black and white men.

Results

Table 1 compares baseline and mortality data for the men for whom income data were available with those for whom such data were not. The latter were more likely to be smokers, had higher levels of blood pressure and had a higher all-cause mortality rate than the former. The age-adjusted relative risk of death for the men without income data, in comparison with those with such data, was 1.12 (95% confidence interval [CI] = 1.02-1.23). With adjustment for smoking, diastolic blood pressure, serum cholesterol, previous heart attack and

Table 1: Baseline data on black men screened between 1973 and 1975, by availability of income data for zipcode area: MRFIT

	Income data available	Income data not available
Number of men	20,224	3,266
Mean age (years)	45.3	46.0
Cigarette smokers (%)	45.8	57.2
Mean systolic blood pressure (mm Hg)	133.6	136.7
Mean diastolic blood pressure (mg/dl)	86.8	90.0
Mean serum cholesterol (mg/dl)	210.0	210.7
Prior hospitalisation for heart attack (%)	1.4	1.4
Medication for diabetes (%)	3.2	3.6
Age-adjusted death rate (per 10,000 person years)	103.0	118.3

medication for diabetes, this relative risk was reduced to 1.02 (95% CI = 0.93-1.12).

The characteristics of the 20,224 black men for whom income data were available are presented in Table 2 according to income tertile. The group in the highest income tertile was lower in terms of mean age, blood pressure, prevalence of cigarette smoking and drug treatment for diabetes, and higher in terms of mean serum cholesterol level, than those in the two lower income tertiles. Stratification based on income was related to other ecologically defined demographic characteristics in the zipcode areas, including percentage unemployed, percentage below the poverty line, percentage in professional or managerial occupations and average years of schooling.

All-cause mortality

During the 16 years of follow-up, 2,937 deaths were identified among the 20,224 black men in this cohort. Mortality rates and relative risk estimates, according to income (categorised into 10 groups), are presented in Table 3. The association was continuous, with no evidence of a threshold. The regression coefficient for each $10,000 lower

Table 2: Characteristics of black men screened, by level of median family income for zipcode of residence and characteristics of zipcode areas of residence

	Income ($) (approximate tertile)[a]		
	<12,333 (n=6,698)	12,333-16,300 (n=6,744)	>16,300 (n=6,782)
Characteristics of men screened			
Mean age (years)	45.9	45.4	44.7
Mean systolic blood pressure (mm Hg)	135.0	133.8	132.0
Mean diastolic blood pressure (mm Hg)	87.8	86.9	85.9
Mean serum cholesterol (mg/dl)	208.7	210.0	211.4
Cigarette smokers (%)	51.9	49.6	45.0
Cigarettes per day for smokers (mean)	18.4	18.3	19.0
Prior hospitalisation for heart attack (%)	1.4	1.5	1.3
Medication for diabetes (%)	3.6	3.4	2.7
Population characteristics of zipcode areas[a]			
Unemployment (%)	5.2	4.9	4.3
Average years of schooling	13.0	13.5	14.1
Managerial or professional occupations (%)	6.0	7.8	11.5
Below the poverty line (%)	21.6	13.6	6.6
Median family income ($)			
White households	16,408	18,686	23,838
Black households	10,189	14,262	21,494

[a] Based on data from the 1980 US Census.

Table 3: All-cause mortality among black men screened, by level of median family income for zipcode of residence

Income ($)	Number of men	Number of deaths	Age-adjusted rate[a]	Age-adjusted relative risk (95% CI)	Age- and risk factor-adjusted relative risk (95% CI)
≤7,500	423	84	137.2	2.05 (1.45, 3.00)	1.92 (1.34, 2.76)
7,501-10,000	2,245	393	120.5	1.97 (1.45, 2.67)	1.80 (1.33, 2.45)
10,000-12,500	4,255	720	116.9	1.88 (1.39, 2.53)	1.70 (1.26, 2.30)
12,501-15,000	4,787	740	107.8	1.71 (1.27, 2.31)	1.59 (1.18, 2.14)
15,001-17,500	2,615	326	89.9	1.43 (1.05, 1.94)	1.36 (1.00, 1.85)
17,501-20,000	2,267	283	89.8	1.41 (1.03, 1.92)	1.34 (0.99, 1.83)
20,001-22,500	1,900	228	86.8	1.40 (1.02, 1.93)	1.34 (0.97, 1.84)
22,501-25,000	757	83	86.5	1.38 (0.97, 1.99)	1.34 (0.93, 1.92)
25,001-27,500	371	32	65.4	1.08 (0.69, 1.70)	1.07 (0.68, 1.68)
27,501+	604	48	57.2	1.00 (no reference)	1.00 (no reference)

[a] By direct method to age distribution of all men screened per 10,000 person years.

Note: Family income levels were based on data from the 1980 US Census. Risk factors were diastolic blood pressure, serum cholesterol level, cigarettes per day, prior hospitalisation for heart attack, and medication for diabetes. CI = confidence interval.

income increment, adjusted for age, translated into a relative risk of mortality of 1.35 (95% CI: 1.24-1.46). Further adjustment for smoking behaviour, diastolic blood pressure, serum cholesterol, history of heart attack and medication for diabetes, reduced this relative risk to 1.29 (95% CI: 1.19-1.40).

The relationship of income with all-cause mortality was examined separately for smokers and non-smokers and according to age at screening (those 35 to 44 years old versus those 45 to 57 years old). For the men who reported smoking cigarettes at the time of screening, the age-adjusted relative risk associated with a $10,000 lower income was 1.29 (95% CI: 1.16-1.43). After adjustment for serum cholesterol, diastolic blood pressure, cigarettes smoked per day, history of heart attack and medication for diabetes this relative risk was 1.27 (95% CI: 1.14-1.41). For men who reported that they were not currently smoking cigarettes, the corresponding relative risks are 1.31 (95% CI: 1.16-1.49) in the age-adjusted analysis and 1.29 (95% CI: 1.14-1.47) after adjustment for the other risk factors. The inverse association between income and mortality risk was also similar for the men aged 35 to 44 years old at screening and the men aged 45 to 57 years old. For the younger men the age-adjusted relative risk of mortality for a $10,000 lower income was 1.33 (95% CI: 1.15-1.54); for the older men, it was 1.36 (95% CI: 1.23-1.49).

Cumulative mortality over the follow-up period reveals no tendency for the rates of mortality to converge (Figure 1). Cumulative mortality at 10 years for men in the lower, middle and upper tertile were 8.1%, 6.4%, and 5.0% respectively. Corresponding percents for 15 years were 15.9, 13.4 and 10.1.

Figure 1: Cumulative mortality among black men screened, for three income categories

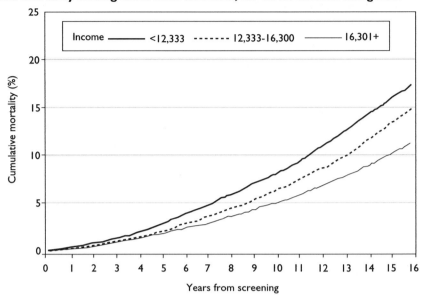

Within each clinical centre, men were screened from a number of zipcode areas. Thus, there was a considerable range in income among the black men screened, not only between centres but within centre (Table 4). This permitted an estimate of the relationship between income and mortality to be obtained for each centre (Table 4 and Figure 2). In Table 4, adjusted relative estimates of all-cause mortality are given for each centre. These estimates compare mortality for those with income below the median for that centre with those above the median. Nineteen of the 22 clinical centres had relative estimates which exceed one. Figure 2 plots adjusted relative risk estimates and 95% confidence intervals of all-cause mortality corresponding to a $10,000 lower income. These estimates were similar for the 22 clinical centres.

Cause-specific mortality

Mortality data for specific causes of death are presented in Table 5. The strongest associations with income were for noncardiovascular, noncancer causes of death, such as chronic obstructive pulmonary disease, infection, AIDS, diabetes, digestive diseases and accidents and violence. The association between income and cancer deaths was relatively weak. Among cardiovascular causes, the gradient between risk of death from haemorrhagic stroke and income was particularly steep. There was also a significant association between income and coronary heart disease mortality.

Table 5 also displays the effect of adjustment for blood pressure,

Figure 2: Relative risk of death associated with a $10,000 lower income among black men screened in each of 22 clinical centres

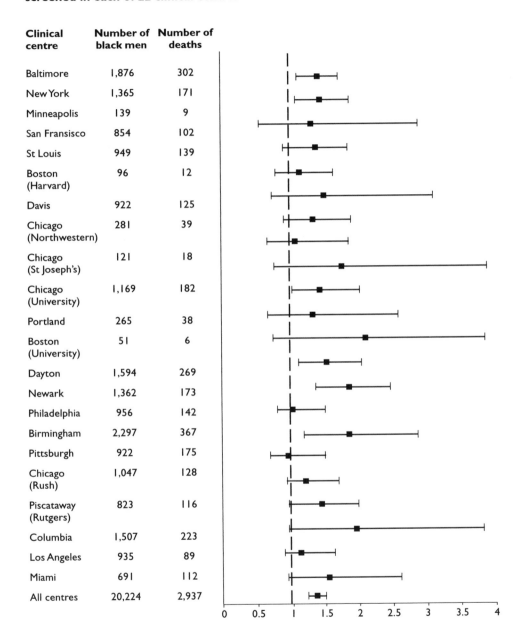

Clinical centre	Number of black men	Number of deaths
Baltimore	1,876	302
New York	1,365	171
Minneapolis	139	9
San Fransisco	854	102
St Louis	949	139
Boston (Harvard)	96	12
Davis	922	125
Chicago (Northwestern)	281	39
Chicago (St Joseph's)	121	18
Chicago (University)	1,169	182
Portland	265	38
Boston (University)	51	6
Dayton	1,594	269
Newark	1,362	173
Philadelphia	956	142
Birmingham	2,297	367
Pittsburgh	922	175
Chicago (Rush)	1,047	128
Piscataway (Rutgers)	823	116
Columbia	1,507	223
Los Angeles	935	89
Miami	691	112
All centres	20,224	2,937

Table 4: Income and all-cause mortality among black men screened, by clinical centre

Clinical centre	Number of black men	Number of zipcode areas[a]	Median income ($)	Range in income for zipcode areas ($)	Relative risk of death[b] (lower versus higher income zipcode areas [%% CI])
Baltimore	1,878	83	15,245	5,000-40,101	1.48 (1.17, 1.86)
New York	1,365	182	14,000	5,000-50,000	1.47 (1.08, 1.99)
Minneapolis	139	20	20,720	8,629-40,631	2.52 (0.63, 10.1)
San Francisco	854	100	15,727	7,451-50,000	1.53 (1.02, 2.28)
St Louis	949	55	14,061	6,661-35,926	1.27 (0.91, 1.78)
Boston (Havard)	96	35	19,065	8,552-50,000	3.02 (0.89, 10.1)
Davis	922	39	14,686	6,956-34,500	1.02 (0.71, 1.45)
Chicago (Northwestern)	281	50	15,956	5,280-50,000	0.77 (0.41, 1.46)
Chicago (St Joseph's)	121	44	15,520	5,280-50,000	2.21 (0.83, 5.91)
Chicago (University)	1,169	52	18,750	5,280-37,781	1.33 (1.00, 1.78)
Portland	265	33	13,750	5,000-39,625	1.51 (0.75, 3.04)
Boston (University)	51	16	18,158	5,000-30,873	2.60 (0.47, 14.3)
Dayton	1,594	59	13,211	5,000-38,756	1.46 (1.14, 1.87)
Newark	1,362	147	15,813	7,239-50,000	1.65 (1.23, 2.24)
Philadelphia	956	119	14,971	5,244-50,000	1.17 (0.84, 1.63)
Birmingham	2,297	60	11,656	5,491-36,239	1.26 (1.03, 1.55)
Pittsburgh	922	70	13,886	5,000-27,652	0.81 (0.60, 1.09)
Chicago (Rush)	1,047	83	18,750	5,280-50,000	1.07 (0.76, 1.52)
Rutgers	823	162	17,893	7,189-40,247	1.17 (0.82, 1.69)
Columbia	1,507	64	13,000	7,157-26,692	1.33 (1.02, 1.73)
Los Angeles	935	140	17,143	7,409-50,000	0.98 (0.64, 1.49)
Miami	691	49	11,824	5,000-42,500	1.05 (0.72, 1.53)

[a] Total adds to more than 1,376 because some centres screened from the same zipcode areas.
[b] Risk of death for those with income below median for clinical centre versus those above median adjusted for age.

serum cholesterol level, smoking behaviour, history of heart attack and treatment for diabetes on income–associated relative risks of mortality. While these adjustments tended to somewhat attenuate the magnitude of the elevated risk in the low income tertile, this effect was generally not marked.

Income distributions for black and white men in the MRFIT screening study cohort were distinctly different (Table 6), but the associations of income with major causes of death were similar for black and white men with few exceptions (Table 7). The income–all-cause mortality gradient was steeper for black than white men ($p=0.03$ after adjustment for risk factors).

Among specific causes the largest difference between black and white men was for noncancer, noncardiovascular disease mortality, for which the income–mortality gradient was also steeper for black than for white men. For lung cancer, there was a suggestion ($p=0.08$)

Table 5: Number of deaths, age-adjusted mortality rates, and relative risk estimates, adjusted for age and other risk factors, for black men screened, by tertile of median family income of zipcode of residence

Cause of death (ICD-9 Codes)	<12,333				12,333-16,300				≥16,300				Adjusted regression coefficient[a] × 10,000	p
			Relative risk				Relative risk				Relative risk			
	Number of deaths	Age-adjusted rate	Adjusted for age	Adjusted for age and other risk factors	Number of deaths	Age-adjusted rate	Adjusted for age	Adjusted for age and other risk factors	Number of deaths	Age-adjusted rate	Adjusted for age	Adjusted for age and other risk factors		
All CVD (390-459)	474	48.8	1.34***	1.26**	378	39.7	1.06	1.03	336	36.8	1.00	1.00	-0.2242	0.0004
Coronary heart disease (410-14, 429.2)	282	29.1	1.33**	1.25*	226	23.8	1.04	1.00	216	23.6	1.00	1.00	-0.2327	0.004
Stroke (430-8)	60	6.2	1.09	1.02	43	4.5	0.88	0.77	40	4.4	1.00	1.00	-0.2683	0.17
Intracranial haemorrhage (431-2)	27	2.8	2.37*	2.16*	12	1.2	1.00	0.96	11	1.2	1.00	1.00	-0.7564	0.03
Nonhaemorrhagic stroke (433-8)	31	3.2	0.86	0.81	27	3.0	0.79	0.77	24	2.8	1.00	1.00	-0.1456	0.56
Other CVD	132	13.6	1.48*	1.41*	109	11.4	1.26	1.23	80	8.7	1.00	1.00	-0.1831	0.14
Cancer (140-209)	378	38.9	1.27**	1.19*	360	37.7	1.22*	1.18	279	31.1	1.00	1.00	-0.0956	15.0
Digestive (150-9)	102	10.4	1.28	1.25	105	10.9	1.37*	1.36	78	8.8	1.00	1.00	-0.0847	0.49
Lung (162)	146	15.1	1.28	1.15	129	13.5	1.16	1.09	97	10.5	1.00	1.00	-0.0447	0.67
Other cancer	130	13.4	1.24	1.19	126	13.4	1.18	1.15	104	11.8	1.00	1.00	-0.1687	0.13
Non CVD, noncancer	298	30.4	2.02***	1.93***	251	25.9	1.71***	1.66***	149	15.3	1.00	1.00	-0.5840	<0.001
Infection (1-139)	24	2.5	2.40*	2.43*	25	2.5	2.37*	2.39*	13	1.2	1.00	1.00	-0.7846	0.008
AIDS (42-4)	11	1.1	4.73***	4.90**	10	0.9	3.53*	3.63*	5	0.4	1.00	1.00	-1.5046	0.001
Diabetes (250)	25	2.6	2.30*	2.28*	27	2.9	2.45*	2.36*	12	1.2	1.00	1.00	-0.8685	0.005
Respiratory (460-519)	61	6.3	2.31***	2.17**	44	4.6	1.75*	1.70*	26	2.7	1.00	1.00	-0.4755	0.02
Chronic obstructive pulmonary disease (490-6)	34	3.5	4.64***	4.41***	22	2.3	3.34**	3.27**	7	0.6	1.00	1.00	-1.0608	.002

Table 5: contd.../

Cause of death (ICD-9 Codes)	Income tertile ($)												
	<12,333				12,333-16 300				≥16,300					
			Relative risk				Relative risk				Relative risk			
	Number of deaths	Age adjusted rate	Adjusted for age	Adjusted for age and other risk factors	Number of deaths	Age adjusted rate	Adjusted for age	Adjusted for age and other risk factors	Number of deaths	Age adjusted rate	Adjusted for age	Adjusted for age and other risk factors	Adjusted regression on coefficient[a] × 10,000	p
Digestive disease (5207-9)	42	4.3	2.21*	2.02*	28	3.0	1.46	1.38	17	1.9	1.00	1.00	-0.6311	0.02
Accidents and violence (800-999)	93	9.3	1.88***	1.80**	76	7.6	1.61*	1.56*	51	5.0	1.00	1.00	-0.5899	0.0003
Suicide (950-9, 980-9)	11	0.1	0.78	0.71	12	1.3	0.83	0.79	12	1.2	1.00	1.00	-0.1433	0.67
Homicide (960-9)	40	0.0	2.43**	2.36*	24	2.3	1.64	1.63	16	1.6	1.00	1.00	-0.8020	0.005
Other non-CVD, noncancer	53	0.5	1.56	1.49	51	5.2	1.44	1.40	30	3.3	1.00	1.00	-0.4266	0.04
All-causes	1,161	19.2	1.44***	1.36***	1003	104.7	1.25***	1.21***	773	84.1	1.00	1.00	-0.2559	<0.0001

[a] Diastolic blood pressure, serum cholesterol level, cigarettes per day, prior hospitalisation for heart attack, and medication for diabetes.
ICD-9 = International Classification of Diseases, Ninth Revision; CVD = cardiovascular disease. *p <0.05; **p <0.01, ***p<0.001.

Table 6: Distribution of black and white householder median family income for zipcode of residence among black and white men screened

Income ($)	Black men		White men	
	Number	%	Number	%
≤10,000	2,628	13.0	397	0.1
10,000-12,499	4,278	21.2	892	0.3
12,500-14,999	4,799	23.7	4,480	1.5
15,000-17,499	2,529	12.5	11,729	3.9
17,500-19,999	2,285	11.3	32,200	10.7
20,000-22,499	1,963	9.7	60,502	20.1
22,500-24,999	762	3.8	56,458	18.8
25,000-27,499	376	1.9	45,311	15.1
27,500-29,999	221	1.1	36,580	12.2
30,000-32,499	146	0.7	25,265	8.4
32,500+	237	1.2	26,871	8.9
Total	20,224	100.0	300,685	100.0

Note: Family income levels were based on data from the 1980 US Census.

Table 7: Relative risks of selected causes of death, adjusted for age and other risk factors, associated with a $10,000 lower median family income of zipcode of residence for black and white men screened

Cause of death	Black men		White men		p for difference in income–mortality association in black and white men after age adjustment[a]	p for difference in income–mortality association in black and white men after risk factor adjustment[a]
	Age-adjusted relative risk	Age- and risk factor-adjusted relative risk	Age-adjusted relative risk	Age- and risk factor-adjusted relative risk		
All causes	1.35	1.29	1.26	1.18	0.12	0.03
Cardiovascular disease	1.31	1.25	1.26	1.17	0.53	0.38
Coronary heart disease	1.32	1.26	1.25	1.16	0.86	0.65
Stroke	1.40	1.31	1.26	1.17	0.31	0.89
Cancer	1.15	1.10	1.21	1.15	0.50	0.81
Lung cancer	1.13	1.05	1.40	1.27	0.08	0.30
Noncancer, non-cardiovascular disease	1.86	1.79	1.36	1.28	0.001	0.001
Respiratory	1.70	1.61	1.56	1.44	0.88	0.71
Suicide	0.93	0.87	1.17	1.11	0.74	0.79
Homicide	2.29	2.23	2.10	2.00	0.89	0.87

[a] p value associated with $10,000 lower median family income and black/white interaction term. *Note:* Risk factors were diastolic blood pressure, serum cholesterol level, medication for diabetes, prior hospitalisation for a heart attack, and cigarettes per day.

that the income–mortality association was steeper for white men than black men when only age adjustment was made; after adjustment for the other risk factors, the significance level of this difference was reduced.

Discussion

The socioeconomic mortality differentials among black men screened for the MRFIT were similar in magnitude to those seen among white men.[12] Within the limitations of the smaller number of deaths, these differentials were seen for a wide variety of causes of death. The associations between socioeconomic position and mortality risk among the black participants are subject to the same potential biases discussed with regard to the white men in Chapter Five.[12] As with the white men, the range in income within each centre for the men screened and the similarity of the associations between income and mortality in each clinical centre provides evidence against the possibility that recruitment of men with both different average incomes and different mortality risks at the various screening centres underlies the observed relationships. The socioeconomic differentials in all-cause mortality rates observed in the NLMS[9] are similar to those in the MRFIT cohort, indicating that the findings are generalisable. The NLMS also has data on black women, among whom the association between family income and mortality was similar to that seen in men.

The issues surrounding the use of an ecological index of socioeconomic position, discussed with regard to white men in the accompanying chapter,[12] are also germane to consideration of the associations seen among black men. In the US there is substantial segregation of white people and black people, especially in metropolitan areas,[13,14] but cutting across this segregation is a gradient of increasing median family income of zipcode area for both groups.

Although the range of income is smaller for black men than for white men, an inverse association between mortality and income is observed in both groups.

The association between mortality risk and income was not confined to the poorest members of the cohort; instead it persisted over the full range of income studied. This was also seen among white men in this study,[12] for whom the average level of income was considerably higher, in keeping with the situation in the US generally.[15] The continuous association between socioeconomic position and mortality risk is a robust finding that has been demonstrated for many populations, both historical and contemporary.[16-19] The existence of such a graded relationship requires explanations which go beyond attribution to living in absolute poverty during adult life.

The mortality differentials by income group showed no sign of decline over a 16-year follow-up period. As discussed in Chapter Five, this argues against an explanation based on the postulate that poor health leads to declining socioeconomic position. The absence of an association between history of myocardial infarction or use of medication for diabetes at screening and income may reflect selection occurring during recruitment to the cohort. Morbidity — including overall measures such as the rating of general health status as less than good and the experience of limitation of activity due to poor health — is more prevalent among lower income black men than higher income black men.[20,21] As well as being related to a shorter expectation of life, low income is accompanied by poorer health status while alive.

Cigarette smoking was strongly associated with mortality risk and was more common among the lower income men. Similar gradients between income and all-cause mortality risk were found for smokers and non-smokers. Adjustment for smoking behaviour and the other cardiovascular disease risk factors measured at baseline produced a moderate degree of attenuation of the associations between income and mortality from coronary heart disease and cancer. The lack of data regarding lifetime exposure to the measured factors, together with the absence of any data regarding obesity, exercise patterns, alcohol use and diet, renders quantification of the attribution of differentials to known risk factors problematic. However, finding socioeconomic differentials for causes of death that are not the outcomes of such known risk factors suggests that additional factors need to be invoked to account for the full spectrum of the income—mortality associations.

The rate of non-coverage by health insurance is higher among those with low household incomes,[20] therefore access to, and availability of, healthcare for lower income men will, on average, be inferior to that of the higher income men. It has been demonstrated that lacking health insurance is a marker of increased mortality risk.[22] In the Hypertension Detection and Follow-up Program (HDFP), which enrolled a large proportion of its white and black participants from relatively poor inner-city areas, higher mortality rates with lower levels of education were seen in the group randomised to receive usual medical care in the community.[23] Referral to the specially established HDFP clinical centres led to a reduction in mortality from cardiovascular disease, the target of the blood pressure lowering intervention. A reduction in noncardiovascular disease mortality (and consequently all-cause mortality) was also seen,[24] however, suggesting that there may have been more general consequences of rendering health care accessible. Furthermore, in the group of participants assigned to receive treatment at the clinical centres, the association between socioeconomic position and mortality risk was markedly attenuated.

The lesser access to medical care that accompanies lower income may explain some of the socioeconomic differentials in mortality risk. Causes of death that cannot be prevented by medical care show similar socioeconomic gradients to potentially preventable causes, however. This should be considered together with the evidence that modifiable risk factors, such as smoking, elevated blood pressure and serum cholesterol, do not fully account for the association between mortality and income. This does not diminish the value of efforts to expand access to health care or to oppose the cynical targeting of minority and poor populations in the marketing of health-damaging products, such as cigarettes.[25] It does, however, emphasise the conclusion of Adler and colleagues that there is 'no easy solution' – in terms of the simple application of current knowledge of disease aetiology and health promotion practice – to the continued existence of socioeconomic inequalities in health.[26]

What is clear is that certain processes that are intimately and robustly linked to material wellbeing have a consistent impact on health status. Comparison of the findings for black men and white men screened for the MRFIT demonstrates that, in general, the association between income and mortality risk is similar in the two groups. The use of 'race'/ethnicity as, in part at least, a proxy for socioeconomic position in some studies has tended to obscure the fact that the dependence of mortality risk on socioeconomic position among black people is at least as strong as among white people in the US. These MRFIT data, added to the findings of other recent investigations,[3,8,27,28] emphasise the importance of focusing on socioeconomic position as a determinant of mortality among black people, as well as between black and whites people.

The economic and social structure that produces a marked gradation of income for black US citizens produces the same for white citizens, but at higher average income levels. Explanations of two of the striking demographic mortality differentials in the US (the higher mortality risk with lower socioeconomic position, and the higher mortality rates for black citizens than for white citizens) should focus on the common underlying factor, the lower levels of wealth and the reduction in life chances, for the groups at higher levels of mortality risk. This does not, however, mean that the increased mortality experience of black people can be simply and completely 'explained' by lower average socioeconomic position.[6,29] First, there needs to be detailed consideration of the forces – including institutional and 'everyday' racism[6,29,30] – that maintain the average socioeconomic position of black people well below that of white people in the US. Second, these same forces can ensure that even within a given socioeconomic strata, the lifetime social circumstances for black citizens in the US can be unfavourable compared to those of white citizens.

Acknowledgements

The principal investigators and senior staff of the clinical, coordinating and support centres, the National Heart, Lung, and Blood Institute project office, and members of the MRFIT Policy Advisory Board and Mortality Review Committee are listed in a previous report (*Journal of the American Medical Association*, 1982, vol 248, pp 1465-77). The mortality follow-up of the men screened for the MRFIT and data analysis for this report were supported by an NIH research grant, R01 HL28715.

References

[1] Cooper, R., Steinhauer, M., Miller, W., David, R. and Schatzkin, A. (1981) 'Racism, society and disease: an exploration of the social and biological mechanisms of differential mortality', *International Journal of Health Services*, vol 11, pp 389-414.

[2] Otten, M.W., Teutsch, S.M., Williamson, D.F. and Marks, J.S. (1990) 'The effects of known risk factors on the excess mortality of black adults in the US', *Journal of the American Medical Association*, vol 263, pp 845-50.

[3] Sorlie, P., Rogot, E., Anderson, R., Johnson, N.J. and Backlund, E. (1992) 'Black–white mortality differences by family income', *Lancet*, vol 340, pp 346-50.

[4] Rogers, R.G. (1992) 'Living and dying in the USA: sociodemographic determinants of death among blacks and whites', *Demography*, vol 29, pp 287-303.

[5] Polednak, A.P. (1993) 'Poverty, residential segregation, and black/white mortality ratios in urban areas', *Journal of Health Care for the Poor and Underserved*, vol 4, pp 363-73.

[6] Krieger, N., Rowley, D.L., Herman, A.A., Avery, B. and Phillips, M.T. (1993) 'Racism, sexism, and social class: implications for studies of health, disease, and well-being', *American Journal of Preventive Medicine*, vol 9, suppl, pp 82-122.

[7] Krieger, N. (1992) 'The making of public health data: paradigms, policies, and policy', *Journal of Public Health Policy*, vol 13, pp 412-27.

[8] Cooper, R.S. (1993) 'Health and social status of blacks in the US', *Annals of Epidemiology*, vol 3, pp 137-44.

[9] Rogot, E., Sorlie, P.D., Johnson, N.J. and Schmitt, C. (1993) *A mortality study of 1.3 million persons by demographic, social, and economic factors: 1979-1985 follow-up*, US National Longitudinal Mortality Study, Washington, DC: National Institute of Health.

[10] Neaton, J.D., Grimm, R.H. and Cutler, J.A. (1987) 'Recruitment of participants for the Multiple Risk Factor Intervention Trial (MRFIT)', *Controlled Clinical Trials*, vol 8, pp 41S-53S.

[11] Neaton, J.D., Kuller, L.H., Wentworth, D. and Borhani, N.O. (1984) 'Total and cardiovascular mortality in relation to cigarette smoking, serum cholesterol concentration, and diastolic blood pressure among black and white males followed for up to five years', *American Heart Journal*, vol 108, pp 759-69.

[12] **Davey Smith, G., Wentworth, D., Stamler, R., Neaton, J.D. and Stamler, J. (1996) 'Socioeconomic differentials in mortality risk among men screened for the Multiple Risk Factor Intervention Trial: Part I – results for 300,685 white men', *American Journal of Public Health*, vol 86, pp 486-96.**

[13] Massey, D.S. and Denton, N.A. (1987) 'Trends in residential segregation of blacks, Hispanics, and Asians: 1970-1980', *American Sociological Review*, vol 52, pp 802-25.

[14] Massey, D.S. and Denton, N.A. (1988) 'Suburbanization and segregation in the US metropolitan areas', *American Journal of Sociology*, vol 94, pp 592-626.

[15] Hacker, A. (1992) *Two nations. Black and White, separate, hostile, unequal*, New York, NY: Ballantine Books.

[16] Morrison, A.S., Kirshner, J. and Molho, A. (1977) 'Life cycle events in 15th century Florence: records of the Monte Delle Doti', *American Journal of Epidemiology*, vol 106, pp 487-92.

[17] **Davey Smith, G., Carroll, D. and Rankin, S. (1992) 'Socioeconomic differentials in mortality: evidence from Glasgow graveyards', *British Medical Journal*, vol 305, pp 1554-7.**

[18] Goldblatt, P. (1990) 'Mortality and alternative social classifications', in P. Goldblatt (ed) *Longitudinal study: Mortality and social organisation*, London: HMSO, pp 163-92.

[19] **Davey Smith, G., Shipley, M.J. and Rose, G. (1990) 'The magnitude and causes of socioeconomic differentials in mortality: further evidence from the Whitehall Study',** *Journal of Epidemiology and Community Health*, **vol 44, pp 265-70.**

[20] US Department of Health and Human Services (DHHS) (1990) *Health status of the disadvantaged: Chartbook 1990*, Washington, DC: DHHS.

[21] Ries, P. (1990) 'Health of black and white Americans, 1985-1987', *Vital and Health Statistics, Series 10*, vol 171, pp 1-92.

[22] Franks, P., Clancy, C.M. and Gold, M.R. (1993) 'Health insurance and mortality: evidence from a national cohort', *Journal of the American Medical Association*, vol 270, pp 737-41.

[23] Hypertension Detection and Follow-up Program Cooperative Group (1987) 'Education level and 5-year all-cause mortality in the HDFP', *Hypertension*, vol 9, pp 641-6.

[24] Hypertension Detection and Follow-up Program Cooperative Group (1979) 'Five-year findings of the HDFP', *Journal of the American Medical Association*, vol 242, pp 2562-77.

[25] Davis, R.M. (1987) 'Current trends in cigarette advertising and marketing', *New England Journal of Medicine*, vol 316, pp 725-32.

[26] Adler, N.E., Boyce, W.T., Chesney, M.A., Folkman, S. and Syme, S.L. (1993) 'Socioeconomic inequalities in health: no easy solution', *Journal of the American Medical Association*, vol 269, pp 3140-5.

[27] Navarro, V. (1990) 'Race or class versus race and class: mortality differentials in the US', *Lancet*, vol 336, pp 1238-40.

[28] Pappas, G., Queen, S., Hadden, W. and Fisher, G. (1993) 'The increasing disparity in mortality between socioeconomic groups in the US, 1960-1986', *New England Journal of Medicine*, vol 329, pp 103-9.

[29] Davey Smith, G. and Egger, M. (1992) 'Socioeconomic differences in mortality in Britain and the US', *American Journal of Public Health*, vol 82, pp 1079-81.

[30] Essed, P. (1991) *Understanding everyday racism: An interdisciplinary theory*, Newbury Park, CA: Sage Publications.

7

Individual social class, area-based deprivation, cardiovascular disease risk-factors and mortality: the Renfrew and Paisley study

George Davey Smith, Carole Hart,
Graham Watt, David Hole
and Victor Hawthorne

Abstract

Objective: To investigate the associations of individual and area-based socioeconomic indicators with cardiovascular disease risk factors and mortality.

Design: Prospective study.

Setting: The towns of Renfrew and Paisley in the West of Scotland.

Participants: 6,961 men and 7,991 women included in a population-based cardiovascular disease screening study between 1972 and 1976.

Main outcome measures: Cardiovascular disease risk factors and cardiorespiratory morbidity at the time of screening; 15-year mortality rates from all-causes and cardiovascular disease.

Results: Both the area-based deprivation indicator and individual social class were associated with generally less favourable profiles of cardiovascular

Journal of Epidemiology and Community Health,
1998, vol 52, pp 399-405

disease risk factors at the time of the baseline screening examinations. The exception was plasma cholesterol concentration, which was lower for men and women in manual social class groups. Independent contributions of area-based deprivation and individual social class were generally seen with respect to risk factors and morbidity. All-cause and cardiovascular disease mortality rates were both inversely associated with socioeconomic position whether indexed by area-based deprivation or social class. The area-based and individual socioeconomic indicators made independent contributions to mortality risk.

Conclusions: Individually assigned and area-based socioeconomic indicators make independent contributions to several important health outcomes. The degree of inequalities in health that exist will not be demonstrated in studies using only one category of indicator. Similarly, adjustment for confounding by socioeconomic position in aetiological epidemiological studies will be inadequate if only one level of indicator is used. Policies aimed at reducing socioeconomic differentials in health should pay attention to the characteristics of the areas in which people live as well as the characteristics of the people who live in these areas.

Introduction

The association between social class, morbidity and mortality is well established.[1,2] Area-based indices of socioeconomic position, often referred to as 'deprivation indices', have also been related to morbidity and mortality for the people to whom these indices are applied.[3-8] The choice of the use of an individually assigned marker of socioeconomic position or an area-based indicator is often made on the pragmatic grounds of data availability. The use of census-level and individual-level socioeconomic data have been shown to lead to associations of a similar magnitude between socioeconomic position and a variety of health measures, with the suggestion that area-based measures slightly underestimated the strength of the associations when compared to the associations of individually based socioeconomic measures and health.[4]

In some,[4,5] but not all,[6] studies the use of larger geographical areas for the assignment of socioeconomic position leads to little, if any, attenuation in the magnitude of associations with health measures. This is surprising if area-based measures are considered merely to be proxy measures of individual socioeconomic position, as the level of misclassification would be expected to be greater when the size of area is larger. There are conceptual reasons as to why area-based measures may not simply function as indicators of individual socioeconomic position. Areas with a high level of socioeconomic disadvantage may also be disadvantaged with respect to transport, retail outlets, leisure facilities, environmental pollution and social disorganisation, in ways that influence health independently of the socioeconomic characteristics of the individuals living in these areas.[12] The demonstration of area-based effects would be important in emphasising the need to focus health promotion initiatives on the broader characteristics of places where disadvantaged people live, rather than simply on the individuals who live in these areas themselves.

The suggestion that the characteristics of area of residence have a particular influence on mortality risk is supported by two investigations which have examined both individual and area-based measures.[13-14] A study based on the Office for National Statistics (ONS) Longitudinal Study – a follow-up of a 1% sample of the 1971 England and Wales Census – indicated little influence of area-based deprivation once individual socioeconomic indicators had been taken into account.[15] This study had several limitations, however. First, no data on health status, health-related behaviours or physiological risk factors were available. Second, the individual socioeconomic indicators were essentially the ones which were used to construct the area-based measure. There would therefore be strong correlations between individual and area-based measures as an automatic consequence of the nature of the data that were used.

The most commonly used individual socioeconomic indicator in British studies is the Registrar General's occupational social class. In this present study we investigate the independent contributions of occupational social class and deprivation level of area of residence to cardiovascular disease risk factors and mortality, using the screening and mortality follow-up data of a large population-based health survey carried out in the West of Scotland between 1972 and 1976.

Methods

The Renfrew/Paisley general population study was carried out between 1972 and 1976 involving residents of the towns of Renfrew and Paisley who were aged 45-64 years. Full details of the study methodology have been reported previously.[7] A response rate of 80% was obtained. A questionnaire was completed by each participant and this was checked when the participant attended a screening examination. The questionnaire recorded smoking habit, occupation, respiratory and cardiovascular symptoms. Social class was determined by regular occupation, according to the Registrar General's classification.[8] In the case of retired men, the last full-time occupation was taken. For housewives and retired women, husbands' or fathers' occupations were used. Participants were classified as non-manual if they were in social classes I, II or IIIN and manual if in social classes IIIM, IV or V. Blood pressure, forced expiratory volume (FEV_1) in one second, height and weight were measured and an electrocardiogram was taken at the screening examination. A non-fasting blood sample was also taken to measure plasma cholesterol concentration.

The six-lead electrocardiogram (leads I, II, III, aVR, aVL and aVF) was taken with the subject sitting. Criteria for myocardial ischaemia on ECG were based on the Minnesota coding scheme. Any of the following codes were considered evidence of ischaemia, encompassing diagnoses of definite myocardial infarction, myocardial ischaemia and left bundle branch block: 1.1-1.3, 4.1-4.4, 5.1-5.3, 7.1. Angina was considered present if the definite or possible criteria of the Rose Angina Questionnaire were met.[9]

FEV_1 relative to the predicted value was used to estimate impairment. Predicted values of FEV_1 were obtained from linear regressions on age and height:

$$\text{Predicted } FEV_1 \text{ for men} = -1.9302 - (0.0290 \times \text{age [years]}) + (0.0373 \times \text{height [cm]})$$
$$\text{Predicted } FEV_1 \text{ for women} = -0.2662 - (0.0289 \times \text{age [years]}) + (0.0238 \times \text{height [cm]})$$

Coefficients were derived from a regression for the 878 men and 2,796 women who had never smoked and who responded 'no' to questions about bronchitis, breathing difficulties, and asthma. The FEV_1 score (%) was calculated as a percentage of actual FEV_1/predicted FEV_1.

The home address at the time of screening was retrospectively postcoded, enabling deprivation category as defined by Carstairs and Morris to be ascertained, using 1981 Census data.[10] Deprivation category varies from 1 (least deprived) to 7 (most deprived) and is calculated from the deprivation score which is based on four variables derived from census data – male unemployment, overcrowding, car ownership and proportion in social classes IV and V.

Both postcode sector and enumeration district deprivation categories were analysed, with the results being very similar. As the postcode sector deprivation category has been more often used in previous work, we have reported on these results here. Fourteen postcode sectors were represented in the study population.

Some addresses could not be postcoded and assigned a deprivation category and some participants had given insufficient information on occupation to assign a social class. The analyses were therefore performed on 6,961 (from 7,058) men and 7,991 (from 8,353) women with complete data. Participants were flagged at the National Health Service Central Register in Edinburgh and notification of deaths had been received for a 15-year follow-up period.[11] Cause of deaths were coded to International Classification of Diseases, Ninth Revision (ICD-9),[12] and cardiovascular disease (CVD) mortality consisted of deaths coded to ICD-9 390-459.

Age-adjusted means for continuous variables were calculated using PROC GLM of the SAS system,[13] with tests for trend being obtained with the PROC REG program. Categorical variables were age-standardised by the direct method, using the male and female study populations as the standard, and tests for trend were obtained with the PROC LOGIST program. Age-adjusted mortality rates were calculated using a person years at risk based lifetable approach and age standardisation was by the direct method. Trend tests were obtained through proportional hazards regression using PROC PHREG, with the age and deprivation score or social class coded as continuous variables. Adjustments were made using social class at six levels and deprivation score, both as continuous variables. Proportional hazards coefficients and their standard errors were calculated using Cox's model.

Adjustment for age and other risk factors was performed by including terms for these in the models. Adjustment for smoking was for the number of cigarettes smoked per day, together with a term for ex-smokers. Exponentiated hazards coefficients were taken as indicators of relative rates of mortality.

Results

No postcode sectors in Renfrew and Paisley were in deprivation category 2 and few participants lived in deprivation categories 1 and 7, the majority living in categories 4 and 5. Tabulation of social class derived from occupation with deprivation category showed that each

Table 1: Deprivation category by social class

Social class	Deprivation category						Total (%)	
	1	3	4	5	6	7		
Men								
I	76	83	72	78	38	2	349	(5.0)
II	126	200	234	290	108	13	971	(13.9)
IIIN	81	166	195	274	102	14	832	(12.0)
IIIM	85	348	607	1,144	528	98	2,810	(40.4)
IV	43	152	341	631	326	70	1,563	(22.5)
V	5	30	61	148	130	62	436	(6.3)
Total (%)	416 (6.0)	979 (14.1)	1,510 (21.7)	2,565 (36.8)	1,232 (17.7)	259 (3.7)	6,961	
Women								
I	41	47	45	44	13	3	193	(2.4)
II	152	235	311	370	158	31	1,257	(15.7)
IIIN	206	307	423	665	325	48	1,974	(24.7)
IIIM	59	191	324	558	287	71	1,490	(18.6)
IV	60	157	473	892	486	138	2,206	(27.6)
V	13	75	160	317	237	69	871	(10.9)
Total (%)	531 (6.6)	1,012 (12.7)	1,736 (21.7)	2,846 (35.6)	1,506 (18.8)	360 (4.5)	7,991	

deprivation category had representatives from each social class (Table 1). There were small numbers of men and women from social class I living in deprivation category 7 and small numbers from social class V living in deprivation category 1.

Table 2 shows the baseline risk factors by deprivation category and social class. Clear relations were seen between height, FEV_1, cholesterol concentration, smoking, bronchitis, angina and deprivation

Table 2: Age-adjusted means and proportions of baseline characteristics by deprivation category and social class

	All	\multicolumn{6}{Deprivation category}							Trend test adjusted for age	Trend test adjusted for age and social class
	All	1	3	4	5	6	7		
Men									
Diastolic BP (mm Hg)	86.1	85.3	87.0	84.5	87.1	84.8	87.9	p=0.13	p=0.12
Non-manual	86.0	85.4	86.7	84.0	87.9	84.0	88.0		
Manual	86.1	85.1	87.3	84.8	86.8	85.1	87.9		
Cholesterol (mmol/l)	5.87	5.83	5.97	5.97	5.80	5.79	5.92	p=0.0025	p=0.34
Non-manual	6.00	5.85	6.07	6.12	5.92	5.96	6.14		
Manual	5.81	5.77	5.88	5.90	5.76	5.75	5.89		
Height (cm)	169.5	171.4	171.1	170.1	169.2	168.3	166.7	p=0.0001	p=0.0001
Non-manual	171.5	171.9	172.1	171.9	171.0	170.6	166.7		
Manual	168.7	170.4	170.2	169.2	168.6	167.7	166.7		
Body mass index (kg/m²)	25.9	25.9	25.7	25.8	26.0	26.0	25.4	p=0.83	p=0.67
Non-manual	25.9	25.7	25.8	25.9	26.0	26.3	25.5		
Manual	25.8	26.4	25.6	25.7	25.9	25.9	25.4		
FEV, score (%)	88.6	94.9	91.6	88.9	88.1	86.9	78.1	p=0.0001	p=0.0001
Non-manual	92.9	96.9	93.9	93.0	92.0	89.7	84.8		
Manual	86.7	90.6	89.5	86.8	86.8	86.3	77.3		
% current smokers	58.6	46.9	48.8	57.5	61.3	62.8	72.0	p=0.0001	p=0.0001
Non-manual	49.7	44.3	44.1	49.1	53.7	53.5	75.4		
Manual	62.6	53.1	52.9	61.5	63.8	65.2	72.1		
% ex-smokers	24.7	32.2	29.8	25.4	23.1	22.3	16.2	p=0.0001	p=0.0001
Non-manual	29.3	33.1	33.0	30.2	26.6	26.0	16.2		
Manual	22.6	29.5	27.3	23.1	22.0	21.4	16.3		
% MRC bronchitis	5.9	3.0	4.2	6.3	6.1	6.5	9.3	p=0.0001	p=0.022
Non-manual	3.1	2.5	2.5	3.3	3.7	3.3	1.9		
Manual	7.1	3.7	5.5	7.9	6.9	7.3	10.5		
% angina	17.6	12.4	15.9	17.3	18.1	18.1	27.8	p=0.0001	p=0.0003
Non-manual	14.3	11.8	13.4	12.9	15.8	16.2	42.9		
Manual	19.2	13.6	17.9	19.5	18.8	18.6	28.6		
% ECG ischaemia	10.5	6.9	11.2	10.8	11.3	9.2	11.3	p=0.24	p=0.17
Non-manual	10.9	8.2	14.2	11.5	11.3	6.1	37.6		
Manual	10.3	3.9	8.7	10.4	11.2	10.0	11.2		

cont.../

Table 2: cont.../

	All		3	4	5	6	7	Trend test adjusted for age	Trend test adjusted for age and social class
		Deprivation category							
		I	3	4	5	6	7		
Women									
Diastolic BP (mm Hg)	85.1	85.0	86.3	83.1	86.3	84.5	85.3	*p*=0.60	*p*=0.67
Non-manual	84.3	85.0	85.8	82.2	85.7	82.7	83.9		
Manual	85.7	85.2	87.0	83.8	86.7	85.5	85.7		
Cholesterol (mmol/l)	6.43	6.36	6.49	6.50	6.43	6.35	6.35	*p*=0.007	*p*=0.12
Non-manual	6.50	6.41	6.50	6.61	6.48	6.46	6.51		
Manual	6.38	6.21	6.48	6.41	6.40	6.30	6.31		
Height (cm)	157.7	160.2	158.2	158.1	157.2	157.4	155.8	*p*=0.0001	*p*=0.0001
Non-manual	159.0	160.3	159.1	159.5	158.4	158.2	157.7		
Manual	156.8	159.8	157.0	157.0	156.5	157.0	155.3		
Body mass index (kg/m^2)	25.8	24.8	25.5	25.6	26.0	26.0	25.9	*p*=0.0001	*p*=0.005
Non-manual	25.2	24.7	25.1	25.1	25.5	25.3	24.9		
Manual	26.2	25.4	26.1	26.0	26.3	26.4	26.2		
FEV$_1$ score (%)	92.5	99.3	96.8	93.0	92.4	89.1	81.6	*p*=0.0001	*p*=0.0001
Non-manual	96.7	100.7	98.5	96.8	96.0	94.0	87.3		
Manual	89.3	95.0	94.4	89.9	90.3	86.7	79.9		
% current smokers	46.8	34.3	37.5	45.3	48.9	51.5	60.8	*p*=0.0001	*p*=0.0001
Non-manual	43.1	33.4	37.5	41.9	47.0	47.2	62.0		
Manual	49.9	37.0	38.5	48.3	50.4	53.7	60.2		
% ex-smokers	7.5	11.7	7.8	8.3	6.8	6.9	5.1	*p*=0.0001	*p*=0.003
Non-manual	8.8	11.8	9.5	9.4	7.8	7.6	3.7		
Manual	6.4	11.9	5.1	7.2	6.1	6.6	5.6		
% MRC bronchitis	4.0	1.9	2.4	3.2	3.9	6.1	7.7	*p*=0.0001	*p*=0.0001
Non-manual	2.3	2.0	1.0	2.0	2.6	4.0	5.1		
Manual	5.3	1.2	4.4	4.0	4.8	7.1	8.4		
% angina	16.9	11.4	15.6	14.9	18.2	18.9	19.7	*p*=0.0001	*p*=0.0002
Non-manual	14.0	10.5	13.0	14.3	15.4	15.5	10.0		
Manual	19.1	13.3	19.1	15.3	19.8	20.6	22.7		
% ECG ischaemia	10.0	8.5	9.6	10.1	9.8	10.0	13.1	*p*=0.018	*p*=0.028
Non-manual	9.0	7.2	9.4	8.9	8.6	10.1	12.2		
Manual	10.6	11.6	10.5	10.8	10.5	9.9	13.0		

category for both men and women. Body mass index and ECG ischaemia were associated with deprivation category only for women. With the exception of cholesterol concentration these associations remained after adjustment for social class. Within each deprivation category, manual and non-manual groups had differing levels of risk factors. Male and female manual social class participants had lower cholesterol concentrations, were shorter, had lower FEV$_1$, were more likely to smoke and have bronchitis and angina than the non-manual social class participants. Manual women had higher diastolic blood pressure and body mass index and had more ECG ischaemia than non-manual women. The associations between social class and risk factors were little changed by adjustment for deprivation.

Death rates (Table 3) show trends with deprivation category for all-cause and CVD mortality for men and women. Death rates for men in deprivation category 7 were almost double the rates for men in deprivation category 1. For men and women, all-cause and CVD mortality retained sizeable associations with deprivation after adjustment for social class (Table 4). Adjustment for risk factors attenuated the associations. Social class differences in all-cause and CVD mortality in men and women were attenuated but remained substantial after adjustment for deprivation score (Table 5). Adjustment for risk factors caused greater attenuation of social class differences in mortality than did adjustment for deprivation score. Formal tests of interaction between social class and deprivation score were not statistically significant.

All-cause mortality was further analysed by division of each deprivation category into non-manual and manual social classes. Taking the baseline category as non-manual workers living in deprivation category 1, the risk increased across deprivation category within both non-manual and manual social classes for men (Table 6). Additionally, manual groups had a higher risk than non-manual groups for each deprivation category. For women, manual groups had a higher mortality risk than non-manual groups for each deprivation category and a clear association between deprivation category and mortality was seen among manual, but not non-manual, women.

Table 3: Fifteen-year age-adjusted death rates by deprivation category

			Deprivation category				
	1	3	4	5	6	7	Trend
Men							
All-cause							
No of deaths	107	246	445	801	424	110	
Death rate	165.7	178.8	200.5	218.3	228.8	292.2	p=0.0001
Cardiovascular disease							
No of deaths	59	137	241	436	208	62	
Death rate	98.7	109.6	118.6	132.6	127.1	184.8	p=0.0001
Women							
All-cause							
No of deaths	78	165	291	539	344	75	
Death rate	97.5	114.2	113.5	131.2	147.1	137.6	p=0.0001
Cardiovascular disease							
No of deaths	41	70	140	268	169	38	
Death rate	52.5	53.8	58.8	71.1	76.9	75.2	p=0.002

Table 4: Relative rates (95% CI) of mortality by deprivation category

	1-3	Deprivation category 4-5	6-7	Trend
Men				
All-cause				
Age	I	1.27 (1.12,1.42)	1.47 (1.28,1.68)	p=0.0001
Age + social class	I	1.19 (1.06,1.35)	1.34 (1.17,1.54)	p=0.0001
Age + risk factors[a]	I	1.12 (1.00,1.26)	1.24 (1.08,1.42)	p=0.0008
Cardiovascular disease				
Age	I	1.24 (1.06,1.45)	1.33 (1.11,1.60)	p=0.0001
Age + social class	I	1.19 (1.01,1.40)	1.26 (1.04,1.52)	p=0.0001
Age + risk factors[a]	I	1.12 (0.95,1.31)	1.19 (0.98,1.43)	p=0.019
Women				
All-cause				
Age	I	1.18 (1.03,1.37)	1.40 (1.19,1.64)	p=0.0001
Age + social class	I	1.12 (0.97,1.30)	1.29 (1.10,1.52)	p=0.006
Age + risk factors[a]	I	1.07 (0.93,1.24)	1.16 (0.99,1.36)	p=0.55
Cardiovascular disease				
Age	I	1.28 (1.04,1.58)	1.48 (1.17,1.86)	p=0.0002
Age + social class	I	1.18 (0.96,1.47)	1.33 (1.05,1.69)	p=0.035
Age + risk factors[a]	I	1.15 (0.93,1.42)	1.21 (0.95,1.52)	p=0.60

Table 5: Relative rates (95% CI) of mortality by social class

	I and II	Social class IIIN	IIIM	IV and V	Trend
Men					
All-cause					
Age	I	1.25 (1.06,1.47)	1.40 (1.23,1.60)	1.52 (1.33,1.74)	p=0.0001
Age + deprivation score	I	1.23 (1.04,1.45)	1.32 (1.16,1.51)	1.41 (1.23,1.62)	p=0.0001
Age + risk factors[a]	I	1.13 (0.96,1.34)	1.18 (1.03,1.34)	1.22 (1.06,1.40)	p=0.005
Cardiovascular disease					
Age	I	1.23 (0.99,1.54)	1.35 (1.13,1.60)	1.33 (1.11,1.60)	p=0.002
Age + deprivation score	I	1.21 (0.97,1.52)	1.27 (1.07,1.52)	1.24 (1.03,1.49)	p=0.033
Age + risk factors[a]	I	1.13 (0.90,1.41)	1.20 (1.01,1.44)	1.16 (0.96,1.39)	p=0.13
Women					
All-cause					
Age	I	0.92 (0.77,1.10)	1.38 (1.17,1.64)	1.32 (1.14,1.54)	p=0.0001
Age + deprivation score	I	0.91 (0.77,1.09)	1.35 (1.14,1.60)	1.27 (1.09,1.49)	p=0.0001
Age + risk factors[a]	I	0.93 (0.78,1.11)	1.21 (1.02,1.44)	1.13 (0.97,1.33)	p=0.014
Cardiovascular disease					
Age	I	0.88 (0.68,1.15)	1.44 (1.12,1.84)	1.50 (1.20,1.87)	p=0.0001
Age + deprivation score	I	0.87 (0.67,1.14)	1.40 (1.09,1.79)	1.44 (1.15,1.80)	p=0.0001
Age + risk factors[a]	I	0.90 (0.69,1.17)	1.19 (0.93,1.53)	1.25 (0.99,1.56)	p=0.005

Note for Tables 4 and 5: [a] Risk factors are diastolic, bold pressure, cholesterol, body mass index, FEV_1 score, smoking, angina, ECG ischaemia and bronchitis.

Table 6: Age-adjusted relative risk (95% CI) for all-cause mortality by deprivation category and social class

	Deprivation category					
	I	3	4	5	6	7
Men						
Non-manual	I	1.06 (0.7-,1.44)	1.02 (0.75-1.37)	1.26 (0.95-1.67)	1.43 (1.03-1.98)	1.70 (0.94-3.08)
Manual	1.17 (0.79,1.73)	1.22 (0.92-1.64)	1.47 (1.13-1.92)	1.56 (1.21-2.01)	1.57 (1.21-2.04)	2.28 (1.67-3.11)
Women						
Non-manual	I	1.05 (0.75-1.48)	1.01 (0.73-1.40)	1.18 (0.87-1.59)	1.40 (1.00-1.95)	0.94 (0.49-1.80)
Manual	1.07 (0.65,1.76)	1.47 (1.05-2.06)	1.40 (1.04-1.88)	1.62 (1.23-2.15)	1.77 (1.32-2.36)	1.67 (1.17-2.39)

Discussion

The population covered in this study all reside within the Renfrew district, an area which includes rural, new town and commuter populations. The 0-64 year age band standardised mortality ratio (SMR) in 1980-85 for Renfrew district was 107, with Scotland as the standard.[10] The area covered by the Renfrew and Paisley study represents the more deprived parts of the Renfrew district, and includes the postcode sector with the highest deprivation score in Scotland.[10] This study therefore covers a representative sample from a largely deprived area, and is unusual in this regard for UK epidemiological studies.[14,15,16]

Within this area of high overall deprivation there was still considerable heterogeneity of both individual social class and area-based deprivation measures. Large differences in cardiovascular disease risk factors by individual social class and area-based deprivation are seen. These generally ran in the same direction, with less favourable socioeconomic position, assigned by either individual, or area-based measures, being accompanied by shorter height, worse lung function and higher prevalences of bronchitis and coronary heart disease. The two socioeconomic measures contributed independently to the distribution of these health-related measures. For women, but not men, body mass index was higher in the groups in less favourable social circumstances, in keeping with other data on the social distribution of obesity.[17] Plasma cholesterol levels were higher in the non-manual social class groups in this study, in line with other investigations carried out at around the same time,[14,15] although this direction of association has not previously been reported for women in the UK, for whom data are sparse.

The higher body mass index in women from manual social groups would be expected to lead to higher circulating cholesterol concentrations, and clearly some other factor is involved in determining the distribution of cholesterol concentrations.

A few studies have examined the contribution of individual and area-based socioeconomic characteristics to the distribution of health-related behaviours. Multilevel modelling approaches have generally identified effects of residential area on smoking behaviour and alcohol consumption,[18,19] together with influences on physiological risk factors such as blood pressure and circulating cholesterol concentration which are responsive to health-related behaviours. These area effects tend to be considerably smaller than the effects of individual socioeconomic position, but the categorisation of the areas has not been one that has explicitly focused on their socioeconomic characteristics. A study in Glasgow that investigated health-related behaviours and physical measurements in relation to individual social class and social characteristics of area of residence found that poorer areas contained people who were less likely to consume (and had less access to) healthy foods, less likely to participate in sport, more likely to be smokers, to be shorter, have higher body mass indices and greater waist to hip ratios.[20,21] Our analyses suggest that the inhabitants of deprived areas are more likely to be smokers, have poor lung function, be shorter and, for women, have higher body mass indices, even after the occupational social class of these individuals has been taken into account.

Geographical differences in mortality that are independent of individual socioeconomic characteristics can be seen in international comparisons or in broad geographical differences within a country (for example, North versus South in England and Wales).[22,23] Few investigations of individual and area-based socioeconomic measures in relation to mortality among individuals have been carried out, however. Carstairs and Morris demonstrated consistent gradients in mortality by deprivation level within social class groups, while the reverse was not the case. This suggests that an important area of residence effect exists. In the Scottish Heart Health Study both an area-based deprivation indicator and individual social class were associated with prevalent coronary heart disease, with both remaining significant predictors in a multivariable model.[24] In the US National Longitudinal Mortality Study median family income for census tract of residence and individual family income have been related to mortality. While larger mortality differentials were seen in relation to individual family income, individual and area-based measures made independent contributions to mortality risk among people of working age.[25] In the England and Wales Longitudinal Study an area-based deprivation indicator showed little influence on mortality once the constituents of the indicator had been adjusted for at the individual level. These latter two studies suffer from the conceptual problem of using identical markers at an aggregate and individual level. If specific influences of place type are considered to exist then their particularity may better be indicated by variables other than those considered at the individual level. Indeed a reanalysis of the England and Wales Longitudinal Study using the Craig–Webber area classification demonstrated an independent contribution of area characteristics after individual socioeconomic indicators had been taken into account.[26]

In our data, as in the similar analyses carried out for the Alameda County Study,[27] an independent, but attenuated, association between area-based deprivation and all-cause mortality was seen after adjustment for an extensive array of risk factors. In our data this was only seen for men, while multivariable analyses were only carried out for both sexes combined in the Alameda County Study. It could be considered that misclassification in the risk factor data will lead to under-adjustment and that with better data the already substantial attenuation in the association between area-based deprivation and mortality brought about risk factor adjustment would be even greater. Alternatively, the unequal distribution of risk factors according to socioeconomic characteristics of areas of residence could be considered to mediate between area and health, rather than confound the association. In this case the multivariable adjustments we have carried out could be considered to represent over-adjustment.

In this study, as in the Alameda County Study, data on socioeconomic position in adulthood were available, but data on childhood socioeconomic circumstances were not. In a further study in the West of Scotland, adjustment for a cumulative socioeconomic indicator, based on social circumstances from childhood through to adulthood, led to considerable attenuation of the association between deprivation level of area of residence and mortality among men.[28] Cumulative lifecourse socioeconomic measures will reflect other factors than socially patterned exposures in adulthood. First, there may be direct influences of childhood socioeconomic deprivation on mortality from various causes in adulthood.[28,29] Second, socioeconomic position in adulthood and area of residence may both be influenced by educational achievement and other factors influencing geographical mobility.

Several calls have been made regarding the necessity to consider geography as an additional dimension in studies of variations in health.[27,30]

This call should be extended to one that recognises the need to include a temporal dimension in addition to current social position and residential area of individuals.

Conceptual issues in the use of area-based socioeconomic indicators

When using area-based indicators of socioeconomic position, two forms of bias could be introduced.[31] It could be considered that the area-based measure serves as a proxy indicator of individual socioeconomic circumstances. In this instance the associations between area-based socioeconomic measures and health outcomes would be underestimates of underlying associations between individual socioeconomic position and health, as considerable misclassification of individual socioeconomic circumstances by the area-based measure would occur. The use of larger geographical areas should lead to greater misclassification of individual socioeconomic position and therefore to weaker associations between the area-based indicator and health outcomes than the underlying association between individual socioeconomic position and health. Conversely, there may be specific characteristics of the areas that influence health in other ways than through individual socioeconomic differences. Technically, the residuals from analyses using individual-level data will be correlated with the area-based indicator.[31,32] In this case, if the area-based measure is used as a proxy for individual socioeconomic position it could overestimate, rather than underestimate, the magnitude of individual-level associations. Area-based measures will, however, provide additional information on the socioeconomic characteristics of residents within the area, independent of the individual socioeconomic circumstances of these people.

The empirical findings with respect to these questions have been variable and have depended on the context of studies and the health outcomes under examination.[4,5,6,31] The contextual effects of areas, and the size of areas which determine these effects, will differ in different places and for different health outcomes, so this inconsistency in the literature is not unexpected.

The particular aspects of different areas which may influence health independently of individual social class are currently under investigation.[27,33] A range of such characteristics, including environmental effects, housing conditions, social disorganisation, transport, insecurity about personal safety, the availability of retail and leisure facilities, socially determined health-related behaviours and access to healthcare, have been implicated in this regard. Further investigation of this issue, both qualitative and quantitative, is required if our current understanding is to be taken forward.

Implications and conclusions

A wide range of characteristics of areas that reflect their broader social constitution, while not being simply reducible to the socioeconomic characteristics of the people living in these areas, have been related to mortality. This includes such factors as socioeconomic inequality within the areas, voting patterns at elections, crime rates, education and medical care expenditure and welfare services.[34-37]

However, studies to date – including our own – have tended to use socioeconomic indicators that have essentially the same meaning at aggregate and individual level. Further investigation of a wider range of socioeconomic and sociocultural characteristics of areas should be undertaken.

Individually assigned and area-based socioeconomic indicators make independent contributions to at least some important health outcomes. The use of either indicator alone when attempting to adjust for socioeconomic confounding in aetiological epidemiological studies may leave a substantial degree of residual confounding. Similarly, the use of only one kind of indicator will not fully describe the degree of inequalities in health which exist. Both area-based and individually based socioeconomic data should be collected where possible and social circumstances acting across the lifecourse, rather than just at one stage, require consideration.

References

[1] Davey Smith, G., Bartley, M. and Blane, D. (1990) 'The Black Report on socioeconomic inequalities in health 10 years on', *British Medical Journal*, vol 301, pp 373-7.

[2] Davey Smith, G., Bartley, M. and Blane, D. (1994) 'Explanations for socioeconomic differentials in mortality: evidence from Britain and elsewhere', *European Journal of Public Health*, vol 4, pp 131-44.

[3] Phillimore, P., Beattie, A. and Townsend, P. (1994) 'Widening inequality of health in northern England, 1981-91', *British Medical Journal*, vol 308, pp 1125-8.

[4] Krieger, N. (1992) 'Overcoming the absence of socio-economic data in medical records: validation and application of a census-based methodology', *American Journal of Public Health*, vol 82, pp 703-10.

[5] Carr-Hill, R. and Rice, N. (1995) 'Is enumeration district level an improvement on ward level analysis in studies of deprivation and health?', *Journal of Epidemiology and Community Health*, vol 49, suppl 2, pp 28-9.

[6] Hyndman, J.C.G., Holman, C.D.J., Hockey, R.L., Donovan, R.J., Corti, B. and Rivera, J. (1995) 'Risk classification of social disadvantage based on geographical areas: comparison of postcode and collector's district analyses', *International Journal of Epidemiology*, vol 24, pp 165-76.

[7] Hawthorne, V.M., Watt, G.C.M., Hart, C.L., Hole, D.J., Davey Smith, G. and Gillis, C.R. (1995) 'Cardiorespiratory disease in men and women in urban Scotland: baseline characteristics of the Renfrew/Paisley (MIDSPAN) study population', *Scottish Medical Journal,* vo; 40, pp 102-7.

[8] General Register Office (1966) *Classification of occupations 1966,* London: HMSO.

[9] Hart, C.L., Watt, G.C.M., Davey Smith, G., Gillis, C.R. and Hawthorne, V.M. (1997) 'Pre-existing ischaemic heart disease and ischaemic heart disease mortality in women compared with men', *International Journal of Epidemiology,* vol 26, pp 508-15.

[10] Carstairs, V. and Morris, R. (1991) *Deprivation and health in Scotland,* Aberdeen: Aberdeen University Press.

[11] Watt, G.C.M., Hart, C.L., Hole, D.J., Davey Smith, G., Gillis, C.R. and Hawthorne, V.M. (1995) 'Risk factors for cardiorespiratory and all cause mortality in men and women in urban Scotland: 15 year followup', *Scottish Medical Journal,* vol 40, pp 108-12.

[12] World Health Organisation (1977) *Classification of diseases 9th revision,* Geneva: WHO.

[13] SAS Institute (1991) *SAS language and procedures: Usage 2, version 6,* Cary, NC: SAS Institute.

[14] **Davey Smith, G., Shipley, M.J. and Rose, G. (1990) 'The magnitude and causes of socio-economic differentials in mortality: further evidence from the Whitehall Study',** *Journal of Epidemiology and Community Health,* **vol 44, pp 265-70.**

[15] Pocock, S.J., Shaper, A.G., Cook, D.G., Phillips, A.N. and Walker, M. (1987) 'Social class differences in ischaemic heart disease in British men', *Lancet,* vol 2, pp 197-201.

[16] Smith, W.C.S., Tunstall-Pedoe, H., Crombie, I.K. and Tavendale, R. (1989) 'Concomitants of excess coronary deaths – major risk factor and lifestyle findings from 10,359 men and women in the Scottish Heart Health Study', *Scottish Medical Journal,* vol 34, pp 550-5.

[17] Davey Smith, G. and Brunner, E. (1997) 'Socio-economic differentials in health: the role of nutrition', *Proceedings of the Nutrition Society,* vol 56, pp 75-90.

[18] Duncan, C., Jones, K. and Moon, G. (1993) 'Do places matter? A multilevel analysis of regional variations in health-related behaviour in Britain', *Social Science and Medicine*, vol 37, pp 725-35.

[19] Hart, C., Ecob, R. and Davey Smith, G. (1997) 'People, places and coronary heart disease risk factors: a multilevel analysis of the Scottish Heart Health Study archive', *Social Science and Medicine*, vol 45, pp 893-902.

[20] Ellaway, A. and Macintyre, S. (1996) 'Does where you live predict health related behaviour? A case study in Glasgow', *Health Bulletin*, vol 54, pp 443-6.

[21] Ellaway, A., Anderson, A. and Macintyre, S. (1997) 'Does area of residence affect body size and shape?, *International Journal of Obesity*, vol 21, pp 304-8.

[22] Wilkinson, R. (1996) *Unhealthy societies: The afflictions of inequality*, London: Routledge.

[23] Martin, W.J. (1956) 'The distribution in England and Wales of mortality from coronary disease', *British Medical Journal*, vol I, pp 1523-5.

[24] Woodward, M. (1996) 'Small area statistics as markers for personal social status in the Scottish Heart Health Study', *Journal of Epidemiology and Community Health*, vol 50, pp 570-6.

[25] Anderson, R.T., Sorlie, P., Backlund, E., Johnson, N. and Kaplan, G. (1997) 'Mortality effects of community socioeconomic status', *Epidemiology*, vol 8, pp 42-7.

[26] Ecob, R. and Jones, K. (1998) 'Mortality variations in England and Wales between types of place: an analysis of the ONS Longitudinal Study', *Social Science and Medicine*, vol 47, pp 2055-66.

[27] Kaplan, G.A. (1996) 'People and places: contrasting perspectives on the association between social class and health', *International Journal of Health Services*, vol 26, pp 507-19.

[28] **Davey Smith, G., Hart, C., Blane, D., Gillis, C. and Hawthorne, V.M. (1997) 'Lifetime socio-economic position and mortality: prospective observational study', *British Medical Journal*, vol 314, pp 547-52.**

[29] Wannamethee, S.G., Whincup, P.H., Shaper, G. and Walker, M. (1996) 'Influence of fathers' social class on cardiovascular disease in middle-aged men', *Lancet*, vol 348, pp 1259-63.

[30] Jones, K. and Moon, G. (1993) 'Medical geography: taking space seriously', *Progress in Human Geography*, vol 17, pp 515-24.

[31] Geronimus, A.T., Bound, J. and Neidert, L.J. (1996) 'On the validity of using census geocode characteristics to proxy individual socio-economic characteristics', *Journal of the American Statistical Association*, vol 91, pp 529-37.

[32] Firebaugh, G. (1978) 'A rule for inferring individual-level relationships from aggregate data', *American Sociological Review*, vol 43, pp 557-72.

[33] Sooman, A., Macintyre, S. and Anderson, A. (1993) 'Scotland's health – a more difficult challenge for some? The price and availability of healthy foods in socially contrasting localities in the West of Scotland', *Health Bulletin*, vol 51, pp 276-84.

[34] Kaplan, G.A., Pamuk, E.R., Lynch, J.W., Cohen, R.D. and Balfour, J.L. (1996) 'Inequality in income and mortality in the United States: analysis of mortality and potential pathways', *British Medical Journal*, vol 312, pp 999-1003.

[35] Ben-Shlomo, Y., White, I.R. and Marmot, M. (1996) 'Does the variation in the socio-economic characteristics of an area affect mortality?', *British Medical Journal*, vol 312, pp 1013-14.

[36] Kennedy, B.P., Kawachi, I. and Prothrow-Stith, D. (1996) 'Income distribution and mortality: cross sectional ecological study of the Robin Hood index in the United States', *British Medical Journal*, vol 312, pp 1004-7.

[37] **Davey Smith, G. and Dorling, D. (1996) ' "I'm all right John": voting patterns and mortality in England and Wales, 1981-92', *British Medical Journal*, vol 313, pp 1573-7.**

8

Is control at work the key to socioeconomic gradients in mortality?

George Davey Smith and Seeromanie Harding

Socioeconomic differentials in coronary heart disease (CHD) are substantial and cannot be accounted for by conventional cardiovascular risk factors.[1] It has been suggested that a particular form of job stress – that associated with a low degree of control over activity at work – is a major contributor to such socioeconomic differentials. Statistical adjustment for self-reported job control has been found to essentially abolish the socioeconomic gradient in CHD incidence.[2] There are, however, serious questions regarding collinearity in such analyses: low control over work is virtually synonymous with low socioeconomic position and an exploration of the associations between different work characteristics and cardiovascular disease risk demonstrates that these associations may be dependent on the social patterning of the work characteristic in question.[3]

Historical considerations lend support to a sceptical view of a specific causal contribution of low job control to the social distribution of CHD. Earlier this century, when most women were not in formal employment, the socioeconomic gradient in CHD was much steeper for women than for men.[1] Similarly the social gradient of CHD among people who are beyond working age is the same as that of those of working years. We have further explored this issue by analysing the association between socioeconomic position, as indexed by car access, and mortality in the Longitudinal Study, a follow-up of 1% of the population of England and Wales from the 1981 Census.[4]

The analyses relate to men and women of working age at the time of the 1981 Census. All-cause and CHD mortality according to household car access (0, 1, or more) in 1981 was examined for those who were in full- or part-time employment and those who were

Lancet, 1997, vol 350, pp 1369-70

seeking work or waiting to take up a job. The mortality differentials according to car access (Table 1) are similar for those in work and for those not working.

What is clear is that socioeconomic differentials are not specific to people in work, for whom low job control could be a plausible mechanism for the increased CHD risk. The hypothesis could be expanded to say that it is control over the contingencies of life in general, rather than at work in particular, which is important. However, if job control explains the socioeconomic gradient in those who are at work, this suggests that there is no independent influence of control during the non-working part of the lives of employed people, while this is of major importance in non-employed people. This seems unlikely. Furthermore, the expanded hypothesis becomes more difficult to test or to implement in intervention programmes.

In the first Whitehall Study,[5] not owning a car was associated with a 49% higher risk of all-cause mortality. Adjustment for employment grade left a significant increase in mortality risk of 28%, just as adjustment for employment grade in the Whitehall II Study left a residual significant influence of job control. Because we have no reason to believe that non-car ownership is a cause of increased mortality, we treat it as a sensitive indicator of socioeconomic position; the same could well be true of job control.

Table 1: Hazard ratios for mortality between 1981 and 1994 from all causes and CHD

	Hazard ratio (95% CI)	
	Employed 1981	**Not employed 1981**
Men		
All-cause		
No car	1.00	1.00
Car	0.70 (0.67-0.73)	0.70 (0.63-0.77)
CHD		
No car	1.00	1.00
Car	0.78 (0.73-0.85)	0.70 (0.59-0.83)
Women		
All-cause		
No car	1.00	1.00
Car	0.69 (0.64-0.75)	0.81 (0.61-1.07)
CHD		
No car	1.00	1.00
Car	0.61 (0.50-0.75)	0.72 (0.37-1.40)

References

[1] Davey Smith, G. (1997) 'Socioeconomic differentials', in D. Kuh and Y. Ben-Shlomo (eds) *A life course approach to chronic disease epidemiology*, Oxford: Oxford University Press, pp 242-73.

[2] Marmot, M.G., Bosma, H., Hemingway, H., Brunner, E. and Stansfeld, S. (1997) 'Contribution of job control and other risk factors to social variations in coronary heart disease incidence', *Lancet*, vol 350, pp 235-9.

[3] Carroll, D., Davey Smith, G. and Bennett, P. (1996) 'Some observations on health and socioeconomic status', *Journal of Health Psychology*, vol 1, pp 23-39.

[4] Goldblatt, P. (1990) *Longitudinal study: Mortality and social organisation*, London: HMSO.

[5] **Davey Smith, G., Shipley, M.J. and Rose, G. (1990) 'Magnitude and causes of socioeconomic differentials in mortality: further evidence from the Whitehall Study', *Journal of Epidemiology and Community Health*, vol 44, pp 265-70.**

Section II
Voting and mortality

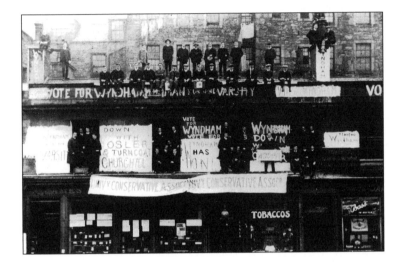

Edinburgh School of Medicine, Chemical Laboratories: students on the
roof and out of the windows during an election.
The Wellcome Library, London. Reproduced with permission.

9

"I'm all right, John": voting patterns and mortality in England and Wales, 1981-92

George Davey Smith and Daniel Dorling

Abstract

Objective: To investigate the association between voting patterns, deprivation, and mortality across England and Wales.

Design: Ecological study.

Setting: All the electoral constituencies of England and Wales.

Main outcome measures: Combined and gender-specific standardised mortality ratios.

Results: For the years surrounding the three elections of 1983, 1987 and 1992 overall standardised mortality ratios showed substantial negative correlations of –0.74 to –0.76 with Conservative voting and substantial positive correlations of 0.73 to 0.77 with Labour voting (all p<0.0001). Correlations were higher for male than female mortality. Conservative voting was strongly negatively correlated (r=–0.84) with the Townsend deprivation score, while Labour voting was positively correlated (r=0.74) with this. Labour and Conservative voting explained more of the variance in mortality than did the Townsend score. In multiple regression analyses for the 1992 Election Labour voting (p<0.0001), Conservative voting (p<0.0001), the Townsend score (p=0.016), and abstentions (p=0.032) were all associated with mortality. Labour and Conservative voting explained 61% of the variance in mortality between constituencies; when Townsend score and abstentions were added this increased to 63%.

Conclusions: Conservative and Labour voting are at least as strongly associated with mortality as is a standard deprivation index. Voting patterns

British Medical Journal, 1996, vol 313, pp 1573-7

may add information above that provided by indicators of material deprivation. People living in better circumstances and who have better health, who are least likely to require unemployment benefit and free school meals or to rely on a state pension in old age, and who are most able to opt out of state-subsidised provision of transport, education, and the NHS, vote for the party that is most likely to dismantle the welfare state.

Introduction

Differences in mortality in residential areas have been analysed for over 150 years in Britain.[1] William Farr considered these differences to show the "comparative salubrity of every part of England and Wales".[1] Later investigators took geographical differences to reflect a wide range of factors, including the influence of altitude, climate, migration, water constituents, specific occupational factors, pollution, and the long-term effects of development during early life.[2] Although these studies have been primarily concerned with the causes of disease, the more general issue of differences in area reflecting socioeconomic disparities has remained a constant theme.[3-8] This is reflected in the development of a series of deprivation indices, which are increasingly being used for health services resource allocation and planning.[9] They generally use census variables such as car ownership, overcrowding, occupational social class, unemployment, the prevalence of lone-parent families, and housing tenure to produce a single score which reflects the degree of material deprivation in an area.

When water hardness is being related in areas to rates of ischaemic heart disease, for example, a causal association between the exposure and the disease is hypothesised.[10] The use of deprivation indices, on the other hand, does not assume a direct causal relation between material deprivation and health outcomes. The deprivation indices are, however, strongly related to mortality and statistically account for a considerable proportion of the variance in mortality between areas, rendering them useful for demonstrating the size of socioeconomic inequalities in health for health service planning and for investigating the degree of inequity in the distribution of health service resources.

Other aspects of the sociocultural constitution of areas, those that cannot be indexed by census variables, may help to explain geographical variations in mortality. One measure, which has been little studied in this regard, is voting behaviour. There are major differences in voting patterns between different social groups, but voting also reflects aspects of the ideology, history, and composition of populations that are not simply reducible to social class. We report the relation between voting and mortality in England and Wales around the time of the last three General Elections.

Methods

The electoral data are the results of the General Elections of 1983, 1987 and 1992 for each constituency in England and Wales. For the purposes of comparison, the Liberal Party, Social Democratic Party, the Alliance, and the Liberal Democrats are treated as a single party throughout this time, which for ease of reference we will call Liberal. There are 561 constituencies in this dataset, the two newly created Milton Keynes constituencies of 1992 being treated as one constituency to maintain historical continuity.

The full postcode of the usual residence of people who had died was used to assign each death in England and Wales to a local government ward, which in turn could then be assigned to the parliamentary constituency in which the person had lived. The deaths were divided into three groups by year of death: 1981-85, 1986-89, and 1990-92. Mortality data coded to constituency are currently available only up to the end of 1992. The all age mortality data in each period used population data from the 1981 and 1991 Censuses corrected for under-enumeration.[11] (Mid-year 1983 and end-year 1987 constituency population profiles were estimated from the two census sources for the first two periods.) Standardised mortality ratios (SMRs) were calculated separately for males and females and for both groups together in each constituency using the overall age-specific death rates for England and Wales for the periods under consideration. SMRs for constituencies in the three time periods were then compared to the corresponding proportions of the electorate voting for each political party in the General Elections of 1983, 1987 and 1992.

The Townsend deprivation score for each constituency was calculated using 1981 and 1991 Census data. This index is based on car ownership, unemployment, overcrowded housing, and housing tenure and reflects levels of material deprivation.[12] Initial analyses computed simple correlations between SMRs and the percentage of the population voting for the major parties or abstaining. Correlations between Townsend deprivation scores and voting behaviour were also computed. Regression analyses then examined the influence of voting patterns and Townsend deprivation scores on SMRs.

Results

Table 1 shows the voting patterns for England and Wales in the three elections. The distribution of votes is only indirectly reflected in the distribution of seats won in British elections, but it is the distribution of votes as indicators of political allegiance which interests us here, not which party won each seat. We are also interested in what proportion of the electorate chose not to vote in each area and the associations between this indicator of political apathy and mortality.

Table 1: General Election figures for England and Wales

Election	Total votes	Overall	Minimum	Maximum	No of seats won[a]
1983					
Conservative	12,211,280	32.38	6.29	48.61	376
Labour	7,466,474	19.80	1.92	53.51	168
Liberal	7,088,222	18.80	5.28	45.11	15
Abstentions	10,625,773	28.18	18.82	48.37	
Electorate	37,707,619	100.00	100.00	100.00	
1987					
Conservative	13,047,000	34.21	5.93	51.42	366
Labour	8,770,926	23.00	4.42	58.60	179
Liberal	6,771,607	17.75	4.61	40.97	13
Abstentions	9,309,140	24.41	15.62	44.56	
Electorate	38,139,406	100.00	100.00	100.00	
1992					
Conservative	13,297,554	34.79	5.98	52.88	325
Labour	10,414,196	27.24	3.72	61.71	222
Liberal	5,643,192	14.76	3.11	42.38	11
Abstentions	8,332,388	21.80	7.03	46.12	
Electorate	38,225,759	100.00	100.00	100.00	

[a] In 1983 two seats were won by Plaid Cymru and total number of seats was 561; in 1987 three seats were won by Plaid Cymru and total number of seats was 561; in 1992 four seats were won by Plaid Cymru and an additional constituency in Milton Keynes was added, raising the number of seats in England and Wales to 562.

In Table 2 the correlations between voting pattern and mortality are presented for the years around each General Election. SMRs showed large positive correlations with Labour voting, smaller positive correlations with abstentions, large negative correlations with Conservative voting, and smaller negative correlations with Liberal voting. The magnitude of positive and negative correlations was greater for male than for female mortality in all cases. The only noticeable change between the elections is the increase over time in the strength of the association of abstention rate with both male and female SMRs.

Figure 1 shows maps of voting patterns in the 1992 Election and maps of mortality for the period around this Election; the degree to which voting and death coincide geographically is evident. Scatter plots of SMRs and voting are shown in Figure 2. Outliers in these scatter plots are labelled, as is Basildon, where the Conservative victory in 1992 was seen as crucial. The result in Basildon was announced early after the polls closed and showed the trend that was to be seen across the country of a secure Conservative victory. Basildon – popularly considered to be inhabited entirely by the species 'Essex person' – was in 1992 considered to be an unlikely Conservative seat, although its position in Figure 2 shows it to be entirely typical.

Table 2: Correlations between voting and SMRs

Election	Overall	Men	Women
1983			
Conservative	−0.76	−0.81	−0.65
Labour	0.76	0.79	0.67
Liberal	−0.49	−0.52	−0.42
Abstentions	0.36	0.43	0.27
1987			
Conservative	−0.75	−0.80	−0.64
Labour	0.77	0.80	0.68
Liberal	−0.52	−0.54	−0.45
Abstentions	0.37	0.43	0.28
1992			
Conservative	−0.74	−0.79	−0.61
Labour	0.73	0.75	0.63
Liberal	−0.50	−0.53	−0.42
Abstentions	0.54	0.62	0.40

Note: All $p < 0.0001$.

Voting patterns were also strongly related to the Townsend deprivation score, which is in turn positively associated with mortality. In Table 3 the Townsend score in 1981 and 1991 is related to the voting and mortality data associated with the closest General Election (1983 and 1992). There has been a moderate degree of attenuation in the strength of correlations between 1983 and 1992, with the exception of the association between the Townsend score and the abstention rate, which has increased greatly.

The contribution of the Townsend score, together with voting data, to the statistical explanation of variation in mortality between constituencies is summarised in Table 4. Around both the 1983 and 1992 Elections, Labour and Conservative voting accounted for more of the variance in mortality than did the Townsend score. In multiple regression analyses for 1983 Labour voting ($p<0.0001$), the Townsend score ($p<0.0001$), and Conservative voting ($p=0.012$) were all associated with mortality. Abstentions were not significantly related to mortality once Labour and Conservative voting and the Townsend score were included in the regression.

In 1992 Labour and Conservative voting and the Townsend score were all associated with mortality ($p<0.0001$). When abstentions were included in the four independent variable model, Labour voting ($p<0.0001$), Conservative voting ($p<0.0001$), the Townsend score ($p=0.016$), and abstentions ($p=0.032$) were all associated significantly with mortality, although the addition of abstentions did not increase

Figure 1: Maps of Labour and Conservative voting in 1992, with maps of high mortality (SMR in white areas <100) and low mortality areas in 1990-92 (SMR in white areas >100)

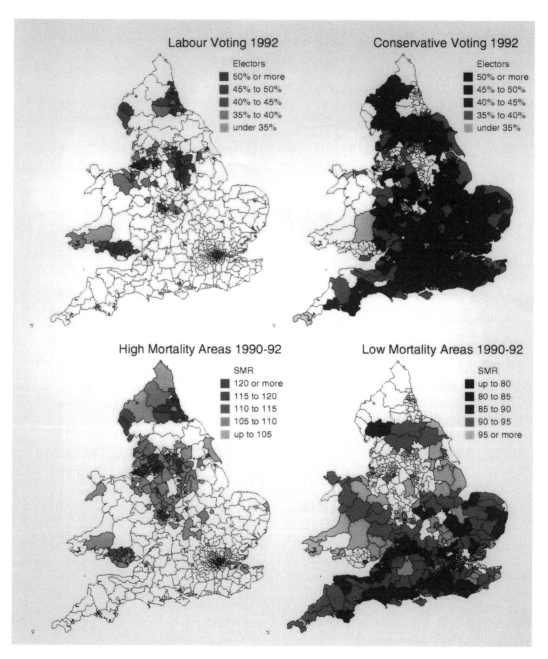

Figure 2: Scatterplots of Conservative and Labour voting in 1992 against all age SMRs for 1990-92

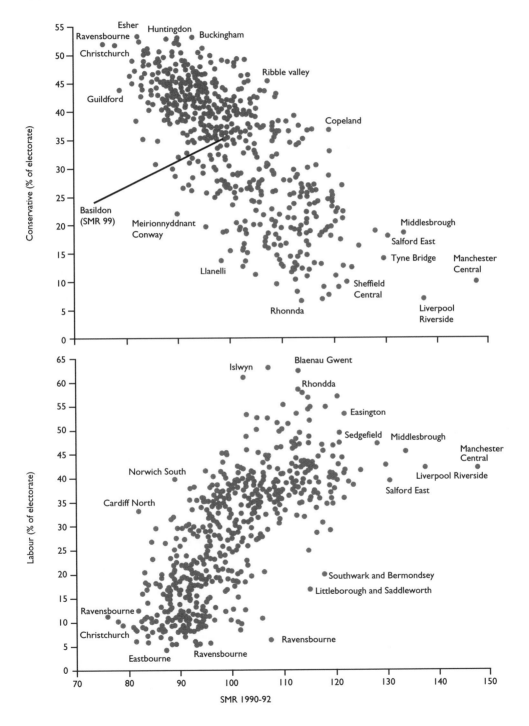

Table 3: Correlations between voting patterns, mortality and Townsend deprivation score

	Townsend 1981 (with election 1983 and mortality 1981-85)	Townsend 1991 (with election 1992 and mortality 1990-92)
Conservative	−0.84	−0.77
Labour	0.74	0.61
Liberal	−0.55	−0.49
Abstentions	0.66	0.84
SMR:		
Overall	0.74	0.67
Men	0.81	0.77
Women	0.60	0.50

Note: All $p<0.0001$.

Table 4: Variances in mortality accounted for by voting and deprivation variables alone and in combination (%)

	1983	1992
Townsend score	54	45
Labour vote	58	53
Conservative vote	58	55
Townsend score and Labour vote	64	61
Townsend score and Conservative vote	61	57
Labour and Conservative vote	62	61
Townsend score and Labour and Conservative vote	65	63

the proportion of variance explained. In all of these analyses the direction of the association between each variable and mortality remained the same as in the univariable case.

Discussion

Voting and mortality across England and Wales

We found that voting patterns can supplement the list of socioeconomic and environmental factors that are strongly associated with mortality.[13] Conservative and Labour voting show associations of equal size with mortality, but in opposite directions. In line with studies of deprivation,[6,14,15] voting is more strongly associated with male than female all-cause mortality. One explanation for this is that mortality from breast cancer – a major contributor to all-cause mortality in women – shows an opposite direction of association with deprivation than other major causes of death.[16] Interestingly, limiting long-standing illness shows larger correlations with a variety of area-based deprivation indices for women than men.[15]

The correlations between voting and mortality were generally of remarkably similar size for the periods surrounding the three most recent elections, even though the geographies of both mortality and voting were slowly changing. The only exception to this relates to abstentions, for which the positive correlations with mortality were greater around 1992 than around 1987 or 1983. Abstentions can be viewed as an indicator of apathy and, more strongly, social disintegration. Abstention rates rose dramatically during the 1980s in particularly poor parts of the country, places where death rates have traditionally been high and where over recent years mortality trends have been unfavourable.[8,12] This reflects the geographical polarisation of the poorest groups in society that took place during the 1980s.[17,18]

Mortality data have been standardised using information about the population drawn from the last two population censuses, and this is known to be deficient in inner-city areas for 1991. To compensate for the undercount in these areas we have included estimates for the number of people not enumerated in each constituency in each age and sex group in 1991. The two constituencies with the highest death rates (Manchester Central and Liverpool Riverside) also experienced some of the highest rates of under-enumeration in the 1991 Census. The places where people are most likely to die young are also the places where people are most difficult to count when alive.

The problems of assessing the political preferences of people living in different areas have risen in recent years. In particular, as a direct result of the introduction of the community charge (poll tax) a large number of people were compelled to exclude themselves from the electoral register for the General Election of 1992.[19] We have not included estimates of the number of adults who were eligible to vote but were excluded from the electoral register in each constituency in our analysis. The two constituencies which saw the highest decrease in voter registrations (of over 30% between 1979 and 1992) were, again, Manchester Central and Liverpool Riverside. These constituencies also saw some of the highest increases in abstentions among those adults who did choose to remain on the electoral register between 1987 and 1992 (increases of 7 and 10 percentage points respectively). If we had included estimates of non-registration in our correlations, the relation between lack of support for the ruling political party and high rates of mortality would have been even stronger. The places where adults are most likely to die are the places where people are least likely to choose (or be registered) to vote.

Could high mortality among Labour voters accentuate Conservative majorities?

To date, studies of voting in Britain have not considered general mortality as a factor in explaining electoral patterns. This is despite easily recognised regularities such as traditional Labour support being extremely high among workers in occupations associated with high mortality and poor health, such as mining. Neither has the direct effect of mortality on voting been considered. If Labour voters die at a younger age than Conservative voters on average, then they will be alive to vote at fewer elections per lifetime. The recent Conservative strategy of encouraging increasing socioeconomic inequality, which has in turn produced increasing socioeconomic differentials in mortality[20] and increases in death rates among some groups living in the most deprived areas,[8,12,21-23] will in turn consolidate the Conservative electoral advantage by hastening (in relative and, for some groups, absolute terms) the death of those who would oppose them at the polls.

Voting and deprivation

The somewhat smaller correlations between the Townsend score and mortality in these data compared with other studies that have investigated deprivation and mortality[7,14,16] reflect our use of the all ages SMRs rather than the truncated age groups (such as 16-64) in other investigations. The strength of the association between area-based deprivation and mortality is attenuated at older ages. The increasing average age of the population may account for the decrease in magnitude of correlation between the Townsend score and mortality between 1983 and 1992, since deaths at older ages – which are less strongly related to deprivation[14] – will contribute more to the SMRs for 1992 than 1983. The same phenomenon may account for the attenuation in the size of correlations between voting behaviour and mortality over time.

As with all investigations using area-based socioeconomic indicators, it could be argued that our data are prone to suffer from the ecological fallacy.[24] This postulates that while phenomena may be associated at the ecological level – for example, areas with high Conservative voting have low mortality – this may not be seen at the individual level – for example, people who vote Conservative may not have lower mortality. We cannot address this problem in this study. Indeed, due to the confidential nature of voting in Britain it is unlikely that such data exist. The partial exception to this relates to the study of mortality of Members of Parliament (MPs). In a mortality study of male MPs elected in 1945, Labour MPs had a 25% higher death rate than non-Labour (mainly Conservative) MPs.[25]

Area-based indicators may capture contextual effects of areas that are not simple aggregates of the characteristics of people living in the areas.[26] Socioeconomically disadvantaged areas may suffer, for instance, from poor leisure facilities, transport, housing conditions, and environmental conditions and have few retail outlets, all of which influence health in ways that are independent of the socioeconomic position of the individual residents.[26] Areas with high socioeconomic inequality have higher mortality and worse profiles with respect to other health indicators, regardless of the overall socioeconomic level.[27,28]

Conclusions

Although the fiscal and social policies of the Conservative and Labour parties have converged greatly over the past 17 years, voting choice remains strongly influenced by individual circumstances. Conservative voters tend to be richer and live in more affluent areas, they are less likely to require unemployment benefit, their children are less likely to receive free school meals, they are less likely to be reliant on a state pension in old age, and, if wealthy enough, they can afford to opt out of much state-subsidised provision (ranging from public transport to education and the NHS). Conservative voters may therefore assume it is sensible for them to support a party that will improve their already (generally) privileged economic situation through apparent tax reductions, while dismantling the components of the welfare state that are most needed by others. Such "I'm all right, Jack" thinking is shortsighted. Across nations overall life expectancy is more favourable in countries with redistributive taxation and with leftist governments committed to greater social expenditure.[29,30] Richard Wilkinson, among others, has argued that in societies with greater socioeconomic inequality life expectancy is lower and several indicators of poor health throughout life – from birth weight, child growth, and general morbidity to risk of death from many causes – are less favourable than in more equal societies.[31] Of particular concern is that the increases in socioeconomic inequality in Britain, which now places the country in the unenviable position of being one of the most inequitable industrialised countries in the world, will have adverse influences on the health and wellbeing of children, which will in turn undermine the future health of the nation.[32]

Acknowledgements

We thank Rosemary Greenwood for help with transferring datasets, Anne Rennie for help with preparing the typescript, and the bar staff at the *Penny Farthing*, where most of this chapter was written.

References

[1] Britton, M. (1990) 'Introduction', in M. Britton (ed) *Mortality and geography: A review in the mid-1980s*, London: HMSO, pp 1-3.

[2] Britton, M. (ed) (1990) *Mortality and geography: A review in the mid-1980s*, London: HMSO.

[3] Engels, F. (1987) (first published 1845) *The condition of the working class in England*, Harmondsworth: Penguin.

[4] Woolf, B. (1947) 'Studies on infant mortality: Part II: social aetiology of still births and infant deaths in county boroughs of England and Wales', *British Journal of Social Medicine*, vol 1, pp 73-125.

[5] Martin, W.J. (1956) 'Distribution in England and Wales of mortality from coronary disease', *British Medical Journal*, vol 1, pp 1523-5.

[6] Charlton, J. (1996) 'Which areas are healthiest?', *Population Trends*, no 83, pp 17-24.

[7] Eames, M., Ben-Shlomo, Y. and Marmot, M.G. (1993) 'Social deprivation and premature mortality: regional comparison across England', *British Medical Journal*, vol 307, pp 1097-102.

[8] McCarron, P.G., Davey Smith, G. and Womersley, J.J. (1994) 'Deprivation and mortality in Glasgow: changes from 1980 to 1992', *British Medical Journal*, vol 309, pp 1481-2.

[9] Spencer, N. and Janes, H. (eds) (1992) *Uses and abuses of deprivation indices*, Warwick: University of Warwick.

[10] Pocock, S.J., Shaper, A.G., Cook, D.G., Packham, R.F., Lacey, R.F. and Powell, P. et al (1980) 'British regional heart study: geographic variations in cardiovascular mortality, and the role of water quality', *British Medical Journal*, vol 1, pp 1243-9.

[11] Simpson, S. (1994) 'Coverage of the Great Britain Census of population and housing', *Journal of the Royal Statistical Society*, vol 157A, pp 313-16.

[12] Phillimore, P., Beattie, A. and Townsend, P. (1994) 'Widening inequality of health in Northern England 1981-91', *British Medical Journal*, vol 308, pp 1125-8.

[13] Britton, M., Fox, A.J., Goldblatt, P., Jones, D.R. and Rosato, M. (1990) 'The influence of socioeconomic and environmental factors on geographic variation in mortality', in M. Britton (ed) *Mortality and geography: A review in the mid-1980s*, London: HMSO, pp 57-78.

[14] Carstairs, V. and Morris, R. (1991) *Deprivation and health in Scotland*, Aberdeen: Aberdeen University Press.

[15] Bentham, G., Eimermann, J., Haynes, R., Lovett, A. and Brainard, J. (1995) 'Limiting long term illness and its associations with mortality and indicators of social deprivation' *Journal of Epidemiology and Community Health*, vol 49, suppl 2, pp S57-64.

[16] Ben-Shlomo, Y. and Davey Smith, G. (1991) 'Deprivation in infancy or in adult life: which is more important for mortality risk?', *Lancet*, vol 337, pp 530-4.

[17] Philo, C. (ed) (1995) *Off the map: The social geography of poverty in the UK*, London: Child Poverty Action Group.

[18] Dorling, D. and Woodward, R. (1996) 'Social polarisation 1971-91: a microgeographical analysis of Britain', *Progress in Planning*, vol 45, pp 67-122.

[19] Smith, J. and McLean, I. (1994) 'The poll tax and the electoral register', in A. Heath, R. Jowell and J. Curtice (eds) *Labour's last chance? The election and beyond*, Dartmouth: Aldershot.

[20] Davey Smith, G. and Egger, M. (1993) 'Socioeconomic differentials in wealth and health', *British Medical Journal*, vol 307, pp 1085-6.

[21] McLoone, P. and Boddy, F.A. (1994) 'Deprivation and mortality in Scotland, 1981 and 1991', *British Medical Journal*, vol 309, pp 1465-70.

[22] Dorling, D. (1997) *Changing life chances in Britain*, York: Joseph Rowntree Foundation.

[23] Phillimore, P. and Beattie, A. (1994) *Health and inequality: The Northern Region, 1981-91*, Newcastle: University of Newcastle-upon-Tyne.

[24] MacRae, K. (1994) 'Socioeconomic deprivation and health and the ecological fallacy', *British Medical Journal*, vol 309, pp 1478-9.

[25] Pincherle, G. (1969) 'Mortality of Members of Parliament', *British Journal of Preventive and Social Medicine*, vol 23, pp 72-6.

[26] Macintyre, S., MacIver, S. and Sooman, A. (1993) 'Area, class and health: should we be focusing on places or people?', *Journal of Social Policy*, vol 22, pp 213-34.

[27] Kaplan, G.A., Pamuk, E.R., Lynch, J.W., Cohen, R.D. and Balfour, J.L. (1996) 'Inequality in income and mortality in the US: analysis of mortality and potential pathways', *British Medical Journal*, vol 312, pp 999-1003.

[28] Ben-Shlomo, Y., White, I.R. and Marmot, M. (1996) 'Does the variation in the socioeconomic characteristics of an area affect mortality?', *British Medical Journal*, vol 312, pp 1013-14.

[29] Lena, H.F. and London, B. (1993) 'The political and economic determinants of health outcomes: a cross-national analysis', *International Journal of Health Services*, vol 23, pp 585-602.

[30] Gough, I. and Thomas, T. (1994) 'Why do levels of human welfare vary among nations?', *International Journal of Health Services*, vol 24, pp 715-48.

[31] Wilkinson, R. (1996) *Unhealthy societies*, London: Routledge.

[32] **Davey Smith, G. (1996) 'Income inequality and mortality: why are they related?', *British Medical Journal*, vol 312, pp 987-8.**

10

Association between voting patterns and mortality remains

George Davey Smith and Daniel Dorling

In Chapter Nine we presented data on the association between voting patterns and mortality in England and Wales during the 1983, 1987, and 1992 British General Elections.[1] There was a strong negative association between voting Conservative and mortality and a strong positive association between voting Labour and mortality; there was a weaker negative association between voting Liberal Democrat and mortality and a weaker positive association between abstention and mortality. The 1997 General Election, in which a Labour government was elected with a large majority, was interpreted as reflecting a breakdown of traditional voting loyalties.[2,3] We analysed the results of the 1997 General Election in England and Wales with the exception of two seats: Tatton, in which an independent candidate stood against a Conservative alleged to have taken money in return for asking questions in Parliament, and West Bromich West, where the speaker of the House of Commons was unopposed. We used mortality data for 1990-92; these are the most recent data from the 1991 Census for which estimates of the population at risk of death were available. In Table 1 we have added our findings for the 1997 Election to the results from previous elections.

The correlations between voting Conservative, Labour, or Liberal Democrat and mortality have changed little. There is a weak negative correlation between voting for the Referendum Party and mortality; the Referendum Party fielded candidates in 547 constituencies and won 2.7% of the vote. The main change over time is the continuing strengthening of the positive correlation between abstaining and mortality. The 60% variance in mortality explained by the voting data is virtually identical with the 61% explained by voting in the 1992 Election. Correlations in the analysis for the 1997 Election may be weakened by the fact that the mortality data are taken from six years before the election. The main change is that for the 1997 Election, voting for Labour and abstaining are the most important variables in explaining the variance in mortality in multiple regression analyses,

British Medical Journal, 1997, vol 315, pp 430-1

Table 1: Correlation between party voted for and mortality (1983-97)

Election year	Overall SMR	Male SMR	Female SMR
1983			
Conservative	−0.76	−0.81	−0.65
Labour	0.76	0.79	0.67
Liberal Democrat	−0.49	−0.52	−0.42
Abstentions	0.36	0.43	0.27
1987			
Conservative	−0.75	−0.80	−0.64
Labour	0.77	0.80	0.68
Liberal Democrat	−0.52	−0.54	−0.45
Abstentions	0.37	0.43	0.28
1992			
Conservative	−0.74	−0.79	−0.61
Labour	0.73	0.75	0.63
Liberal Democrat	−0.50	−0.53	−0.42
Abstentions	0.54	0.62	0.40
1997			
Conservative	−0.72	−0.79	−0.58
Labour	0.66	0.69	0.57
Liberal Democrat	−0.49	−0.52	−0.41
Referendum	−0.27	−0.29	−0.22
Abstentions	0.61	0.69	0.47

Note: All SMRs *p*<0.0001.

while in the 1992 Election Labour and Conservative voting contributed most to the analyses.

Frank Dobson, the Labour health secretary after the 1997 Election, has stated that "Labour will tackle the underlying causes of bad health and if we succeed we will be able to use the slogan 'Vote Labour, live longer'".[4] Increasingly it is young adults living in places where few people vote who die youngest. Perhaps the new Labour government should concentrate on socially excluded groups, who may not contribute to electoral success but nevertheless require the most from an administration that offered to lead us away from 18 years of selfishness under the Conservative government.

References

[1]   **Davey Smith, G. and Dorling, D. (1996) "'I'm all right, John": voting and mortality in England and Wales, 1981–92', *British Medical Journal*, vol 313, pp 1573-7.**

[2]   Cornford, J., Dorling, D. and Tether, B. (1995) 'Historical precedent and British electoral prospects', *Electoral Studies*, vol 14, pp 123-42.

[3]   Pattie, C., Johnston, R., Dorling, D., Rossiter, D., Tunstall, H. and MacAllister, I. (1997) 'New Labour, new geography? The electoral geography of the 1997 British general election', *Area*, vol 29, pp 253-9.

[4]   Hall, C. (1997) 'NHS change will take years, says Dobson', *Daily Telegraph*, 20 May, p 9.

11

Analysis of trends in premature mortality by Labour voting in the 1997 General Election

Daniel Dorling, George Davey Smith and Mary Shaw

Mortality relates to voting patterns within areas: mortality is higher the greater the proportion of the electorate who vote Labour or abstain and the converse is the case with regard to the percentage of the electorate who vote Conservative.[1] This reflects the socioeconomic characteristics of individuals who vote for these parties, with Labour being identified with the working class and the Conservatives with the middle class. In the 1997 Election, Labour was returned to office after 18 years in opposition. The government has released targets for reducing health inequalities and made it clear that such a reduction is a principal policy aim.[2] These targets may be difficult to meet for two reasons. Firstly, factors influencing inequalities in adult health act from an early age onwards and may not respond rapidly to social change;[3] secondly, there has as yet been no reduction in social inequality (as indexed by income inequality) under the Labour government.[4] Here we use premature mortality as an indicator of which population groups have fared best under the present government.

Methods and results

The mortality data are from the Office for National Statistics' digital records of all deaths in England and Wales and the equivalent records from the General Register Office for Scotland.[1] The full postcode of the usual residence of the deceased was used to assign each death to one of the 641 parliamentary constituencies to reflect where the deceased usually lived. The death data were provided for single years.

British Medical Journal, 2001, vol 322, pp 1336-7

Standardised mortality ratios (SMRs) and directly age-standardised mortality for the age range 0-64 years were calculated using rates for England and Wales.

Because there was no census at the end of the 1990s, population by age group and gender must be estimated. The Office for National Statistics and the General Register Office produced mid-year population estimates for 1999 and earlier years at the local and unitary authority district levels. To maintain a geographical base consistent with previous studies of Britain's health gap, these district-level estimates were interpolated to the electoral ward level and then aggregated to parliamentary constituencies. The interpolation was based on population estimates for 1996, which were available at electoral ward level, and was carried out such that for each age-sex group $W_{1999} = W_{1996} + P_{1996} \times (D_{1999} - D_{1996})$, where W and D are the ward and district level population, P is the proportion of D resident in W, and the subscript is the year. The district level population for 1996-99 for each age-sex group is from the mid-year estimates of the Office for National Statistics and the General Register Office.

Table 1 shows the SMRs for two periods according to the percentage of the vote for Labour in 1997. SMRs rose by 0.8% reflecting the relatively smaller fall in mortality in Scotland compared with that in England and Wales. The absolute change in mortality nationally fell by 1.8% when mortality for all of Britain was directly standardised by age and sex to the population in England and Wales.

Table 1: SMRs for 1995-96 and 1998-99, and change in SMRs between these time periods, according to percentage of the Labour vote in 1997 (parliamentary constituencies ranked by Labour votes and divided into 10 equal population groups on the basis of percentage of the vote which was for Labour)

10% groups	% Labour vote (of all 1997 voters)	SMR 1995-96	SMR 1998-99	Change %	Change in absolute mortality rate (%)
First	72	126	127	1.1	−2.2
Second	64	120	124	3.9	+0.5
Third	59	113	115	2.3	−0.6
Fourth	55	108	110	2.1	−0.8
Fifth	51	103	105	2.0	−0.8
Sixth	46	97	98	0.3	−2.8
Seventh	39	89	89	0.7	−2.4
Eighth	30	85	85	0.6	−1.9
Ninth	22	81	81	−0.4	−3.4
Tenth	14	86	84	−2.0	−4.9
Total[a]	44	101	101	0.8	−1.8

[a] SMRs are 101 because the rates used for standardisation are for England and Wales, and rates are higher in Scotland. SMRs rose by 0.8% reflecting the relatively smaller fall in mortality in Scotland as compared to England and Wales over the period. Absolute change in mortality showed a national fall of 1.8% when mortality (for all of Britain) was directly age-sex standardised to the English and Welsh population.

In absolute terms, mortality has improved for all but one of the tenths, although mortality has tended to improve most in areas with the fewest Labour voters. However, the absolute mortality of people living in the tenth with the second highest percentage of Labour voters has actually risen over this period. In relative terms, mortality worsened in eight of the tenths, and it worsened most in the areas with higher proportions of Labour voters (with the exception of the tenth with the highest percentage of Labour voters). The correlation between the percentage of the Labour vote and (directly age-sex standardised) absolute change in mortality is 0.13 (p=0.002). The equivalent correlation with the change in SMR is also 0.13 (p=0.001).

Comment

Labour's slogan during the 1997 campaign was: 'Things can only get better'. We have shown that in absolute terms things got better for most areas, but improvement was smaller in areas with a higher percentage of Labour voters. In relative terms things got worse for people in constituencies in which a high proportion of people voted Labour, while things got better for people in constituencies where people generally voted Conservative. This mirrors trends in income inequality, which has increased throughout the period of the Labour government: the Gini coefficient for the distribution of adjusted post-tax income increased from 38 in 1997-98, to 39 in 1998-99, and 40 in 1999-2000.[4] Where Labour has improved the life chances of poorer people in Britain they have tended to only just move these people above various 'poverty lines'.[5] It is possible that this trend accounts for the absolute rise in mortality for those younger than age 65 experienced by people living in the tenth with the second highest percentage of Labour voters. Time, and the continued monitoring of the performance of the government through statistics, will tell.

References

[1] **Davey Smith, G. and Dorling, D. (1996) '"I'm all right, John": voting and mortality in England and Wales, 1981–92', *British Medical Journal*, vol 313, pp 1573-7.**

[2] Department of Health (accessed 11 May 2001) *Health inequalities* (www.doh.gov.uk/healthinequalities/).

[3] Davey Smith, G., Gunnell, D. and Ben-Shlomo, Y. (2001) 'Life-course approaches to socioeconomic differentials in cause-specific adult mortality', in D. Leon and G. Walt (eds) *Poverty, inequality and health: An international perspective*, Oxford: Oxford University Press, pp 88-124.

[4] Lakin, C. (2001) 'The effects of taxes and benefits on household income, 1999-2000', *Economic Trends*, vol 569, pp 35-74.

[5] Sutherland, H. and Piachaud, D. (2001) 'Reducing child poverty in Britain: an assessment of government policy 1997-2001', *The Economic Journal*, vol 111, pp 85-101.

Section III
The Whitehall Study

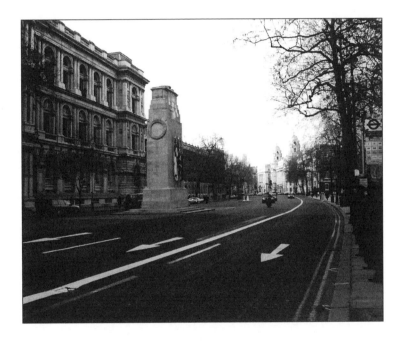

Whitehall, London. Photograph: Mary Shaw.

Magnitude and causes of socioeconomic differentials in mortality: further evidence from the Whitehall Study

George Davey Smith, Martin J. Shipley
and Geoffrey Rose

Abstract

Study objective: The aim was to explore the magnitude and causes of the differences in mortality rates according to socioeconomic position in a cohort of civil servants.

Design: This was a prospective observational study of civil servants followed up for 10 years after baseline data collection.

Setting: Civil service office in London.

Participants: 11,678 male civil servants were studied, aged 40-64 at baseline screening between 1967 and 1969. Two indices of socioeconomic position were available on these participants – employment grade (categorised into four levels) and ownership of a car.

Measurement and main results: Main outcome measures were all-cause and cause-specific mortality, with cause of death taken from death certificates coded according to the Eighth Revision of the International Classification of Diseases (ICD). Employment grade and car ownership were independently related to total mortality and to mortality from the major cause groups. Combining the indices further improved definition of mortality risk and the age-adjusted relative rate between the highest grade

Journal of Epidemiolgy and Community Health,
1990, vol 44, pp 265-70

car owners and the lowest grade non-owners of 4.3 is considerably larger than the social class differentials seen in the British population. Factors potentially involved in the production of these mortality differentials were examined. Smoking, plasma cholesterol concentration, blood pressure and glucose intolerance did not appear to account for them. The pattern of differentials was the same in the group who reported no ill health at baseline as it was in the whole sample, which suggests that health selection associated with frank illness was not a major determinant. The contribution of height, a marker for environmental factors acting in early life, was also investigated. Whereas adjustment for employment grade and car ownership attenuated the association between short stature and mortality, height differences within employment grade and car ownership groups explained little of the differential mortality.

Conclusion: The use of social class as an index of socioeconomic position leads to underestimation of the association between social factors and mortality, which may be reflected in public health initiatives and priorities. Known risk factors could not be shown to account for the differentials in mortality, although the degree to which this can be explored with single measurements is limited.

Introduction

Since the 1911 Census the classification of occupations into the Registrar General's social classes has been the basis for the examination of socioeconomic differentials in mortality rates.[1] As the inventor of this system made clear, it was intended to categorise people according to their degree of material wellbeing among other factors.[2,3] Since then information generated from the analysis of mortality according to the Registrar General's social classes has been used to support the notion that lower living standards are associated with higher death rates.[3-5]

The appropriateness of the Registrar General's social classes for examining socioeconomic differences in mortality has been questioned and defended from several standpoints.[6-9] This categorisation is imprecise with regard to income – within class variation in income is greater than that between classes.[10] Other factors within the social environment will also be distributed more unevenly than the Registrar General's social class categorisation would suggest. Thus estimates from social class analysis will attenuate the underlying associations between material and social wellbeing and mortality.[11] The OPCS Longitudinal Study has explored this by combining other indicators of socioeconomic position – housing tenure and occupancy, possession of household amenities, car ownership, and level of education – with the Registrar General's social classes in the examination of mortality and cancer registration rates.[12-14] When these classifications were combined, independent effects were seen. This suggests that the effects of socioeconomic environment upon health are not adequately characterised by the use of social class categories alone. Better discrimination is achieved by combining indicators of socioeconomic position.

Complementary findings have come from follow-up of a cohort study of civil servants, the Whitehall Study, in which employment grade has served as the marker of socioeconomic position.[15-17] The differences in 10-year mortality rates between grades were considerably greater than the Decennial Supplements suggested.[10]

It is of interest to see if further refinement of categorisation in the Whitehall Study leads to increases in differentials. The availability of data regarding car ownership allows this to be examined. Having access to a car was the strongest independent predictor of mortality among men who could be assigned to a social class in the Longitudinal Study.[18] Thus the combination of employment grade and car ownership provides a test of the hypothesis that more precise classification of socioeconomic position increases the mortality differentials observed.

The present study examines the independent and combined effects of employment grade and car ownership on mortality. The 10-year follow-up data are examined, as mortality over this period corresponds best with the Decennial Supplements, which only cover men aged 64 years and under. Analyses are repeated after excluding men sick at the time of screening, to allow the effects of selection to be explored. The degree to which differences in smoking, blood pressure, plasma cholesterol concentration and glucose tolerance can explain mortality differentials is also examined.

It has been postulated that factors acting during early life are related to the risk of cardiovascular disease in adulthood.[19] Height is influenced both by genetic factors and by childhood environment.[20,21] Short stature is associated with higher mortality risk in the Whitehall Study,[17] a finding in line with other investigations which have related markers of early environmental conditions to mortality.[22,23] The possible role of conditions in childhood, as indexed by height, in the generation of socioeconomic position differentials in mortality in adulthood is investigated in the present cohort.

Methods

In the Whitehall Study 18,403 men aged 40–64 were examined between 1967 and 1969.[24] Measurements included height, weight, blood pressure, a six lead electrocardiogram, plasma cholesterol concentration and a glucose tolerance test. A questionnaire was completed regarding age, civil service employment grade, smoking habits and health status.

The electrocardiogram was coded according to the Minnesota

system,[25] and was regarded as positive for ischaemia if Q/QS items (codes 1.1-3), ST/T items (codes 4.1-4 or 5.1-3), or left bundle branch block (code 7.1) were present. Subjects with blood glucose two hours after a post-fasting 50g glucose load >11.1mmol/litre (>200mg/ 100ml) or with previously diagnosed diabetes constituted the diabetic group; non-diabetic subjects with glucose concentrations above the 95th centile point (5.4-11.0mmol/litre; 96-199mg/100ml) formed the group with impaired glucose tolerance, and other subjects were designated as being normoglycaemic.

The questionnaire used in the study was modified at various times, the details of car ownership and employment grade having been obtained from the 11,678 subjects who were seen in the middle period of the survey. This group forms the basis for the analysis. Employment grade was categorised as administrative, professional or executive, clerical and 'other grades' (men in messenger and other unskilled manual jobs). Smoking has been categorised according to cigarette use as 'current smoker', 'ex-smoker' and 'never smoker'. The 409 men who smoked pipes or cigars only have been excluded from the analyses that involve smoking status.

Data were missing for car ownership (5), blood pressure (3), cholesterol (556), glucose tolerance (90), body mass index (2), and smoking status (3). Subjects were only excluded from the analyses for which their specific data were missing.

Records from over 99% of subjects were traced and flagged at the National Health Service Central Registry. Death certificates coded according to the eighth revision of the International Classification of Diseases (ICD) were obtained, and this almost complete mortality follow-up provides the basis for this analysis. Mortality has been classified as being due to cardiovascular disease (ICD codes 390-458), neoplasms – virtually all cancers (ICD codes 140-239), or other causes. For seven deaths the cause was unknown. These have been included in all-cause mortality, but have been excluded from analyses of cause-specific mortality. Mortality causes have also been classified according to whether smoking is considered to play a role in their aetiology.[26-29] The causes deemed to be smoking-related, with their ICD codes are: malignant neoplasms of the lip (ICD 140), tongue (141), mouth and pharynx (143-9), oesophagus (150), pancreas (157), respiratory system (160-3), and urinary system (188-9); hypertensive disease (400-4); ischaemic heart disease (410-14); pulmonary heart disease (426); cerebrovascular disease (430-8); diseases of the arteries, arterioles and capillaries (440-8); pneumonia (480-6); bronchitis and emphysema (491-2); and peptic ulcer (531-4).

Mortality rates have been calculated using person years at risk. These rates and also all means and proportions have been standardised for age at entry by the direct method, using the study population as the standard. Adjustment for other major risk factors and calculation of confidence intervals for the relative risks was done using Cox's proportional hazards regression model.[30] The associations between employment grade and risk factors were examined by fitting a trend term for grade in a regression model of the variable of interest, while adjusting for age and car ownership. These were computed using multiple regression for the continuous variables and log linear models for the discrete factors.

Results

Seventy-two per cent of the study population owned a car, percentages falling from 91% (600/658) in administrators, through 82% (6,877/

Table I: Age-adjusted 10-year mortality rates with their standard errors and number of deaths, by employment grade and car ownership status

		Car owner					
		Yes			No		
	Employment grade	Rate[a]	SE[b]	No of deaths	Rate	SE	No of deaths
All causes	Administrative	4.4	(1.0)	21	4.9	(2.9)	3
	Professional or executive	8.5	(0.4)	496	10.7	(0.9)	147
	Clerical	10.8	(1.2)	79	14.2	(1.2)	165
	Other	11.9	(2.1)	42	18.8	(2.0)	133
	Total[c]	9.2	(0.4)	638	11.9	(0.6)	448
Cardiovascular disease	Administrative	3.3	(0.9)	14	1.5	(1.5)	1
	Professional or executive	4.9	(0.3)	281	5.7	(0.7)	79
	Clerical	5.8	(0.9)	42	7.4	(0.9)	85
	Other	6.7	(1.6)	23	9.8	(1.4)	73
	Total[c]	5.2	(0.3)	360	6.3	(0.5)	238
Cancer	Administrative	1.1	(0.4)	7	3.5	(2.4)	2
	Professional or executive	2.6	(0.2)	156	3.3	(0.5)	45
	Clerical	3.2	(0.7)	24	4.6	(0.7)	54
	Other	3.7	(1.1)	14	4.6	(0.9)	33
	Total[c]	2.9	(0.2)	201	3.7	(0.4)	134
Other causes	Administrative	0.0	–	0	0.0	–	0
	Professional or executive	1.0	(0.1)	57	1.5	(0.3)	21
	Clerical	1.7	(0.5)	13	2.2	(0.5)	25
	Other	0.9	(0.4)	4	4.2	(1.0)	26
	Total[c]	1.1	(0.1)	74	1.8	(0.2)	72
Non-smoking related cause	Administrative	0.7	(0.3)	5	1.7	(1.7)	1
	Professional or executive	2.2	(0.2)	134	2.7	(0.4)	39
	Clerical	2.9	(0.6)	21	3.9	(0.6)	43
	Other	1.9	(0.7)	9	3.7	(0.9)	25
	Total[c]	2.2	(0.2)	169	3.4	(0.3)	108

[a] Rates per 1,000 person years; [b] SE= standard error of the rates; [c] adjusted for employment grade and age.

117

8,387) in professionals/executives and 39% (665/1,712) in clerical staff, to 34% (307/916) among other grades. The small number of administrators without a car produces only imprecise estimates of rates.

Table 1 presents age-standardised 10-year mortality rates according to employment grade and car ownership. Each is independently and consistently related to all-cause mortality rates. The relationship is also seen for the major groups of causes and for causes unrelated to smoking, although there is some loss of consistency, perhaps due to the small number of deaths in some categories.

After adjusting for age, the relative mortality rate associated with not owning a car was 1.49 (95% CI: 1.4-1.7); adjusting for employment grade reduces this to 1.28 (1.1-1.5). Compared to the professional or executives, the age-adjusted relative mortality rates for the administrators, clerical and other grades were 0.51 (0.3-0.8), 1.43 (1.2-1.7), and 1.64 (1.4-2.0) respectively. After adjusting for car ownership these became 0.52 (0.3-0.8), 1.29 (1.1-1.5) and 1.46 (1.2-1.8). Thus, while car ownership and grade are associated, much of their associations with mortality are independent of one another.

Employment grade and car ownership were related to indicators of health status and to risk factors for cardiovascular disease. Age-adjusted values according to employment grade and car ownership are presented in Tables 2 and 3. Independent associations were examined, and after adjusting for car ownership, lower work grade was significantly associated ($p<0.05$) with higher systolic blood pressure and body mass index, lower plasma cholesterol concentration and shorter height, and higher prevalence of smoking, glucose intolerance or being diabetic, and having disease at baseline (abnormal

Table 2: Means and standard errors for major risk factors (age-adjusted) by employment grade and car ownership

		Employment grade							
		Administrative		Professional or executive		Clerical		Other	
		Mean	SE	Mean	SE	Mean	SE	Mean	SE
Systolic blood pressure	Car owner	133.3	(0.94)	135.2	(0.25)	136.0	(0.83)	137.2	(1.21)
(mm Hg)	No car	133.8	(2.43)	136.8	(0.52)	135.9	(0.68)	136.2	(1.12)
Diastolic blood	Car owner	84.0	(0.61)	84.2	(0.71)	84.2	(0.58)	86.5	(0.92)
pressure (mm Hg)	No car	83.8	(1.83)	84.8	(0.35)	84.6	(0.4)	84.5	(0.72)
Plasma cholesterol	Car owner	5.32	(0.06)	5.22	(0.02)	5.23	(0.05)	5.12	(0.08)
concentration (mmol/litre)	No car	5.37	(0.17)	5.23	(0.03)	5.27	(0.05)	5.05	(0.07)
Body mass index (kg/m²)	Car owner	24.5	(0.12)	24.8	(0.03)	24.8	(0.12)	25.5	(0.21)
	No car	24.8	(0.33)	24.6	(0.08)	24.5	(0.11)	24.8	(0.17)
Height (m)	Car owner	1.784	(0.003)	1.764	(0.001)	1.744	(0.003)	1.754	(0.005)
	No car	1.768		1.755	(0.002)	1.737	(0.002)	1.722	(0.004)

Table 3: Prevalence (age-adjusted) of risk factors by employment grade and car ownership

		Administrative		Professional or executive		Clerical		Other	
		%	n	%	n	%	n	%	n
Car owner	Non-smokers	27	(166)	21	(1,421)	15	(94)	15	(41)
	Ex-smokers	43	(221)	43	(2,788)	34	(230)	30	(94)
	Current smokers	30	(162)	37	(2,417)	51	(327)	55	(161)
No car	Non-smokers	23	(13)	20	(299)	17	(162)	13	(69)
	Ex-smokers	30	(17)	34	(488)	29	(308)	20	(131)
	Current smokers	48	(26)	46	(671)	54	(559)	67	(396)
Car owner	No disease at entry	83	(504)	79	(5,517)	79	(520)	81	(235)
	Disease at entry	17	(96)	21	(1,360)	21	(145)	19	(72)
No car	No disease at entry	81	(47)	77	(1,175)	74	(762)	70	(389)
	Disease at entry	19	(11)	23	(335)	26	(285)	30	(220)
Car owner	Normoglycaemic	94	(565)	93	(6,407)	91	(601)	88	(263)
	Glucose intolerant or diabetic	5	(32)	7	(422)	9	(58)	12	(42)
No car	Normoglycaemic	96	(56)	92	(1,385)	91	(933)	91	(535)
	Glucose intolerant or diabetic	4	(2)	8	(140)	9	(84)	9	(65)

Above data grouped under heading: **Employment grade**

electrocardiogram, angina, intermittent claudication, dyspnoea, or being under medical care for hypertension or heart disease).

Independently of employment grade, non-ownership of a car was significantly associated with lower height and body mass index, higher systolic blood pressure, and higher prevalence of smoking and disease at baseline.

Smoking, pre-existing disease, and other risk factors might therefore account for the socioeconomic differences in mortality. Table 1 shows that these differences are seen for mortality from causes not related to smoking. Within subjects who had never smoked, the same consistent pattern of all-cause mortality rates by grade and car ownership as exists in the whole cohort is seen, although this is based on only 114 deaths. Furthermore, excluding the 22% of subjects with disease at baseline examination has little effect on the pattern of mortality differentials.

Relative rates were calculated with the largest group – professional or executive grade car owners – as the baseline category. Relative rates for cardiovascular disease and all-causes were adjusted for age, smoking (category and number of cigarettes smoked), systolic blood pressure, plasma cholesterol concentration, and glucose intolerance. Relative rates for neoplasms and other causes were adjusted for age and smoking. The independent associations of grade and car ownership

Table 4: Adjusted relative rates[a] for 10-year mortality for major causes of death by employment grade and car ownership status (95% CI)

		Employment grade			
		Administrative	Professional or executive	Clerical	Other
All causes	Car owner	0.60 (0.4-0.9)	1.0 –	1.26 (1.0-1.6)	1.19 (0.9-1.6)
	No car	0.71 (0.2-2.2)	1.21 (1.0-1.5)	1.45 (1.2-1.7)	1.60 (1.3-2.0)
Cardiovascular disease	Car owner	0.71 (0.4-1.2)	1.0 –	1.16 (0.8-1.6)	1.13 (0.7-1.7)
	No car	0.40 (0.1-2.9)	1.12 (0.9-1.5)	1.27 (1.0-1.6)	1.53 (1.2-2.0)
Cancer	Car owner	0.59 (0.3-1.3)	1.0 –	1.21 (0.8-1.9)	1.33 (0.8-2.3)
	No car	1.37 (0.3-5.5)	1.16 (0.8-1.6)	1.60 (1.2-2.2)	1.40 (0.9-2.1)
Other causes	Car owner	0.0 –	1.0 –	1.80 (1.0-3.3)	1.02 (0.4-2.8)
	No car	0.0 –	1.48 (0.9-2.4)	2.00 (1.2-3.2)	2.84 (1.7-4.7)

[a] For all-causes and cardiovascular disease relative rates are adjusted for age, systolic blood pressure, cholesterol concentration, smoking status, and glucose intolerance. For cancer and 'other' causes relative rates are adjusted for age and smoking status.

Table 5: Relative rates for the lowest two tertiles of height versus the top tertile, with various adjustments

		Adjusted for:	
	Age	Age, grade, and car ownership	Age, grade, car ownership, risk factors[a]
All causes			
Height <173cm	1.41	1.28	1.26
173cm ≤ Ht ≤ 178cm	1.14	1.11	1.11
Cardiovascular			
Height <173cm	1.57	1.44	1.39
173cm ≤ Ht ≤ 178cm	1.20	1.18	1.18
Cancer			
Height <173cm	1.01	0.92	0.92
173cm ≤ Ht ≤ 178cm	0.96	0.93	0.93
Other causes			
Height <173cm	2.36	1.91	1.89
173cm ≤ Ht ≤ 178cm	1.66	1.55	1.56

[a] Risk factors are (i) for all causes and cardiovascular disease: systolic blood pressure, cholesterol concentration, smoking status and number of cigarettes per day, glucose intolerance; (ii) for neoplasms and other causes: smoking status and number of cigarettes per day.

with mortality rates are not greatly affected by these adjustments (Table 4).

Height, which is inversely associated to all-cause mortality, coronary heart disease and non-CHD mortality in this cohort,[17] was related to employment grade and car ownership. The relative mortality rates for the lowest two tertiles of height versus the top tertile are shown in Table 5. Lower height is significantly ($p<0.05$) related to increased rates of all-cause, cardiovascular, and noncardiovascular non-cancer mortality, but not to mortality from cancers. Adjusting for grade and car ownership reduced the strength of, but did not abolish, the associations between height and mortality.

Adjustment for grade and car ownership together resulted in greater reduction in the relative rates than did adjustment for just one of these factors.

Additional adjustment for risk factors had little effect on the size of the relative rates. Conversely, adjustment for height left the relative mortality rates by employment grade and car ownership status virtually unchanged.

Discussion

Mortality differentials according to civil service employment grade are enhanced by the combination of this measure with details of car ownership. Over the follow-up period, at the end of which the cohort was aged 50-74, the mortality rate ratio for 'other' grades without a car compared to administrators with a car was 4.3. For clerical staff without a car the corresponding ratio was 3.2. Clerical workers and administrators both fall into non-manual social class groups. In the 1971 Decennial Supplement[10] the mortality rate ratios for group III non-manual compared to group I were 1.4 in the five-year age band 40-44, remaining approximately at this level in the bands 45-49 and 50-54, falling to 1.2 in the bands 55-59 and 60-64 (the oldest available). Clearly categorisation by employment grade and car ownership in these civil servants produces groups with greater differentials in mortality than does the Registrar General's social class system.

In addition to having been used in the Longitudinal Study and the present study, car ownership has served as an indicator of material wellbeing in a complementary series of investigations. In a study of regional mortality rate variation in the North of England, social class composition of the areas accounted for only a part of the variance in rates.[31] A composite indicator of deprivation, which combined car ownership, unemployment rates, house ownership, and overcrowding, accounted for a greater portion of the variance. Car ownership and unemployment were the most important of the four measures of deprivation in this respect. Similarly car ownership, together with other indices of deprivation, can statistically account for the mortality differences between Scotland and England/Wales,[32] which are partially independent of social class.

Such studies have led to the proposal that composite measures of deprivation may better reveal the relationship between socioeconomic position and health than does analysis by social class alone.[33]

In these studies car ownership has been taken to be a proxy measure of income. Among these civil servants it is probable that within any employment grade the car owners earn more, in relation to their needs, than do those without cars. Needs will vary with factors such as family size and number of dependants. Car ownership may index both absolute and relative income level and thus usefully complement grade (and social class) in the process of socioeconomic stratification. It is not possible to separate out those who choose not to have a car despite adequate resources from those who could not afford to run a car. Clearly the consequences of not owning a car may be very different in these two groups.

Explanations which have been advanced for the social class inequalities in mortality are that they are artefactual or that they are due to health selection, health-related behaviours, or material factors.[34]

The major artefact explanation suggests that differential recording of social class at Census and at death causes numerator/denominator bias which leads to apparent differentials in the Decennial Supplements. Cohort studies such as the present one and the Longitudinal Study are not subject to this bias.

The selection hypothesis postulates that when people become unhealthy they tend to move into lower social class groups.[35,36] Data on changes in civil service employment grade or car ownership were not available in the present study. Excluding subjects with identifiable disease at the start of the study did not greatly influence the mortality differentials, so grade mobility or selective recruitment of such people is unlikely to be an adequate explanation. Furthermore, such exclusions overcompensate for possible selection, since differential prevalence rates of disease in these middle-aged men will reflect socioeconomic factors over their lifecourses. Other studies, including the Longitudinal Study, suggest that selective social mobility cannot account for inequalities in mortality by social class.[37-39]

Of the health-related behaviours, the role of smoking was investigated through separated analyses for smoking-unrelated causes of death, through analysis of mortality among subjects who had never smoked, and through controlling for smoking in proportional hazards models. While smoking is clearly an important cause of mortality, and the higher prevalence of smoking among men without cars and the lower grades will contribute to their increased mortality, it is not a sufficient explanation. Plasma cholesterol concentrations were unrelated to car ownership and were higher among the higher grades.

Other dietary factors and health-related behaviours could not be examined.

In the British Regional Heart Study much of the social class differentials in ischaemic heart disease incidence were accounted for by smoking and blood pressure differences (the manual groups had lower mean cholesterol levels than the non-manual groups).[40] It was suggested that the inaccuracy inherent in using single measurements of risk factors as proxy measures of lifetime exposure may produce the residual associations between social class and ischaemic heart disease incidence after adjustment for risk factors. The use of imprecise measures of exposure will, of, course prevent full adjustments to be made, but it is also the case that the use of crude markers of socioeconomic position may mask considerably stronger underlying relationships between socioeconomic position and ischaemic heart disease incidence. The impression in both measurements of risk factors and in the indexing of socioeconomic position must be taken into account if this question is to be explored further.

We can say little about specific aspects of the material and social conditions of life for which employment grade and car ownership are proxy measures. It has been postulated that deprivation around infancy and childhood increases later risk of mortality from cardiovascular disease.[19] Height in adulthood reflects conditions in early life and both higher grade and car ownership are associated with greater height. Men without cars and subjects in lower employment grades may therefore have experienced more deprivation in early life. Height was unrelated to mortality from cancers, a finding in line with those of a study which related birth weight and growth in the first year of life to mortality in adulthood.[22]

The differentials in mortality for all cancers combined, which do not appear to be related to early life deprivation, were similar to those for cardiovascular disease and other causes. (However, see Chapter Thirteen for further exploration of differentials in site-specific cancers.) Furthermore, controlling for height had little effect upon the mortality differentials by grade and car ownership status from all causes and from the major cause groups. On the other hand, the relationship between height and mortality is partially accounted for by socioeconomic position in adulthood. Thus material conditions in childhood, to the extent to which they are indexed by adult height, seem to explain little of the mortality differentials related to socioeconomic position. Conversely, the association between height and mortality is partially due to the relationship between height and socioeconomic position in adult life. In the present data set, socioeconomic position in adult life was categorised into groups which were powerful discriminators of mortality risk. In studies which use less precise indices, relationships between markers of early life experience and mortality may suffer from residual confounding by adult socioeconomic position.

The potential explanations for the mortality differentials cannot be evaluated fully in the present data. However, the similarity of the differentials across the major cause groups renders a single explanation unlikely. Low social class similarly increases risk from most major causes of death.[10,41] When attempting to account for the association between socioeconomic position and death rates from any particular cause, this general relationship must also be considered.

Men in the Whitehall Study were mainly from non-manual social class groups. In 1968, 49% of the population of Britain had access to a car,[42] whereas 72% of the subjects in this study were car owners. The study sample were therefore a relatively privileged group; in 1972, 18% of unskilled and 31% of semi-skilled manual workers had cars,[43] compared to 34% of the 'other grade' civil servants. It is probable that the range of material wellbeing within this sample does not match that seen in the general population, yet the mortality gradients are considerably greater than those seen in analysis by social class. This could reflect well-stratified recruitment of higher mortality cohorts into lower civil service grades, and within these grades into lower income jobs, leading to less car ownership.

This may be part of the explanation of the current findings, but it is also likely that grade and car ownership produce better classification of the socioeconomic position of subjects than does the Registrar General's social class system, which in turn leads to greater mortality differentials. A host of factors in the social environment may influence health but are only poorly indexed by social class – earnings, wealth possession, social status, education, position in the labour market, chance of unemployment, housing quality, hours and conditions of work, and expenditure on housing, heating and clothing.[44] The roughness of the Registrar General's social class categorisation was recognised at the time of its inception,[45] and other studies have shown that refinements produce larger differentials. The use of social class in conjunction with other indices of socioeconomic position is advisable, for if inequalities in health are underestimated, the degree to which public health policy takes account of them will be inadequate.

References

[1] Stevenson, T.H.C. (1923) 'The social distribution of mortality from different causes in England and Wales, 1910-12', *Biometrika*, vol 15, pp 382-400.

[2] Stevenson, T.H.C. (1928) 'The vital statistics of wealth and poverty', *Journal of the Royal Statistical Society*, vol 91, pp 207-20.

[3]   Registrar General (1923) *Mortality of men in certain occupations in the three years 1910, 1911 and 1912*, Supplement to the 75th Annual Report of the Registrar General for England and Wales, Part 4, London: HMSO.

[4]   Logan, W.P.D. (1954) 'Social class variations in mortality', *British Journal of Preventive Social Medicine*, vol 8, pp 128-37.

[5]   Department of Health and Social Security (1980) *Inequalities in health*, London: HMSO.

[6]   Leete, R. and Fox, A.J. (1977) 'Registrar-General's social classes: origins and uses', *Population Trends*, vol 8, pp 1-7.

[7]   Jones, I.G. and Cameron, D. (1984) 'Social class analysis: an embarrassment to epidemiology', *Community Medicine*, vol 6, pp 37-46.

[8]   Alderson, M. (1984) 'A comment on social class analysis', *Community Medicine*, vol 6, pp 1-3.

[9]   Fox, A.J. and Jones, D.R. (1985) 'Authors' reply', *Journal of Epidemiology and Community Health*, vol 39, pp 275-6.

[10] Office of Population Censuses and Surveys (1978) *Occupational mortality, decennial supplement 1970-72*, DS no 1, London: HMSO.

[11] Morris, J.N. (1979) 'Social inequalities undiminished', *Lancet*, no I, pp 87-90.

[12] Fox, A.J. and Goldblatt, P. (1982) *Socioeconomic differentials in mortality 1971-75*, Office of Population Censuses and Surveys Series LS1, London: HMSO.

[13] Leon, D. (1988) *Social distribution of cancer 1971-75*, Office of Population Censuses and Surveys Series LS3, London: HMSO.

[14] Moser, K.A., Pugh, H.S. and Goldblatt, P.O. (1988) 'Inequalities in women's health: looking at mortality differentials using an alternative approach', *British Medical Journal*, vol 296, pp 1221-4.

[15] Marmot, M.G., Rose, G., Shipley, M. and Hamilton, P.J.S. (1978) 'Employment grade and coronary heart disease in British civil servants', *Journal of Epidemiology and Community Health*, vol 32, pp 244-9.

[16] Rose, G. and Marmot, M.G. (1981) 'Social class and coronary heart disease', *British Heart Journal*, vol 45, pp 13-19.

[17] Rose, G., Marmot, M.G. and Rose, G. (1984) 'Inequalities in death – specific explanations of a general pattern?', *Lancet*, vol 1, pp 1003-6.

[18] Goldblatt, P.O. (1987) *Mortality differences at working ages: The use of generalised linear models to compare measures*, Social Statistics Research Unit Working Paper No 53, London: City University.

[19] Forsdahl, A. (1977) 'Are poor living conditions in childhood and adolescence an important factor for arteriosclerotic heart disease?', *British Journal of Preventive Social Medicine*, vol 31, pp 91-4.

[20] Rona, R.J. (1981) 'Genetic and environmental factors in the control of growth in childhood', *British Medical Bulletin*, vol 37, pp 265-72.

[21] Kuh, D. and Wadsworth, M. (1989) 'Parental height: childhood environment and subsequent adult height in a National Birth Cohort', *International Journal of Epidemiology*, vol 18, pp 663-8.

[22] Barker, D.J.P., Winter, P.D., Osmond, C., Margetts, B. and Simmonds, S.J. (1989) 'Weight in infancy and death from ischaemic heart disease', *Lancet*, vol 2, pp 577-80.

[23] Nystrom Peck, A.M. and Vagero, D.H. (1989) 'Adult body height, self-perceived health and mortality in the Swedish population', *Journal of Epidemiology and Community Health*, vol 43, pp 380-4.

[24] Reid, D.D., Brett, G.Z., Hamilton, P.J.S., Jarrett, R.J., Keen, H. and Rose, G. (1974) 'Cardiorespiratory disease and diabetes among middle-aged male civil servants', *Lancet*, vol 1, pp 469-73.

[25] Rose, G.A. and Blackburn, H. (1968) *Cardiovascular survey methods*, Geneva: WHO.

[26] Doll, R. and Peto, R. (1976) 'Mortality in relation to smoking: 20 years' observations on male doctors', *British Medical Journal*, vol 2, pp 1523-36.

[27] Shinton, R. and Beevers, G. (1989) 'Meta-analysis of relation between cigarette smoking and stroke', *British Medical Journal*, vol 298, pp 789-94.

[28] Hammond, E.C. (1966) 'Smoking in relation to the death rates of one million men and women', in W. Haenzel (ed) *Epidemiological approaches to the study of cancer and other chronic diseases*, Bethesda, MD: National Cancer Institute, pp 127-204.

[29] International Agency for Research in Cancer (IARC) (1986) *Tobacco smoking*, Monographs on the evaluation of the carcinogenic risk of chemicals to humans, vol 38, Lyon: IARC.

[30] Cox, D.R. (1972) 'Regression models and life-tables', *Journal of the Royal Statistical Society Series B – Statistical Methodology*, vol 34, pp 187-220.

[31] Townsend, P., Phillimore, P. and Beattie, A. (1988) *Health and deprivation: Inequality and the north*, London: Croom Helm.

[32] Carstairs, V. and Morris, R. (1989) 'Deprivation: explaining differences in mortality between Scotland and England and Wales, *British Medical Journal*, vol 299, pp 886-9.

[33] Carstairs, V. and Morris, R. (1989) 'Deprivation and mortality: an alternative to social class?', *Community Medicine*, vol 11, pp 210-19.

[34] Blane, D. (1985) 'An assessment of the Black Report's explanations of health inequalities', *Sociology of Health and Illness*, vol 7, pp 423-5.

[35] Stern, J. (1983) 'Social mobility and the interpretation of social class mortality differentials', *Journal of Social Policy*, vol 12, pp 27-49.

[36] Illsley, R. (1986) 'Occupational class, selection and the production of inequalities in health', *Quarterly Journal of Social Affairs*, vol 2, pp 151-65.

[37] Goldblatt, P. (1988) 'Changes in social class between 1971 and 1981: could these affect mortality differential among men of working age?', *Population Trends*, vol 51, pp 9-17.

[38] Goldblatt, P. (1989) 'Mortality by social class, 1971-85', *Population Trends*, vol 56, pp 6-15.

[39] Wilkinson, R.G. (1986) 'Occupational class, selection and inequalities in health: a reply to Raymond Illsley', *Quarterly Journal of Social Affairs*, vol 2, pp 415-22.

[40] Pocock, S.J., Shaper, A.G., Cook, D.G., Phillips, A.N. and Walker, M. (1987) 'Social class differences in ischaemic heart disease in British men', *Lancet*, vol 2, pp 197-201.

[41] Office of Population Censuses and Surveys (1986) *Occupational mortality decennial supplement 1979-80; 1982-3*, London: HMSO.

[42] Central Statistical Office (1971) *Social trends no 2, 1971*, London: HMSO.

[43] Office of Population Censuses and Surveys (1974) *General household survey for 1972*, London: HMSO.

[44] Reid, I. (1989) *Social class differences in Britain: Life-chances and life-styles*, Glasgow: Fontana Press.

[45] Stocks, P. (1928) 'Discussion on Dr Stevenson's Paper', *Journal of the Royal Statistical Society*, vol 91, pp 225-6.

13

Confounding of occupation and smoking: its magnitude and consequences

George Davey Smith and Martin J. Shipley

Introduction

The potential reduction in mortality that could be achieved through reductions in smoking behaviour has often been calculated on the assumption that smokers would reduce their mortality rate to that of the ex-smokers in the population if they quit, or would have the mortality rates of lifetime non-smokers if they had never started smoking.[1-3] In a recent contribution to this journal, Sterling and Weinkam[4] have pointed out that since smoking is strongly related to occupation and to socioeconomic position, these assumptions do not hold. The smoking group within a population will over-represent the working class, whose mortality exceeds that of the middle classes independently of smoking. Thus a more appropriate comparison would be between the mortality rates of smokers, ex-smokers and non-smokers within the same socioeconomic groups.

In this chapter we demonstrate the effects of making such appropriate comparisons when predicting the benefits of non-smoking. We use data from the Whitehall Study of London civil servants, in which both occupational grade and smoking have been shown to be strongly associated with mortality rates.[5,6] The extent of confounding due to the relationship between smoking and employment grade is examined.

Data, methods and results

The data used for the calculations come from the Whitehall Study of London civil servants.[5] Employment grade and smoking behaviour data were available for 16,930 men aged 40-64, who were examined

Social Science and Medicine, 1991, vol 32, pp 1297-300

between 1967 and 1969. Employment grade was categorised as administrative, professional or executive, clerical, and 'other grades' (mainly men in messenger and other manual jobs). The participants in this study were largely white collar employees – only 'other grades' includes blue collar workers.

Smoking behaviour has been categorised according to cigarette use as 'current smoker', 'ex-smoker' and 'never smoker'. Participants who only smoked a pipe or cigars have been excluded from these analyses. Mortality records were provided by the NHS Central Registry, with 1,670 deaths occurring over a 10-year follow-up period.

Risk of mortality over this 10-year follow-up period has been calculated, standardised for age at entry by the direct method, using the study population as the standard. The risk of death is presented in terms of deaths per 10 years per 100 men.

Age-adjusted 10-year mortality risks according to employment grade and smoking status are presented in Figure 1. There is a gradient such that mortality risk increases with lower employment grade, independent of smoking status. Similarly, increased mortality risk among smokers is seen, independent of employment grade. Smokers among the administrative grade have a mortality risk which approximated that of never smokers in the clerical grade. Similarly, smokers among the professional or executive grade had a risk of mortality which approximated that of never smokers in the 'other grade'. In these observational data, smoking and being in an employment grade two levels beneath the actual grade were related with approximately the same elevation in mortality risk. The effect of grade and smoking behaviour were mixed, since smoking varied according to employment grade, as shown in Figure 2. Higher grade

Figure 1: Ten-year mortality risk by smoking behaviour and employment grade

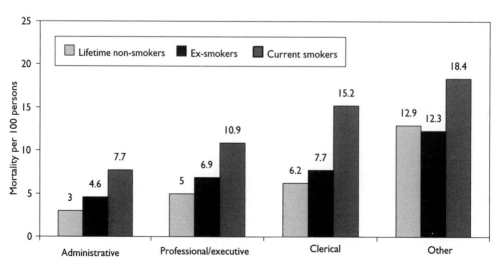

participants are less likely to smoke and more likely to be ex-smokers or lifetime non-smokers than the lower grades.

In the Whitehall Study, 69% of men fall into the professional/ executive employment grade, thus the actual study sample is not representative of a population in which the size of the socioeconomic groups are roughly equivalent. We have applied the Whitehall Study data to a hypothetical population containing equal numbers of subjects within each socioeconomic group. For ease of exposition we have used a population of 4,000 men − 1,000 in each employment grade. Table 1 shows the number of men in this hypothetical population with respect to employment grade and smoking status.

The number of deaths within this population which could have been avoided if all current smokers quit, or if they had never started smoking, are now calculated. For the purpose of this demonstration it is assumed that the mortality risk differences with smoking behaviour seen in the observational data are, with the exception of the confounding by employment grade, due to the smoking behaviour itself.

Applying the grade and smoking status specific mortality risk to our hypothetical population, and summing the deaths across the four grade categories, gives overall (crude) 10-years mortality risk per 100 persons of 5.8 for lifetime non-smokers, 7.4 for ex-smokers and 14.1 for current smokers. Over 10 years the apparent reduction in mortality risk for smokers who quit would be 6.7 (ie 14.1-7.4) per 100 persons, the equivalent value being 8.5 (ie 14.1-5.6) per 100 persons if smoking had never been started. Applying these mortality risk reductions to our population containing 1,870 current smokers suggests that 125

Figure 2: Smoking behaviour by employment grade

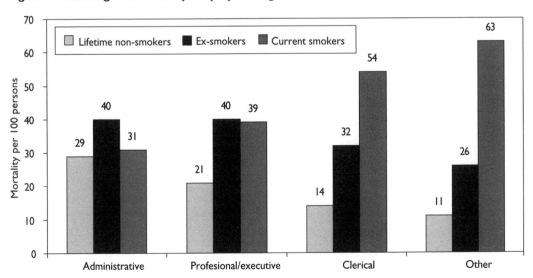

Table 1: Employment grade and smoking status structure of hypothetical population

	Lifetime non-smokers	Ex-smokers	Current smokers	Total
Administrative	290	400	310	1,000
Professional/executive	210	400	390	1,000
Clerical	140	320	540	1,000
Other	110	260	630	1,000

deaths (ie 6.7 multiplied by 1,870/100) could have been prevented if all smokers quit, or 159 lives saved (ie 8.5 multiplied by 1,870/100) if smoking had not commenced, over a 10-year period.

However, if individuals quit smoking, their mortality risk would not fall to the overall mortality risk of ex-smokers within the population, but to that of ex-smokers within their employment grade. Similarly if people never commenced smoking, their mortality risk would not be the overall mortality risk of never smokers with the population, but would be that of never smokers within their employment grade. We have therefore repeated these calculations allowing the mortality risk of smokers to be reduced to that of ex-smokers or lifetime non-smokers within their own employment grade. The calculations performed above have been repeated for each employment grade group separately. These results have been combined to produce counts for the whole population. If all 1,870 smokers quit, the number of lives saved would be 103; if smoking was never started, the number would be 126. Thus, taking into account the association between smoking and employment grade leads to reduced estimates of the contribution of smoking to mortality.

An alternative approach is to examine the risk which could become attached to an exposure solely due to its relationship with socioeconomic position. We have calculated the mortality risk that would be associated with an exposure related with grade to the same degree as smoking, but by itself not a cause of increased mortality. To do this we have applied the employment grade specific mortality risks for current smokers and never smokers to a hypothetical population with the same percentages of men in each employment grade as is true for current smokers and never smokers in the study sample. The 10-year mortality risk would be 12.5 per 100 persons for the exposed, and 9.6 per 100 persons for the unexposed, a risk ratio of 1.30.

Discussion

In this example we have examined the extent to which the confounding of occupational grade and smoking could distort estimates of the effects of the latter. We show that this confounding leads to overestimation of the number of deaths in our hypothetical population that could be attributed to smoking by approximately a quarter. The true extent of confounding may well be greater than this, however. Car ownership serves as an additional marker of socioeconomic position, discriminating within employment grades. In the Whitehall Study, mortality risk is independently related to car ownership and to employment grade (Figure 3).[6]

The two markers of socioeconomic position are both associated with smoking behaviour, with car owners being less likely to smoke within each grade (Figure 4). Thus the confounding of the smoking–mortality relationship by socioeconomic position will not be fully accounted for by examining the contribution of employment grade, as we have done here.

In some studies of smoking and mortality – such as the British doctors study[7] – groups which are relatively homogenous with respect to occupation and socioeconomic circumstances have been investigated. The degree of confounding will be less in studies with homogeneous populations. Indeed the smoking-associated relative risk for coronary heart disease (CHD) in the British doctors study is markedly lower than that seen in the British Regional Heart Study (BRHS), in which the sample included all social classes.[8] In the BRHS smoking was more prevalent in the manual social class groups,[9] and

Figure 3: Ten-year mortality risk by grade and car ownership

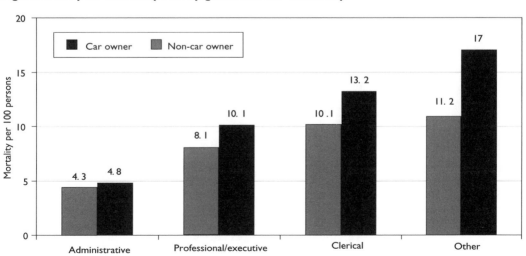

Figure 4: Current smokers by grade and car ownership

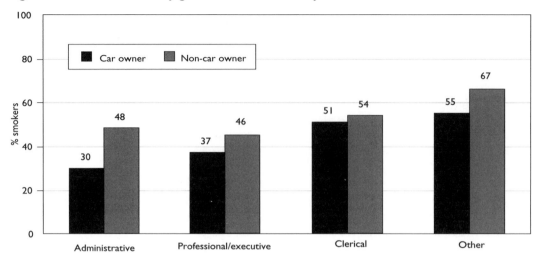

thus positive confounding of the smoking–CHD relationship would be expected.

We have discussed how confounding of smoking behaviour with socioeconomic position could lead to exaggeration of the mortality excess associated with smoking. Misclassification of smoking behaviour could, on the other hand, lead to under-estimation of the relationship between smoking and mortality. One way this could occur is if some smokers claim not to be smokers (or vice versa). Other studies have demonstrated that this is not usually a major problem;[10] nor is there evidence that such misreporting is strongly associated with socioeconomic position. Failure to take account of the duration and quantity of smoking by the participants who quit, that is, the ex-smokers, and not considering the amount smoked by current smokers would also influence some of the estimates of confounding we have given here. However, as Figure 3 demonstrates, use of employment grade will not fully account for socioeconomic differentials in mortality – a considerable residual effect, indexed by car ownership, remains. It is not possible to resolve the issue of the influence of the relative degrees of misclassification of smoking behaviour and socioeconomic position within the present dataset, but it is unlikely that the degree of confounding we demonstrate here represents an overestimate of the true situation.

In our example an exposure would be associated with a 30% increased risk of mortality purely because of its association with employment grade, if it had the same social distribution as smoking. This demonstrates the importance of considering such confounding within observational studies. It has been common, however, for epidemiologists to take only a partial view of this problem. A typical example is provided by the BRHS. When considering social class differentials in CHD risk, the investigators adjusted for smoking behaviour.[9] However, when the association between smoking behaviour and CHD risk was studied in the BRHS it was not considered necessary to adjust for markers of socioeconomic position.[8] This is particularly surprising since confounding by socioeconomic factors could plausibly contribute to the results from this study which were not in accord with previous findings.

In several papers,[4,11,12] Sterling and Weinkam discuss the importance of recognising the confounding of occupation and smoking behaviour. In this brief chapter we have demonstrated that the effect of such confounding within a largely white collar cohort is not trivial. If the range of occupational groups studied was broader, confounding would probably be revealed as being an even more substantial contributor to observed effects. The study of an homogeneous group, such as doctors, is analogous to the consideration of just one employment grade within the present civil service cohort. However, even with civil service employment grades socioeconomic differentials in mortality risk can be demonstrated. While studying homogeneous groups will reduce the magnitude of confounding, it will not necessarily remove it completely.

In the Whitehall Study, occupational levels serve as a much more powerful discriminator of mortality risk than would Registrar General's social class – the usual measure of socioeconomic position used in British studies.[6] Thus statistically 'controlling for' social class could leave most of this elevated risk unaccounted for, and apparently an attribute of the exposure itself.

The extent to which confounding, and residual confounding, can distort associations has frequently been underestimated within both social and biomedical epidemiology.[13] Quantitative estimates of the magnitude of these effects, such as we have presented here, can provide a useful corrective to this tendency.

References

[1] Atkinson, A.B. and Townsend, J.L.B. (1977) 'Economic aspects of reduced smoking', *Lancet*, no II, pp 492-5.

[2] Public Health Service (1979) *Smoking and health*, Washington, DC: Department of Health, Education and Welfare.

[3] Shephard, R.J. (1981) *Ischaemic heart disease and exercise*, London: Croom Helm.

[4] Sterling, T. and Weinkam, J. (1990) 'The confounding of occupation and smoking and its consequences', *Social Science and Medicine*, no 30, pp 457-67.

[5] Reid, D.D., Hamilton, P.J.S., McCartney, P. and Rose, G. (1976) 'Smoking and other risk factors for coronary heart disease in British civil servants', *Lancet*, vol 2, pp 979-84.

[6] **Davey Smith, G., Shipley, M.J. and Rose, G. (1990) 'The magnitude and causes of socioeconomic differentials in mortality: further evidence from the Whitehall Study',** *Journal of Epidemiology and Community Health*, **vol 44, pp 265-70.**

[7] Doll, R. and Peto, R. (1976) 'Mortality in relation to smoking: 20 years' observation on male British doctors', *British Medical Journal*, vol 2, pp 1525-36.

[8] Cook, D.G., Pocock, S.J., Shaper, A.G. and Kussick, S.J. (1986) 'Giving up smoking and the risk of heart attacks: a report from the British Regional Heart Study', *Lancet*, vol 2, pp 1376-80.

[9] Pocock, S.J., Shaper, A.G., Cook, D.G., Phillips, A.N. and Walker, M. (1987) 'Social class differences in ischaemic heart disease in British men', *Lancet*, vol 2, pp 197-201.

[10] Borgers, D. and Junge, B. (1979) 'Thiocyanate as an indicator of tobacco smoking', *Preventive Medicine*, vol 8, pp 351-7.

[11] Sterling, T.D. (1978) 'Does smoking kill workers or does work kill smokers? Or: the mutual relationship between smoking, occupation and respiratory disease', *International Journal of Health Services*, vol 8, pp 437-52.

[12] Sterling, T.D. and Weinkham, J.J. (1978) 'Smoking patterns by occupation, industry, sex and race', *Archives of Environmental Health*, vol 33, pp 313-17.

[13] Davey Smith, G. and Phillips, A. (1990) 'Declaring independence: why we should be cautious', *Journal of Epidemiology and Community Health*, vol 44, pp 257-8.

14

Socioeconomic differentials in cancer among men

George Davey Smith, David Leon, Martin J. Shipley and Geoffrey Rose

Abstract

The relationship between cancer and socioeconomic position is examined for men using data from three sources – the Whitehall Study of London civil servants, the OPCS Longitudinal Study and the Registrar General's Decennial Supplement. Mortality from, or registration for, malignant neoplasms was higher overall in lower socioeconomic groups. There was considerable variation in the strength, and to a lesser extent direction, of the association of specific cancer sites and socioeconomic position within each of the studies. However, between the studies the relationships between socioeconomic and the particular cancers were very similar.

The similarity in results, taken in conjunction with the differences in design and methods of the three studies, makes it very unlikely that these consistent associations are due to artefacts. The heterogeneity in relationships between specific cancer sites and socioeconomic position suggests that no single factor – such as differences in general susceptibility or differences in smoking behaviour – can account for these associations. However, socioeconomic differentials displayed by a particular malignancy do offer clues to its aetiology, and provide an indication of the scope that exists for reducing the burden of cancer within a population.

Introduction

The relationship between cancer rates and socioeconomic position has been investigated for many years, primarily as a source of aetiological hypotheses. The early studies which treated cancer as a

International Journal of Epidemiology,
1991, vol 20, pp 339-45

single condition[1,2] soon gave way to site-specific investigations[3,5] which were notable in providing some of the earliest systematic evidence that environmental factors were important in the aetiology of a number of cancers. In the 1950s cancer incidence rates were used for the first time in explicit attempts to throw light on the still obscure aetiology of a range of malignancies.[6,7] In addition to the underlying role of specific environmental factors, it was also postulated that lower socioeconomic position may go with an increased predisposition to cancer in general.[8] This latter suggestion is in line with proposals that there is heightened general susceptibility to disease in particular groups.[9-13] Examination of differentials in site-specific cancer rates is necessary to evaluate these hypotheses.

This paper begins with a report of new analyses of differentials in cancer mortality according to employment grade in the Whitehall Study of London civil servants.[14] In this study the differentials in all-cause and in total cancer mortality have been larger than the equivalent social class differences in the British population,[15] which may reflect the fact that the use of civil service employment grade produces groups which are more homogeneous with respect to aspects of material circumstances than those generated by the Registrar General's social classes.

The differentials in site-specific cancer mortality in the Whitehall Study are compared to the socioeconomic differentials in two other datasets; cancer mortality in the latest Registrar General's Decennial Supplement on occupational mortality[16] and cancer registrations in the Office of Population Censuses and Surveys Longitudinal Study.[17,18]

Participants and methods

The Whitehall Study

In the Whitehall Study 18,403 male civil servants aged 40-64 were examined between 1967 and 1969.[14] A questionnaire was completed regarding age, civil service employment grade and smoking habits. In two departments, with a total of 873 subjects, employment grades were not comparable with the rest of the sample. Thus 17,530 subjects remain for this study. In some of the analyses, these men are divided into four employment grades: administrative, professional or executive, clerical, and 'other grades' (men in messenger and other unskilled manual jobs). In other analyses, a dichotomy is made between a 'high' group, composed of the administrative and the professional and executive grades, and a 'low' group, consisting of the remainder. Smoking has been categorised according to cigarette use as 'current smoker', 'ex-smoker' and 'never smoker'. The 409 men who only smoked pipes or cigars have been excluded from the analyses that involve smoking status.

Records from over 99% of subjects were traced and flagged at the National Health Service Central Registry. Death certificates coded according to the Eighth Revision of the International Classification of Diseases (ICD) have been obtained, and this mortality follow-up to 31 January 1987 provides the basis for this analysis. For 10 subjects, cause of death was unknown: these have been excluded from cause-specific mortality analyses.

Mortality due to malignant neoplasms (ICD codes 140-209) has been divided into the following main groups: oesophagus (ICD code 150), stomach (151), colon (153), rectum (154), pancreas (157), trachea, bronchus and lung (162 – referred to as lung cancer), prostate (185), bladder (188), brain (191), unspecified primary (195-9), haematopoietic (200-7) and other (all other codes). Three sites with a small number of deaths were included in the 'other' group for the main analyses, but were also examined separately since they have previously been seen to show associations with socioeconomic position. These were liver and gallbladder (155-6 – referred to as liver), kidney (189) and malignant melanoma (172).

Mortality rates have been calculated using person years at risk. These rates have been standardised for age at entry using the direct method, using five-year age bands and the total population as the standard. Calculation of rate ratios and confidence intervals (CI) used Cox's proportional hazards regression model,[19] with age as a continuous variable and grade as a factor. To validate the presentation of summary measures of the grade effect, formal tests of heterogeneity over age and calendar period were carried out using standard methods.

The Decennial Supplement

Data from microfiche published as part of the 1981 Registrar General's Decennial Supplement on Occupational Mortality in Great Britain[16] were used. Death certificates were coded according to the Ninth Revision of the ICD. For the sites considered here the ICD code groups remain the same as described above, except for unspecified primary (which are ICD 195 and ICD 199 only in ICD-9, codes 196-8 having been dropped) and haematopoietic malignancies (ICD 200-8). Inspection of the bridge coding exercise,[20] in which a sample of deaths were coded according to both ICD-8 and ICD-9, reveals that these changes had no important influence on classification of these groups.

Mortality rates were calculated by social class based on occupation (Table 1) for men aged 20-64. The denominators comprised the number of observed deaths in Great Britain in four peri-censal years

Table 1: The Registrar General's social classes

Social class		Examples of occupations in class
I	Professional occupations	Doctors, engineers, lawyers, surveyors
II	Intermediate occupations	Teachers, nurses
IIIN	Skilled occupations (non-manual)	Cashiers, police officers, commercial travellers
IIIM	Skilled occupations (manual)	Metal workers, butchers, ambulancemen and women
IV	Partly skilled occupations	Bar staff, bus conductors, machine tool operators
V	Unskilled occupations	Labourers, officer cleaners, porters

(1979-80, 1982-83) classified into social class groups based on occupation stated on the death certificate, while the numerators were estimated from the distribution of the population of Great Britain by social class derived from occupation at the 1981 Census.

Standardised mortality ratios (SMRs) were calculated for non-manual and manual workers by aggregating observed and expected deaths for social classes I, II, IIIN and IIIM, IV, V respectively. The magnitudes of the manual to non-manual differentials in cancer mortality were estimated by taking the ratios of the corresponding SMRs.

The Longitudinal Study

The design and methods used in the Office of Population Censuses and Survey Longitudinal Study have been detailed elsewhere.[17,18,21] In summary, the study population is a 1% sample of those enumerated at the 1971 Census of England and Wales. The sample was defined as all those individuals whose date of birth fell on one of four dates of birth spread evenly throughout the year. Nearly 97% (513,072) of these individuals were traced and flagged at the NHS Central Register, providing the basis for the linkage of cancer registrations from the National Cancer Registration Scheme to the census information on study members.

The data described here are from the first five years' follow-up (1971-75) as previously published.[17] Cancer incidence data for 1971-81 has also been published,[18] but were not sufficiently comprehensive to be used in the comparison in our secondary analysis. Census information was used to classify men in the study by five socioeconomic measures: housing tenure, household access to cars, household access to domestic amenities, social class and educational qualifications. Person years at risk were accumulated for each level of each measure, taking into account age at risk and year of follow-up. Indirect standardisation was used to estimate the ratio of the cancer registration rate for any one level of a measure to the rate in an appropriate standard group (Table 2), adjusting for age and calendar period. This was expressed as a standardised registration ratio.

Results

There were 4,031 deaths during the follow-up of the Whitehall Study cohort, of which 1,237 were due to cancer. The age-adjusted mortality rates by employment grade from all-causes, all cancers, specific cancer sites and from causes other than cancer are reported in Table 3, for sites with more than 35 deaths. The age-adjusted relative rates of mortality for the low grades (clerical and other) compared to the high grades (administration, professionals and executives) are also given. For cancer and noncancer mortality, the gradients of the rates across the employment grades and the low/high grade rate ratios are virtually identical. Conversely, while many of the site-specific rate ratios are not statistically significant, there is evidently considerable variation (heterogeneity) in the associations between cancer mortality for specific sites and employment grade (χ^2 for heterogenerity = 45.3, 11 df, $p<0.001$).

The low/high grade rate ratios for sites with less than 35 deaths (excluded from Table 3) were as follows: kidney, 1.4 (27 deaths), liver, 2.9 (18 deaths) and melanoma, 0.5 (7 deaths). Only for liver was the relationship with grade statistically significant.

Mortality from cancers which have consistently been associated with smoking[22,23] have been examined according to smoking behaviour and employment grade. The mortality rate ratios for each smoking and employment grade category compared to those high grade subjects who had never smoked are presented for the aggregate of all smoking related sites in Table 4. In the Whitehall Study, bladder

Table 2: Definition of 'high' and 'low' socioeconomic categories and standard population rates used in the Longitudinal Study (LS)

	Housing tenure	Household access to cars	Access to household amenities	Own social class	Educational qualifications
'High' socioeconomic category	Owner-occupied	Access to one or more cars	Sole use of all amenities	Non-manual social classes	Higher/professional qualifications or A levels
'Low' socioeconomic category	Local authority	No access to cars	One or more amenities missing	Manual social classes IIIM-V	No higher/professional qualifications or A levels
Standard population[a]	All LS males	All LS males	All LS males	All LS men aged 15 and over at Census	All LS men aged 18-70 at Census

[a] Source of standard rates used in calculation of standardised registration ratios.

Table 3: Age-adjusted mortality rates per 1,000 person years (number of deaths) by employment grade in Whitehall Study

	Admin-istrators	Professional or executive	Clerical	Other	χ^2 for trend	Low/high grade rate ratio
All-causes[a]	9.89	12.84	18.00	20.81	137.60	1.48
	(141)	(2322)	(905)	(663)	($p<0.001$)	(1.4-1.6)
All cancers	3.14	3.91	5.30	6.24	45.65	1.48
	(47)	(713)	(265)	(212)	($p<0.001$)	(1.3-1.7)
Specific cancers:						
Oesophagus	0.05	0.11	0.13	0.19	3.07	1.53
	(1)	(21)	(6)	(8)	($p=0.08$)	(0.8-3.1)
Stomach	0.16	0.29	0.46	0.57	9.27	1.85
	(2)	(54)	(24)	(20)	($p=0.002$)	(1.2-2.8)
Colon	0.37	0.43	0.40	0.44	0.30	0.94
	(6)	(74)	(21)	(13)	($p>0.5$)	(0.6-1.4)
Rectum	0.26	0.13	0.13	0.23	0.06	1.07
	(4)	(26)	(6)	(6)	($p>0.5$)	(0.5-2.2)
Pancreas	0.24	0.20	0.25	0.40	0.55	1.37
	(4)	(37)	(14)	(9)	($p=0.5$)	(0.8-2.3)
Lung	0.81	1.15	2.09	2.99	71.79	2.19
	(12)	(207)	(108)	(110)	($p<0.001$)	(1.8-2.7)
Prostate	0.40	0.38	0.23	0.34	2.81	0.60
	(5)	(62)	(11)	(10)	($p=0.1$)	(0.4-1.0)
Bladder	0.16	0.18	0.10	0.23	0.00	0.91
	(2)	(29)	(6)	(8)	($p>0.5$)	(0.5-1.7)
Brain	0.15	0.13	0.13	0.07	0.03	0.91
	(3)	(28)	(6)	(3)	($p>0.5$)	(0.4-1.9)
Unspecified	0.19	0.15	0.43	0.17	3.94	2.39
	(2)	(29)	(20)	(6)	($p=0.05$)	(1.4-4.2)
Haematopoietic	0.21	0.37	0.35	0.26	0.16	0.91
	(4)	(69)	(15)	(10)	($p>0.5$)	(0.6-1.5)
Other	0.13	0.39	0.60	0.34	1.52	1.32
	(2)	(77)	(28)	(9)	($p=0.2$)	(0.8-2.1)
Noncancer	6.70	8.91	12.69	14.44	91.77	1.49
	(93)	(1,603)	(639)	(449)	($p<0.001$)	(1.4-1.6)

[a] Includes 10 deaths in which the specific cause was unknown.

cancer is not associated with either employment grade or smoking. For the other sites, as well as for all smoking-associated cancers, combined, mortality rate ratios within each smoking category are highest in the low employment grade.

From the Decennial Supplement data, cancer sites have been ranked according to the size of the manual/non-manual SMR ratio. All malignant neoplasms taken together have a manual/non-manual SMR ratio of 1.48 (95% CI: 1.3-1.7).

Site-specific ratios are compared to the corresponding low/high grade rate ratio from the Whitehall Study in Table 5. The similarity in

Table 4: Age-adjusted mortality rate ratios[a] and 95% CI (observed number of deaths) by employment grade and smoking status for the aggregate of all smoking-associated cancer sites[b] in the Whitehall Study

	Smoking status		
	Never smoked	Ex-smoker	Current smoker
Employment grade			
High	1.0 (26)	2.1 (119)	4.6 (223)
		1.4-3.2	3.1-6.9
Low	1.4 (11)	2.6 (51)	7.5 (237)
	0.7-2.9	1.6-4.3	5.0-11.3

[a] Relative to those in the high employment grade who had never smoked.

[b] Oral cavity, pharynx, oesophagus, pancreas, larynx, lung, bladder, kidney, unspecified sites.

Table 5: Ranking of cancer sites among men according to relationship with socioeconomic position from the Whitehall Study and the 1981 Decennial Supplement

Whitehall Study[a]		Decennial Supplement[b]	
Site	Low/high mortality rate ratio	Site	Low/high mortality rate ratio
Liver	2.85	Lung	1.97
Unspecified	2.39	Stomach	1.81
Lung	2.19	Unspecified	1.52
Stomach	1.85	Liver	1.51
Oesophagus	1.53	Oesophagus	1.41
Kidney	1.45	Bladder	1.44
Pancreas	1.37	Rectum	1.24
Rectum	1.07	Pancreas	1.23
Colon	0.94	Haematopoietic	1.09
Haematopoietic	0.91	Prostate	1.07
Brain	0.91	Kidney	1.03
Bladder	0.91	Colon	1.00
Prostate	0.60	Brain	0.96
Melanoma	0.54	Melanoma	0.65

[a] Prospective cohort study of cancer mortality. Socioeconomic position based on civil service grade.

[b] Socioeconomic position based on Registrar General's social classes (Table 1).

rank order between the two studies is strong; only for bladder and kidney cancer is there any obvious discrepancy in ranking between the studies. The highest mortality rates are more consistently found in the low socioeconomic position category in the Decennial Supplement data than in the Whitehall Study. In the former only two cancer sites, melanoma and brain, show higher rates among the non-manual group, whereas in the latter study six sites demonstrate higher rates in the higher employment grade group.

In the OPCS Longitudinal Study, for each measure of socioeconomic position a 'high' and 'low' category was defined, as shown in Table 2. The magnitude of the socioeconomic differential in cancer registration rates was estimated by the ratio of the standardised registration ratios in the low to the high category. For all malignant neoplasms taken together, the low to high SRRs were 1.26 for access to household amenities, 1.14 for social class and 1.28 for education.

Within each measure, cancer sites were ranked according to the magnitude of the low/high differential.[17] The ranking of cancer sites was strikingly similar across the five measures, this being formally tested using Friedman's two-way analysis of variance with ranks.[24] The test statistic was highly significant ($\chi^2 = 29.4$, 10 df, $p=0.001$), suggesting that the similarity in the ranking of the differentials was very unlikely to be due to chance. A summary ranking of sites was determined by ordering the sites according to their mean rank across the five measures. This ranking is presented in Table 6, along with the corresponding rank orders from the Whitehall Study and the Decennial Supplement, for the ten cancer sites for which there were data in each study. Friedman's test statistic was highly significant when applied to the date in Table 6 ($\chi^2 = 23.29$, 9 df, $p=0.006$), suggesting that the similarity in ranking of cancer sites seen in the three data sets was unlikely to be due to chance.

Discussion

Rates of death or cancer registration from all malignant neoplasms taken together were highest in lower socioeconomic position groups in each of the three studies examined here. Site-specifically, within each study, there was considerable variation in the strength and direction of the association with socioeconomic position. However, between the three studies, the relationships between socioeconomic position and particular cancers were very similar. This concordance is very striking given that the studies differ considerably in their design, endpoint (death or cancer registration), calendar period of follow-up, age distribution of their populations and the definitions of socioeconomic position employed.

The contrast between the consistency across studies in the

Table 6: Ranking[a] of cancer sites among men according to relationship with socioeconomic position from the Longitudinal Study, the 1981 Decennial Supplement and the Whitehall Study

Longitudinal Study[b]	Decennial Supplement[c]	Whitehall Study[d]
Lung	Lung	Unspecified
Unspecified	Stomach	Lung
Stomach	Unspecified	Stomach
Bladder	Bladder	Pancreas
Rectum	Rectum	Rectum
Pancreas	Pancreas	Colon
Haematopoietic	Haematopoietic	Haematopoietic
Brain	Prostate	Brain
Colon	Colon	Bladder
Prostate	Brain	Prostate

[a] Ranking according to magnitude of low/high rate ratio; those sites with the largest ratio are placed at the top of each column.

[b] Prospective cohort study of cancer incidence. See Table 2 and text for details of socioeconomic classifications used.

[c] Socioeconomic position based on Registrar General's social classes (Table 1).

[d] Prospective cohort study of cancer mortality. Socioeconomic position based on civil service grade.

association between cancer risk and socioeconomic position with the variation in the design and methods between each study makes it unlikely that these associations are artefacts. However, the potential artefactual explanations for these associations need to be considered.

Two of the studies rely on data from death certificates, the imperfections of which are well known.[25,26] If misclassification of cancer is related to socioeconomic position then their association will be distorted. Only one study of level of agreement between autopsy and clinical diagnosis of cause of death has examined the influence of the socioeconomic position of the deceased.[27] Compared with pathologists, the clinicians tended to overdiagnose neoplasms as the underlying cause of death in the non-manual group and to underdiagnose them in the manual group. This would tend towards underestimation of the degree to which lower socioeconomic groups experience higher overall cancer mortality. In this autopsy study,[27] diagnostic disagreements for individual cancer sites by socioeconomic position could not be examined due to small numbers.

Differential misclassification between cancer sited could clearly distort the association of particular cancers with socioeconomic position. A large study from the US[28] of the accuracy of death certificates suggests that misclassification between cancer sites is not great enough to account for the heterogeneity of associations with socioeconomic position reported here.

In the Decennial Supplement, numerator/denominator biases could produce artefactual social class differentials in cancer mortality.[29] However, reports from the Longitudinal Study,[30] which avoids this potential bias, have demonstrated that this does not seriously distort the social class associations with mortality.

The Longitudinal Study data based on the prospective linkage of cancer registrations to census data on individuals avoids both the problems of numerator:denominator bias and biases in death certification. The use of registration data has the further strength that differentials in incidence are not contaminated by any differentials in cancer survival.[18,31] However, during the follow-up period 1971-75 it is known that registration of cancer for England and Wales was incomplete.[32] If completeness of registration varied by socioeconomic category, this could bias the observed differentials; but this is not very plausible, given the heterogeneity in the direction of differentials by cancer site, the highest rate being found sometimes in the 'low' category and sometimes in the 'high' category.

Logan[5] reported that over the whole period from 1911 to 1971, social classes I and II in Britain had the lowest overall cancer mortality rates. Of the sites under investigation here, consistently higher rates were reported for manual workers for stomach and oesophagus malignancies. Smaller and less consistent relationships in the same direction were seen for bladder, rectum and liver malignancies. Lung cancer mortality was highest in social class V over the whole period, but up to and including the 1931 Decennial Supplement social classes I and II had higher rates than social classes III and IV. Only since 1961 has there been an increasing gradient from social class I to social class V, consistent with what is known about the development of socioeconomic differences in smoking habits. For colon, haematopoietic, prostate and brain cancers a gradient of increasing mortality with higher social class groups was seen in the early reports, but this had been markedly attenuated or had disappeared by 1971. Pancreas and kidney cancers have demonstrated no consistent associations with social class. Malignant melanoma mortality has only been reported separately since 1951 and has subsequently shown a positive gradient. While these data are subject to bias, they do further underline the contention that the association between cancer risk and socioeconomic position varies between site and over long periods of time.

Studies of socioeconomic position and cancer outside the UK[33-38] have also produced results similar to those reported here. Lung, stomach and oesophageal cancer have been consistently associated with lower socioeconomic position, with prostate, brain and colon cancer being associated with higher socioeconomic position.

Thus the associations between cancer risk and socioeconomic position are almost certainly real and not artefacts. The observed heterogeneity in the association with specific cancer sites leads to a further conclusion. It has been suggested that increased general susceptibility to disease is seen in lower socioeconomic position groups.[9-13] In terms of cancer mortality, these suggestions are linked to the theory that immune system surveillance prevents the propagation of potentially malignant cells which have been transformed by contact with exogenous carcinogens,[39,40] this immune suppression being related to stresses from the social environment. The heterogeneity in socioeconomic associations with cancer offers no support for such assertions.

The socioeconomic differentials displayed by a particular malignancy do offer clues to its aetiology. Thus the associations of socioeconomic position with colon cancer in countries as different as Columbia[41], New Zealand[42] and Hong Kong[43] have been used to formulate and test aetiological theories.

The investigation of the causes of a particular cancer can benefit from consideration of the socioeconomic position relationships which it displays and any complete aetiological explanation should be consistent with the existence of such relationships. This is particularly true for sites such as the stomach, which show a strong and persistent association with socioeconomic position, yet whose specific aetiology is far from clear.

References

1   Heron, D. (1907) 'Note on class incidence of cancer', *British Medical Journal*, vol 1, pp 621-2.

2   Brown, J.W. and Lal, M. (1914) 'An inquiry into the relation between social status and cancer mortality', *Journal of Hygiene*, vol 14, pp 186-200.

3   Young, M. (1926) 'The variation in the mortality from cancer of different parts of the body in groups of men of different social status', *Journal of Hygiene*, vol 25, pp 209-17.

4   Stevenson, T.H.C. (1928) 'The vital statistics of wealth and poverty', *Journal of the Royal Statistical Society*, vol 91, pp 207-20.

5   Logan, W.P.D. (1982) *Cancer mortality by occupation and social class 1851-1971*, London: HMSO.

6   Clemmesen, J. and Nielsen, A. (1951) 'The social distribution of cancer in Copenhagen, 1943 to 1947', *British Journal of Cancer*, vol 5, pp 159-71.

7   Cohart, E.M. (1954) 'Socioeconomic distribution of stomach cancer in New Haven', *Cancer*, vol 7, pp 455-61.

8   Buell, P., Dunn, J.E. and Breslow, L. (1960) 'Occupational social class risks of cancer mortality in men', *Journal of Chronic Disease*, vol 12, pp 600-21.

9   Thurlow, H.J. (1967) 'General susceptibility to illness: a selective review', *Canadian Medical Association Journal*, vol 97, pp 1397-404.

10 Najman, J.M. (1980) 'Theories of disease causation and the concept of general susceptibility: a review', *Social Science and Medicine*, vol 14A, pp 231-7.

11 Syme, S.L. and Berkman, L.F. (1976) 'Social class, susceptibility and sickness', *American Journal of Epidemiology*, vol 104, pp 1-8.

12 Najman, J.M. and Congalton, A.A. (1979) 'Australian occupational mortality, 1965-67: cause specific or general susceptibility?', *Social Health and Illness*, vol 1, pp 158-76.

13 Susser, M.W., Watson, W. and Hopper, K. (1985) *Sociology in medicine*, Oxford: Oxford University Press.

14 Reid, D.D., Brett, G.Z., Hamilton, P.J.S., Jarrett, R.J., Keen, H. and Rose, G. (1974) 'Cardiorespiratory disease and diabetes among middle-aged male civil servants: a study of screening and intervention', *Lancet*, vol 1, pp 469-73.

15 Marmot, M.G., Shipley, M.J. and Rose, G. (1984) 'Inequalities in death – specific explanation of a general pattern', *Lancet*, vol 1, pp 1003-6.

16 Office of Population Censuses and Surveys (1990) *Occupational mortality: The Registrar General's Decennial Supplement for Great Britain, 1979-1980, 1982-83*, Series LS, no 5, London: HMSO.

17 Leon, D.A. (1990) *Longitudinal study: Socio-demographic differences in cancer survival, 1971-83*, OPCS Series LS, no 5, London: HMSO.

18 Kogevinas, E. (1990) *Longitudinal study: Socio-demographic differences in cancer survival, 1971-83*, OPCS Series LS, no 5, London: HMSO.

19 Cox, D.R. (1972) 'Regression models and life tables', *Journal of the Royal Statistical Society Series B*, vol 34, 187-220.

20 Office of Population Censuses and Surveys (1983) *Mortality statistics: Comparison of 8th and 9th revisions of the International Classification of Disease*, Series DH1, no 10, London: HMSO.

21 Fox, A.J. and Goldblatt, P. (1982) *Longitudinal study: Socio-demographic mortality differentials, 1971-1975*, OPCS Series LS, no 1, London: HMSO.

22 Zaridze, D.G. and Peto, R. (1986) *Tobacco: A major international health hazard*, IARC Scientific Publications, no 74, Lyon: International Agency for Research on Cancer.

23 Hammond, E.C. (1966) 'Smoking in relation to the death rates of one million men and women', in W. Haenszel (ed) *Epidemiological approaches to the study of cancer and other chronic diseases*, National Cancer Institute Mongraph No. 19, Bethesda, MD: US Department of Health, Education and Welfare, pp 127-204.

24 Friedman, M. (1937) 'The use of ranks to avoid the assumption of normality implicit in the analysis of variance', *Journal of the American Statistical Association*, vol 32, pp 675-701.

25 Abramson, J.H., Sacks, M.I. and Cahana, E. (1974) 'Death certification data as an indication of the presence of certain common conditions at death', *Journal of Chronic Disease*, vol 24, pp 417-31.

26 Cameron, H.M. and McGoogan, E. (1981) 'A prospective study of 1152 hospital autopsies: II. Analysis of inaccuracies in clinical diagnosis and their significance', *Journal of Pathology*, vol 133, pp 285-300.

27 Samphier, M.L., Robertson, C. and Bloor, M.J. (1988) 'A possible artefactual component in specific cause mortality gradients', *Journal of Epidemiology and Community Health*, vol 42, pp 138-43.

28 Percy, C., Stanek, E. and Gloeckler, L. (1981) 'Accuracy of cancer death certificates and its effect on cancer mortality statistics', *American Journal of Public Health*, vol 71, pp 242-50.

29 Bloor, M., Samphier, M. and Prior, L. (1987) 'Artefact explanations of inequalities in health: an assessment of the evidence', *Social Health and Illness*, vol 9, pp 231-64.

30 Goldblatt, P. (1989) 'Mortality by social class, 1971-85', *Population Trends*, no 56, pp 6-15.

31 Leon, D.A. and Wilkinson, R.G. (1989) 'Inequalities in prognosis: socioeconomic differences in cancer and heart disease survival', in A.J. Fox (ed) *Health inequalities in European countries*, Aldershot: Gower, pp 280-300.

[32] Swerdlow, A.J. (1986) 'Cancer registration in England and Wales: some aspects relevant to interpretation of the data', *Journal of the Royal Statistical Society Series A: Statistics in Society*, vol 149, pp 146-60.

[33] Kitagawa, E.M. and Hauser, P.M. (1973) *Differential mortality in the US: A study in socioeconomic epidemiology*, Cambridge, MA: Harvard University Press.

[34] Nayha, S. (1977) 'Social group and mortality in Finland', *British Journal of Preventive and Social Medicine*, vol 31, pp 231-7.

[35] Vagero, D. and Persson, G. (1986) 'Occurrence of cancer in socioeconomic groups in Sweden', *Scandinavian Journal of Social Medicine*, vol 14, pp 151-60.

[36] Pukkala, E. and Teppo, L. (1986) 'Socioeconomic status and education as risk determinants of gastrointestinal cancer', *Preventive Medicine*, vol 15, pp 127-38.

[37] Pearce, N.E. and Howard, J.K. (1986) 'Occupation, social class and male cancer mortality in New Zealand, 1974-78', *International Journal of Epidemiology*, vol 15, pp 456-62.

[38] Levi, F., Negri, E., La Vecchia, C. and Te, V.C. (1988) 'Socioeconomic groups and cancer risk at death in the Swiss canton of Vaud', *International Journal of Epidemioliogy*, vol 17, pp 711-17.

[39] Sterling, P. and Eyer, J. (1981) 'Biological basis of stress-related mortality', *Social Science and Medicine*, vol 15E, pp 3-42.

[40] Totman, R. (1987) *Social causes of illness*, London: Souvenir Press.

[41] Haenszel, W., Correa, P. and Cuello, C. (1975) 'Social class differences among patients with large-bowel cancer in Cali, Columbia', *Journal of the National Cancer Institute*, vol 54, pp 1031-5.

[42] Smith, A.H., Pearce, N.E. and Joseph, J.G. (1985) 'Major colo-rectal cancer aetiological hypotheses do not explain mortality trends among Maori and non-Maori New Zealanders', *International Journal of Epidemiology*, vol 14, pp 79-85.

[43] Crowther, J.S., Drasar, B.S., Hill, M.J. et al (1976) 'Faecal steroids and bacteria and large bowel cancer in Hong Kong by socioeconomic groups', *British Journal of Cancer*, vol 34, pp 191-8.

Section IV
Health and lifetime social circumstances: the Collaborative Study

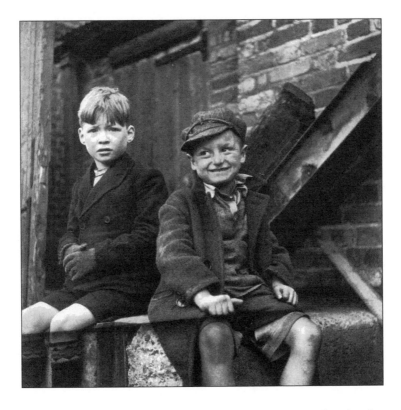

Boys in the 1930s. Photograph by Edith Tudor Hart, reproduced with permission of Wolf Suschitzsky.

15

Lifetime socioeconomic position and mortality: prospective observational study

George Davey Smith, Carole Hart,
David Blane, Charles Gillis and
Victor Hawthorne

Abstract

Objectives: To assess the influence of socioeconomic position over a lifetime on risk factors for cardiovascular disease, on morbidity, and on mortality from various causes.

Design: Prospective observational study with 21 years of follow-up. Social class was determined as manual or non-manual at three stages of participants' lives: from the social class of their father's job, the social class of their first job, and the social class of their job at the time of screening. A cumulative social class indicator was constructed, ranging from non-manual social class at all three stages of life to manual social class at all three stages.

Setting: 27 workplaces in the West of Scotland.

Participants: 5,766 men aged 35-64 at the time of examination.

Main outcome measures: Prevalence and level of risk factors for cardiovascular disease; morbidity; and mortality from broad cause of death groups.

Results: From non-manual social class locations at all three life stages to manual at all stages there were strong positive trends for blood pressure, body mass index, current cigarette smoking, angina, and bronchitis. Inverse

British Medical Journal, 1997, vol 314, pp 547-52

trends were seen for height, cholesterol concentration, lung function, and being an ex-smoker. 1,580 men died during follow-up. Age-adjusted relative death rates in comparison with the men of non-manual social class locations at all three stages of life were 1.29 (95% CI: 1.08-1.56) in men of two non-manual and one manual social class locations; 1.45 (1.21-1.73) in men of two manual and one non-manual social class locations; and 1.71 (1.46-2.01) in men of manual social class at all three stages. Mortality from cardiovascular disease showed a similar graded association with cumulative social class. Mortality from cancer was mainly raised among men of manual social class at all three stages. Adjustment for a wide range of risk factors caused little attenuation in the association of cumulative social class with mortality from all-causes and from cardiovascular disease; greater attenuation was seen in the association with mortality from noncardiovascular, noncancer disease.

Fathers having a manual occupation was strongly associated with mortality from cardiovascular disease: relative rate 1.41 (1.15-1.72). Participants' social class at the time of screening was more strongly associated than the other social class indicators with mortality from cancer and from noncardiovascular, noncancer causes.

Conclusions: Socioeconomic factors acting over the lifetime affect health and risk of premature death. The relative importance of influences at different stages varies for the cause of death. Studies with data on socioeconomic circumstances at only one stage of life are inadequate for fully elucidating the contribution of socioeconomic factors to health and mortality risk.

Introduction

The ubiquitous nature of the association between unfavourable socioeconomic circumstances in adulthood and premature death has been shown in many studies, with various socioeconomic indicators being related to morbidity and mortality.[1-6] It has long been recognised that the effects of poor social circumstances in early life can have lasting influences,[7,8] and studies relating childhood socioeconomic position to later risk of illness and premature death have been performed.[9-12] These studies have generally been inspired by suggestions that the early environment has specific influences which alter later susceptibility to disease. They have yielded somewhat equivocal findings, well illustrated by two reports from the same study coming to opposite conclusions about the relative importance of childhood and adulthood socioeconomic environment in relation to the risk of coronary heart disease.[10,13]

Recently the importance of considering the cumulative effect of socioenvironmental exposures over a lifetime has been recognised.[14-16] The Department of Health's report *Variations in health* concluded that "it is likely that cumulative differential lifetime exposure to health damaging or health promoting physical and social environments is the main explanation for observed variations in health and life expectancy".[17] Few empirical data exist on such cumulative effects, however.

In the National Longitudinal Survey of Older Men in the US education, first occupation, occupation in middle age, and family assets contributed independently to the risk of premature death,[18] but other data on risk factors were not available and patterns for different causes of death have not been examined. We investigated the contributions of indicators of socioeconomic position over the course of a lifetime to the risk of premature death in a large cohort of men in the West of Scotland who had detailed examinations in middle age and for whom 21 years of subsequent mortality follow-up data were available.

Methods

This analysis is based on a cohort of men recruited from 27 workplaces in Glasgow, Grangemouth, and Clydebank between 1970 and 1973. The workplaces included engineering, manufacturing, and petrochemical plants; a publishing house; civil service departments; administrative and professional divisions from British Rail; architectural institutes; legal and dental offices; and banks. Response rates were available for the workplaces from which 87% of the sample was recruited. For these sites, 70% of those invited completed the questionnaire and attended for examination. The achieved sample was 6,022 men and 1,006 women, from which the 5,766 men aged 35-64 at the time of examination are the basis for the present report. The mortality data in the women were not analysed as only 176 women had died.

The examinations used similar procedures to those used for the Renfrew/Paisley study population.[19] An extensive questionnaire, completed by the subject, was checked at the screening examination. These examinations were conducted at clinics established for this purpose at or near the workplaces.

The information collected at baseline examination included:

- *Sociodemographic data:* age, father's occupational social class, the social class of the participant's first regular job, excluding temporary work, and his occupational social class at the time of screening, and whether he drove a car regularly.

- *Medical history:* angina, previous heart attack and intermittent claudication from the Rose questionnaire,[20] respiratory symptoms from the Medical Research Council questionnaire.[21]
- *Health-related behaviours:* detailed smoking history.
- *Physical examination:* height, weight, blood pressure while seated (taken with a London School of Hygiene and Tropical Medicine sphygmomanometer, diastolic pressure being recorded at the disappearance of the fifth Korotkoff sound), lung function measured with the Garthur Vitalograph, serum cholesterol concentration, and six lead electrocardiogram (leads I, II, III, aVR, aVL, and aVF).

Persistent phlegm was defined as usually bringing up phlegm from the chest first thing in the morning on most days for three months during winter each year. 'Infective phlegm' was defined as usually bringing up phlegm from the chest first thing in the morning in winter and having had a period of increased cough and phlegm lasting for three weeks or more in the previous three years. Breathlessness was defined as a positive response to the question: 'Do you get short of breath walking with people of your own age on level ground?' Bronchitis was defined as having persistent and 'infective' phlegm and being breathless.[20]

Angina was considered present if chest pain or discomfort when walking uphill or hurrying was sited in the sternum or the left chest and arm; caused the subject to stop or slow down; went away when the subject stopped or slowed down; and went away in 10 minutes or less.[20]

Forced expiratory volume in one second (FEV_1) was taken as the better of two expirations. To estimate impairment the expected value was obtained from linear regression equations of age and height, in which expected $FEV_1 = -278.06 + 4.33 \times \text{height} - 3.06 \times \text{age}$. Age was measured in years and height in centimetres and the value was divided by 100 to give FEV_1 in litres. The coefficients were derived from a healthy subset of the population who had never smoked and answered no to questions on phlegm and breathlessness and to questions asking whether they had a wheezy or whistling chest and whether their breathing was affected by the weather. The adjusted FEV_1 was calculated as (actual $FEV_1 \div$ expected FEV_1) x 100.

The electrocardiograms were coded according to the Minnesota system.[20] Any of the codes 1.1-1.3, 4.1-4.4, 5.1-5.3 and 7.1, which encompass diagnoses of definite myocardial infarction, myocardial ischaemia, and left bundle branch block, were considered to be evidence of ischaemia.

Data on father's first or current social class were missing in 199 men, who were excluded from the present analyses, which are therefore based on 5,567 participants. The home address at the time of screening was retrospectively given a postcode, enabling an area-based deprivation category at the time of the 1981 census as defined by Carstairs and

Morris to be ascertained.[22] Deprivation category varies from 1 (least deprived) to 7 (most deprived) and is based on four variables derived from Census data at the level of the postcode sector: male unemployment, overcrowding, car ownership, and proportion of residents in social classes IV and V.

We identified men who had died over the 21 years of follow-up by flagging at the NHS Central Registry in Edinburgh, which also provides death certificates coded according to the ninth revision of the International Classification of Diseases (ICD). We calculated mortality using a person years at risk lifetable approach. These rates have been standardised for age by the direct method, with the total study population as the standard. We tested for trends in age-adjusted rates by proportional hazards regression using the PROC PHREG program in the SAS system,[23] with age and the cumulative social class indicator (defined in the 'Results' section) coded as a continuous variable as covariates. We standardised continuous variables for age using the PROC GLM program, with tests for trend for age-adjusted means being obtained with the PROC REG program. We standardised categorical variables for age by a direct method and tested for trends with the PROC LOGIST program.

Proportional hazards coefficients and their standard errors were calculated using Cox's model.[24] Adjustment for age and other risk factors was performed by including terms for these in the proportional hazards models. Exponentiated hazards coefficients were taken as indicators of relative death rates.

Results

Table 1 shows the distribution of social class at different points during the lives of the study population. The largest category consisted of men whose fathers had had manual social class occupations, whose first job had been in a manual social class occupation, and who had a

Table 1: Distribution of social class according to manual or non-manual occupation of study population

Social class at screening	First social class	
	Non-manual	**Manual**
Manual		
Father's social class:		
Non-manual	34	177
Manual	247	2,319
Non-manual		
Father's social class:		
Non-manual	956	165
Manual	923	746

Table 2: Population characteristics according to cumulative social class (values are age-adjusted means or proportions unless stated otherwise)

	Cumulative social class based on occupation					
	All three non-manual (n=956)	Two non-manual, one manual (n=1,122)	Two manual, one non-manual (n=1,170)	All three manual (n=2,319)	Total (n =5,567)	p value for trend
Age at screening (years)[a]	47.5	47.7	48.6	48.6	48.2	<0.0001
Blood pressure (mm Hg):						
Systolic	131.1	132.2	134.1	136.1	134.1	<0.0001
Diastolic	82.4	83.1	84.1	84.7	83.9	<0.0001
Cholesterol (mmol/l)	6.3	6.1	5.8	5.7	5.9	<0.0001
Height (cm)	176.0	174.4	172.6	170.8	172.8	<0.0001
Body mass index (kg/m²)	24.7	25.1	25.4	25.3	25.2	<0.0001
FEV₁ (%)	99.4	98.0	94.0	90.3	94.2	<0.0001
Percentage (no) of subjects:						
With angina	4.4 (39)	5.4 (57)	6.5 (77)	7.5 (176)	6.3 (349)	0.0002
With electrocardio-graphic ischaemia	5.9 (55)	5.2 (57)	6.1 (74)	5.9 (143)	5.9 (329)	0.64
With bronchitis	0.6 (5)	0.5 (6)	2.9 (35)	3.4 (79)	2.2 (125)	<0.0001
Who had never smoked[b]	20.0 (194)	22.1 (254)	18.1 (209)	14.5 (330)	17.7 (987)	<0.0001
Who were current smokers[b]	45.4 (435)	46.8 (522)	55.4 (649)	63.5 (1,471)	55.3 (3,077)	<0.0001
Who were ex-smokers[b]	30.6 (289)	27.7 (306)	22.9 (270)	20.5 (482)	24.2 (1,347)	<0.0001
Average no of cigarettes smoked per day[c]	19.6	18.3	19.2	18.9	19.0	0.58
Percentage (no) of subjects: Who drove cars regularly	69.3 (669)	57.5 (646)	54.3 (632)	40.8 (938)	51.8 (2,885)	<0.0001
Living in area of residence of deprivation category 5-7	18.6 (173)	32.0 (354)	54.3 (638)	66.0 (1,539)	48.6 (2,704)	<0.0001

[a] Not age-adjusted.
[b] Excluding 154 men who smoked a pipe or cigars and two men with missing data.
[c] For current cigarette smokers only.

manual social class occupation at the time of screening. The only group that was particularly small consisted of men with fathers who had had a non-manual social class occupation, whose first job had been in a non-manual social class occupation, and who had a manual social class occupation at the time of screening.

A cumulative social class indicator was constructed by summing the number of occasions in which each participant's class location was manual or non-manual. In Table 2 population characteristics are presented according to this cumulative social class indicator. The men in whom social class was manual on three occasions were on average one year older than the men in whom class was non-manual on all three occasions. After the remaining data on risk factors were adjusted for age, we found that moving from the men who had consistently non-manual social class locations to those who had consistently manual social class locations showed trends of increasing systolic and diastolic blood pressure, body mass index, current cigarette smoking, and prevalence of bronchitis and angina and decreasing cholesterol concentration, height, lung function, and prevalence of never having smoked. The men consistently in manual social class locations were less likely than those consistently in non-manual social class locations to be regular drivers.

Being a regular car driver is taken to be mainly a marker for ownership of a car, which has been used in various studies as an indicator of available income.[3,4] The men consistently in manual social class locations were also more likely to live in a postcode sector with unfavourable socioeconomic characteristics at the time of the 1981 Census.

Table 3: Age-adjusted death rates (per 1,000 person years) over 21 years of follow-up according to cumulative social class[a]

| | Cumulative social class based on occupation | | | |
	All three non-manual	Two non-manual, one manual	Two manual, one non-manual	All three manual
All causes				
Number of deaths	190	280	339	771
Mortality	100.1	123.4	135.1	153.9
Cardiovascular causes				
Number of deaths	84	145	197	388
Mortality	48.3	70.3	84.4	86.6
Cancer				
Number of deaths	73	86	95	247
Mortality	41.8	42.4	45.2	58.0
Noncardiovascular, noncancer causes				
Number of deaths	33	49	47	136
Mortality	19.1	25.7	22.6	34.0

[a] Significance tests for trend across age-adjusted relative rates are given in Table 6.

Over the 21 years of follow-up, 1,580 members of the cohort died. Table 3 shows age-adjusted mortality from all-causes, cardiovascular disease, cancer, and other causes. Mortality increased with the extent to which the men had had manual social class locations at different times in their life. The trends were most consistent for mortality from all-causes and cardiovascular disease; for mortality from cancer the main difference was between men who had had manual social class locations at all three stages of their life compared with the rest.

We fitted proportional hazards models with social class coded as manual or non-manual at the three different stages of life individually and simultaneously. The social class of first occupation was not significantly associated with mortality from all causes or any subcategory of mortality when father's and current social class were taken into account (Table 4). Father's social class and current social class were similarly related to mortality from all-causes, both when treated singularly and when entered in the model with simultaneous adjustment for all social class measures. Within this general picture, mortality from cancer and noncardiovascular, noncancer causes seemed to be more strongly associated with social class at the time of screening than with father's social class; the reverse was the case for mortality from cardiovascular disease.

Two additional indicators of socioeconomic position in adulthood were available: car use and deprivation category of area of residence. Table 5 shows that these indicators are associated with mortality within the strata of cumulative social class. In analyses adjusted only for age, not being a regular car driver was associated with a relative rate of

Table 4: Mortality by social class at three different stages of life (values are age-adjusted relative rates [95% CI], for individual socioeconomic measures above, and then from a model simultaneously examining each social class indicator)

	Father's social class	First social class	Current social class
All-causes			
Individual	1.44 (1.27-1.64)	1.29 (1.16-1.43)	1.40 (1.27-1.55)
Simultaneous	1.28 (1.11-1.47)	1.01 (0.89 -1.16)	1.29 (1.14-1.47)
Cardiovascular causes			
Individual	1.58 (1.32-1.89)	1.35 (1.16-1.56)	1.38 (1.20-1.59)
Simultaneous	1.41 (1.15-1.72)	1.08 (0.90-1.30)	1.20 (1.01-1.43)
Cancer			
Individual	1.26 (1.02-1.56)	1.25 (1.04-1.50)	1.35 (1.13-1.61)
Simultaneous	1.11 (0.87-1.41)	1.04 (0.82-1.31)	1.28 (1.03-1.60)
Noncardiovascular, noncancer causes			
Individual	1.45 (1.07-1.98)	1.18 (0.92-1.53)	1.59 (1.24-2.03)
Simultaneous	1.28 (0.91-1.80)	0.80 (0.58-1.10)	1.67 (1.22-2.28)

Table 5: All-cause mortality by cumulative social class, car driving, and deprivation category of area of residence (values are age-adjusted relative rates [95% CI])

	Cumulative social class			
	All three non-manual	Two non-manual, one manual	Two manual, one non-manual	All three manual
Regular car driver				
Yes	1	1.28 (1.01-1.63)	1.36 (1.08 -1.73)	1.57 (1.27-1.95)
No	1.22 (0.91-1.64)	1.52 (1.19-1.95)	1.76 (1.40-2.21)	2.00 (1.64-2.44)
Deprivation category of area of residence				
1-4	1	1.25 (1.01-1.56)	1.37 (1.09-1.72)	1.70 (1.39-2.09)
5-7	1.06 (0.74-1.52)	1.41 (1.10-1.82)	1.54 (1.25-1.90)	1.74 (1.45-2.09)

mortality of 1.34 (95% CI: 1.21-1.48); inclusion of the cumulative social class indicator reduced this to 1.25 (95% CI: 1.13-1.39).

Living in an area in deprivation categories 5-7 was associated with an age-adjusted relative rate of mortality of 1.21 (1.10-1.34). After inclusion of the cumulative social class indicator this became 1.07 (0.96-1.19).

Table 6 shows relative rates of mortality adjusted for age and risk factors. For mortality from cardiovascular disease and all causes the relative rates were adjusted for age, smoking (number of cigarettes smoked, with an additional adjustment for being an ex-smoker), diastolic blood pressure, serum cholesterol concentration, body mass

Table 6: Relative death rates (95% CI) by cumulative social class, adjusted for age and risk factors

	Cumulative social class				
	All three non-manual	Two non-manual, one manual	Two manual, one non-manual	All three manual	*p* value for trend
All-causes					
Age	1	1.29 (1.08-1.56)	1.45 (1.21-1.73)	1.71 (1.46-2.01)	<0.0001
Age and risk factor[a]	1	1.30 (1.08-1.57)	1.33 (1.11-1.60)	1.57 (1.33-1.85)	<0.0001
Cardiovascular causes					
Age	1	1.51 (1.16-1.98)	1.90 (1.47-2.45)	1.94 (1.53-2.45)	<0.0001
Age and risk factor[a]	1	1.57 (1.20-2.05)	1.78 (1.37-2.31)	1.92 (1.51-2.45)	<0.0001
Cancer					
Age	1	1.04 (0.76-1.42)	1.06 (0.78-1.44)	1.44 (1.11-1.87)	0.001
Age and risk factor[b]	1	1.04 (0.76-1.42)	1.01 (0.74-1.37)	1.34 (1.03-1.75)	0.009
Noncardiovascular, noncancer causes					
Age	1	1.31 (0.84-2.03)	1.16 (0.75-1.82)	1.75 (1.20 -2.56)	0.002
Age and risk factor[b]	1	1.30 (0.83-2.02)	1.02 (0.65-1.60)	1.42 (0.97-2.09)	0.09

[a] Adjusted for age, smoking, diastolic blood pressure, cholesterol concentration, body mass index, adjusted FEV_1, angina, bronchitis, electrocardiographic ischaemia.
[b] Adjusted for age, smoking, body mass index, adjusted FEV_1, and bronchitis.

index, adjusted FEV_1, angina, bronchitis, and electrocardiographic ischaemia. For mortality from cancer and from noncardiovascular, noncancer causes the relative rates were adjusted for age, smoking, body mass index, adjusted FEV_1, and bronchitis. Such adjustment led to some attenuation in the increased risk of death in relation to social class, although for mortality from all-causes, cardiovascular disease, and cancer this attenuation was not great. For mortality from noncardiovascular, noncancer causes more considerable attenuation of the trend of increasing risk of death with cumulative social class group was seen, with the association becoming non-significant at conventional levels.

Discussion

Cumulative socioeconomic disadvantage and mortality

Most of the numerous studies relating socioeconomic position to mortality have used measures of socioeconomic circumstances in adulthood.[1-5] This in part reflects the view that exposures acting at this time have the most impact on the risk of premature death.[8] However, the risk of premature death may reflect the accumulation of environmental insults or the cumulative effects of unfavourable behavioural or psychological factors, which progressively increase susceptibility to disease.[25,26] The few studies that have assessed socioeconomic position throughout life show the strengths of this notion. Thus, in a study based on record linkage of the 1960, 1970 and 1980 Censuses in Norway, particularly high risks of premature death were seen among men who had had limited education and then worked in manual occupations and lived in poor housing.[27,28] Similar findings have come from the National Longitudinal Survey of Older Men in the US.[18]

Our cohort was recruited from workplaces, but the study was initiated at a time of comparatively low unemployment and recruited men from across the social spectrum. The mortality differentials according to social class in our study are similar to those in men of the same age group in Scotland around 1981, the mid-point of the follow-up period. For men aged 55-64 in the general Scottish population the death rates were 66% higher in social classes IV and V than in social classes I and II.[29] In our study the age-adjusted death rate was 61% higher in men of social classes IV and V than in men of social classes I and II. The general population data also show mortality differentials for the main causes of death that are similar in size to those seen in our study. Our workplace sample thus seems to be a reasonable model for studying factors underlying socioeconomic differentials in risk of premature death in the general population, and the non-response rate, which is comparable to that in other such studies, does not seem to have introduced any serious bias. Our findings (a) that socioeconomic position in early and later life contribute separately to the risk of premature death and (b) that the risk can be further differentiated by adding additional adult socioeconomic indicators (use of a car and area based deprivation category) to the cumulative social class indicator are likely to be generalisable to other populations.

The cumulative social class indicator shows graded associations with most of the risk factors and morbidity measures included in our study. Strong associations with mortality were also evident. Adjustment for risk factors measured in adulthood attenuated the association of social class with mortality from cancer and from noncancer, noncardiovascular causes more than it did that with mortality from cardiovascular disease. This may partly reflect the fact that a major risk factor for coronary heart disease – serum cholesterol concentration – was higher in the group with the more favourable socioeconomic experience.

The use of a cumulative social class indicator does not take into account directions of social class change. Thus a participant whose father had had a manual occupation, whose first occupation had been manual, and who had a non-manual occupation at screening would be in the same group as a participant whose father had had a non-manual occupation and who had manual occupations both at labour market entry and at screening. Other studies have suggested that social mobility is not an important contributor to overall mortality differentials,[30] and detailed analyses of our data (to be reported elsewhere) show this too. We repeated the mortality analyses using all combinations of social class and found that the associations of mortality with cumulative social class were generally not dependent on the order in which different social classes came.

Socioeconomic position in childhood and mortality

There has been particular interest in the association between living conditions in childhood and risk of coronary heart disease in adult life. This follows from the work of Forsdahl, who suggested that early deprivation followed by later affluence increased the risk of coronary heart disease, an effect in part mediated by an increase in blood cholesterol concentrations.[31,32] The attribution of increased risk of coronary heart disease to an interaction between poor socioeconomic circumstances in early life and later affluence has received little support from subsequent studies.[9,10,33] Similarly, the suggestion that the effects of deprivation in early life are mediated through high blood cholesterol concentrations in adulthood has not been substantiated in later investigations.[33] In our cohort men with fathers of manual social class had lower, rather than higher, serum cholesterol concentrations than men with fathers of non–manual social class.[34] In contrast to these negative assessments of the Forsdahl hypothesis, the basic notion that unfavourable socioeconomic conditions in childhood predispose to increased risk of coronary heart disease in adulthood has received more support. Most[9,11,13,33,35-37] but not all[10,38] studies have found an association of childhood socioeconomic circumstances with risk of coronary heart disease, which was apparently not purely due to the adverse social conditions in adulthood of those born into poor circumstances.

In a Swedish Census follow-up study men with fathers who had manual occupations had considerably higher risk of dying from coronary heart disease than had those whose fathers had non-manual occupations.[35] For mortality from all-causes this was much less evident, mortality being dependent on social class in adulthood much more than social class in childhood. This particular dependence of the risk of coronary heart disease on socioeconomic circumstances in childhood has also been observed in area-based studies from Finland.[39,40] Our study had similar findings, father's social class being particularly important for mortality from cardiovascular disease but not for mortality from cancer or noncardiovascular, noncancer causes. Analyses of the association between height and cause-specific mortality, in which height is taken to be an indicator of childhood circumstances, show similar specificity.[41] These findings are clearly relevant to the hypothesis that foetal development is associated with the risk of cardiovascular disease in later life[42] as parental social class will influence early development. Socioeconomic factors in childhood will also influence growth, and recent evidence suggests that poor growth in childhood is also associated with higher mortality from cardiovascular disease in adulthood.[43] Studies with data covering all stages of development are needed to determine which stages of development most affect the risk of cardiovascular disease in adulthood.

Conclusions

Our data show a clear cumulative effect of socioeconomic circumstances acting over a lifetime. Combining the cumulative social class index with additional indicators of socioeconomic position in adulthood led to further differentiation of the risk of premature death. This has important implications for studies that try to control for socioeconomic factors when analysing outcomes in relation to socially patterned exposures. Single measures of adult social class, traditionally used in such studies, will not adequately capture the full extent of socioeconomic differentials between groups with different exposures. Statistical adjustment for these single measures will therefore not control for socioeconomic differences, and apparently 'independent' risk relations may remain confounded by factors related to socioeconomic environment.[44]

Specific patterns emerge within the general picture of higher death rates among people with less favourable socioeconomic trajectories during their lives.

Firstly, mortality from cardiovascular disease seems to be more strongly related to cumulative social disadvantage than does that from cancer or noncardiovascular, noncancer causes.

Secondly, whereas social class in adulthood is the more important socioeconomic indicator over a lifetime for differentiating groups with differing risks of mortality from cancer and noncardiovascular, noncancer causes, the socioeconomic environment in childhood seems to be particularly important with respect to mortality from cardiovascular disease. These findings should help direct the attention of disease-specific aetiological research to influences acting both in childhood and in adult life.

The Department of Health's report *Variations in health* has directed attention to the accumulation of socially patterned adverse exposures over a lifetime.[17] Our results add to the, as yet, limited data that show the necessity of such an approach. Any serious attempt to elucidate the contributions of socially distributed risk factors to the risk of disease in adulthood should aim to collect information covering the entire lifespan of study participants.[14]

References

[1] Davey Smith, G., Bartley, M. and Blane, D. (1990) 'The Black Report on socioeconomic inequalities in health 10 years on', *British Medical Journal*, vol 301, pp 373-7.

[2] Moser, K., Pugh, H. and Goldblatt, P. (1990) 'Mortality and the social classification of women', in P. Goldblatt (ed) *Longitudinal study: Mortality and social organisation*, London: HMSO, pp 145-62.

[3] Goldblatt, P. (1990) 'Mortality and alternative social classifications', in P. Goldblatt (ed) *Longitudinal study: Mortality and social organisation*, London: HMSO, pp 163-92.

[4] **Davey Smith, G., Shipley, M.J. and Rose, G. (1990) 'The magnitude and causes of socioeconomic differentials in mortality: further evidence from the Whitehall Study',** *Journal of Epidemiololgy and Community Health*, **vol 44, pp 260-5.**

[5] **Davey Smith, G., Neaton, J.D., Wentworth, D., Stamler, R. and Stamler, J. (1996) 'Socioeconomic differentials in mortality risk among men screened for the Multiple Risk Factor Intervention Trial: Part I – results for 300,685 white men',** *American Journal of Public Health*, **vol 86, pp 486-96.**

[6] Eachus, J., Williams, M., Chan, P., Davey Smith, G., Grainge, M., Donovan, J. and Frankel, S. (1996) 'Deprivation and cause-specific morbidity: evidence from the Somerset and Avon survey of health', *British Medical Journal*, vol 312, pp 287-92.

[7] Burnett, J.C. (1880) 'The prevention of hare-lip, cleft-palate, and other congenital defects: as also of hereditrary disease and constitutional taints by the medicinal and nutritional treatment of their mother during pregnancy', *Homæpathic World*, October, pp 437-51.

[8] Kuh, D. and Davey Smith, G. (1993) 'When is mortality risk determined? Historical insights into a current debate', *Social History of Medicine*, vol 6, pp 101-23.

[9] Burr, M.L. and Sweetnam, P.M. (1980) 'Family size and paternal unemployment in relation to myocardial infarction', *Journal of Epidemiology and Community Health*, vol 34, pp 93-5.

[10] Lynch, J.W., Kaplan, G.A., Cohen, R.D., Kauhanen, J., Wilson, T.W. and Smith, N.L. (1994) 'Childhood and adult socioeconomic status as predictors of mortality in Finland', *Lancet*, vol 343, pp 524-7.

[11] Gliksman, M.D., Kawachi, I., Hunter, D., Colditz, G.A., Manson, J.E., Stampfer, M.J., Speizer, F.E., Willett, W.C. and Hennekens, C.H. (1995) 'Childhood socioeconomic status and risk of cardiovascular disease in middle aged US women: a prospective study', *Journal of Epidemiology and Community Health*, vol 49, pp 10-15.

[12] Elo, I.T. and Preston, S.H. (1992) 'Effects of early-life conditions on adult mortality: a review', *Population Index*, vol 58, pp 186-212.

[13] Kaplan, G.A. and Salonen, J.T. (1990) 'Socioeconomic conditions in childhood and ischaemic heart disease during middle age', *British Medical Journal*, vol 301, pp 1121-3.

[14] Ben-Shlomo, Y. and Davey Smith, G. (1991) 'Deprivation in infancy or adult life: which is more important for mortality risk?', *Lancet*, vol 337, pp 530-4.

[15] Mann, S.L., Wadsworth, M.E.J. and Colley, J.R.T. (1992) 'Accumulation of factors in influencing respiratory illness in members of a national birth cohort and their offspring', *Journal of Epidemiology and Community Health*, vol 46, pp 286-90.

[16] Davey Smith, G., Bartley. M. and Blane, D. (1994) 'Explanations for socioeconomic differentials in mortality: evidence from Britain and elsewhere', *European Journal of Public Health*, vol 4, pp 131-44.

[17] Department of Health (1995) *The health of the nation: Variations in health: What can the Department of Health and the NHS do?*, London: DoH.

[18] Mare, R.D. (1990) 'Socioeconomic careers and differential mortality among older men in the US', in J. Vallin, S. D'Souza and A. Palloni (eds) *Measurement and analysis of mortality: New approaches*, Oxford: Clarendon Press, pp 362-87.

[19] Hawthorne, V.M., Watt, G.M.C., Hart, C.L., Hole, D.J. and Davey Smith, G. et al (1995) 'Cardiorespiratory disease in men and women in urban Scotland: baseline characteristics of the Renfrew/Paisley (Midspan) study population', *Scottish Medical Journal*, vol 40, pp 102-7.

[20] Rose, G.A., Blackburn, H., Gillum, R.F. and Prineas, R.J. (1982) *Cardiovascular survey methods*, Geneva: WHO.

[21] Medical Research Council (1965) 'Definition and classification of chronic bronchitis for epidemiological purposes', *Lancet*, no I, pp 775-9.

[22] Carstairs, V. and Morris, R. (1991) *Deprivation and health in Scotland*, Aberdeen: Aberdeen University Press.

[23] SAS Institute (1991) *SAS language and procedures: Usage 2, version 6*, Cary, NC: SAS Institute.

[24] Cox, D.R. (1972) 'Regression models and life tables', *Journal of the Royal Statistical Society Series B*, vol 34, pp 187-220.

[25] Jones, H.B. (1956) 'A special consideration of the ageing process, disease and life expectancy', *Advances in Biology and Medical Physics*, vol 4, pp 281-337.

[26] Alter, R. and Riley, J. (1989) 'Frailty, sickness and death: models of morbidity and mortality in historical populations', *Population Studies*, vol 43, pp 25-46.

[27] Salhi, M., Caselli, G., Duchêne, J., Egidi, V., Santini, A., Thiltgès, E. and Wunsch, G. (1995) 'Assessing mortality differentials using life histories: a method and applications', in A. Lopez, G. Caselli and T. Valkonen (eds) *Adult mortality in developed countries: From description to explanation*, Oxford: Clarendon Press.

[28] Wunsch, G., Duchêne, J,. Thiltgès, E. and Salhi, M. (1996) 'Socioeconomic differences in mortality: a life course approach', *European Journal of Population*, vol 12, pp 167-85.

[29] Office of Population Censuses and Surveys (1986) *Occupational mortality 1979-1980, 1982-1983*, London: HMSO.

[30] Blane, D., Davey Smith, G. and Bartley, M. (1993) 'Social selection: what does it contribute to social class differentials in health?', *Sociology of Health and Illness*, vol 15, pp 1-15.

[31] Forsdahl, A. (1977) 'Are poor living conditions in childhood and adolescents an important risk factor for arteriosclerotic heart disease?', *British Journal of Preventive and Social Medicine*, vol 31, pp 91-5.

[32] Forsdahl, A. (1978) 'Living conditions in childhood and subsequent development of risk factors for arteriorsclerotic heart disease', *Journal of Epidemiology and Community Health*, vol 32, pp 34-7.

[33] Notkola, V., Punsar, S., Karvonen, M.J. and Haapakaski, J. (1985) 'Socioeconomic conditions in childhood and mortality and morbidity caused by coronary heart disease in adulthood in rural Finland', *Social Science and Medicine*, vol 21, pp 517-23.

[34] Blane, D., Hart, C.L., Davey Smith, G., Gillis, C.R., Hole, D.J. and Hawthorne, W.M. (1996) 'The association of cardiovascular disease risk factors with socioeconomic position during childhood and during adulthood', *British Medical Journal*, vol 313, pp 1434-8.

[35] Vågerô, D. and Leon, D. (1994) 'Effect of social class in childhood and adulthood on adult mortality', *Lancet*, vol 343, pp 1224-5.

36 Gillum, R.F. and Paffenbarger, R.S. (1978) 'Chronic disease in former college students. XVII. Socio-cultural mobility as a precursor of coronary heart disease and hypertension', *American Journal of Epidemiology*, vol 108, pp 289-98.

37 Wannamethee, S.G.,Whincup, P.H., Shaper, G. and Walker, M. (1996) 'Influence of father's social class on cardiovascular disease in middle-aged men', *Lancet*, vol 348, pp 1259-63.

38 Hasle, H. (1990) 'Association between living conditions in childhood and myocardial infarction', *British Medical Journal*, vol 300, pp 512-13.

39 Valkonen, T. (1987) 'Male mortality from ischaemic heart disease in Finland: relation to region of birth and region of residence', *European Journal of Population*, vol 3, pp 61-83.

40 Koskinen, S. (1994) *Origins of regional differences in mortality from ischaemic heart disease in Finland*, NAWH Research Report 41, Helsinki: National Research and Development Centre for Welfare and Health.

41 Leon, D., Davey Smith, G., Shipley, M. and Strachan, D. (1995) 'Height and mortality in London: early life influences, socioeconomic confounding or shrinkage?', *Journal of Epidemiology and Community Health*, vol 49, pp 5-9.

42 Barker, D.J.P. (1995) 'Early nutrition and coronary heart disease', in D.P. Davies (ed) *Nutrition in child health*, London: Royal College of Physicians of London, pp 77-85.

43 Gunnell, D., Davey Smith, G., Frankel, S., Nanchahal, K., Braddon, F.E.M., Pemberton, J. and Peters, T.J. (1998) 'Childhood leg length and adult mortality – follow up of the Carnegie (Boyd-Orr) survey of diet and health in pre-war Britain', *Journal of Epidemiology and Community Health*, vol 52, pp 142-52.

44 Davey Smith, G. and Phillips, A.N. (1992) 'Confounding in epidemiological studies: why "independent" effects may not be all they seem', *British Medical Journal*, vol 305, pp 757-9.

16

Education and occupational social class: which is the more important indicator of mortality risk?

George Davey Smith, Carole Hart,
David Hole, Pauline MacKinnon, Charles
Gillis, Graham Watt, David Blane
and Victor Hawthorne

Abstract

Study objectives: In the UK, studies of socioeconomic differentials in mortality have generally relied upon occupational social class as the index of socioeconomic position, while in the US, measures based on education have been widely used. These two measures have different characteristics; for example, social class can change throughout adult life, while education is unlikely to alter after early adulthood. Therefore, different interpretations can be given to the mortality differentials that are seen. The objective of this analysis is to demonstrate the profile of mortality differentials, and the factors underlying these differentials, which are associated with the two socioeconomic measures.

Design: Prospective observational study.

Setting: 27 work places in the west of Scotland.

Participants: 5,749 men aged 35-64 who completed questionnaires and were examined between 1970 and 1973.

Journal of Epidemiology and Community Health,
1998, vol 52, pp 153-60

Findings: At baseline, similar gradients between socioeconomic position and blood pressure, height, lung function, and smoking behaviour were seen, regardless of whether the education or social class measure was used. Manual social class and early termination of full-time education were associated with higher blood pressure, shorter height, poorer lung function, and a higher prevalence of smoking. Within education strata, the graded association between smoking and social class remains strong, whereas within social class groups the relation between education and smoking is attenuated. Over 21 years of follow-up, 1,639 of the men died. Mortality from all-causes and from three broad cause of death groups (cardiovascular disease, malignant disease, and other causes) showed similar associations with social class and education. For all-cause of death groups, men in manual social classes and men who terminated full-time education at an early age had higher death rates. Cardiovascular disease was the cause of death group most strongly associated with education, while the noncardiovascular noncancer category was the cause of death group most strongly associated with adulthood social class. The graded association between social class and all-cause mortality remains strong and significant within education strata, whereas within social class strata the relation between education and mortality is less clear.

Conclusions: As a single indicator of socioeconomic position, occupational social class in adulthood is a better discriminator of socioeconomic differentials in mortality and smoking behaviour than is education. This argues against interpretations that see cultural rather than material resources as being the key determinants of socioeconomic differentials in health. The stronger association of education with death from cardiovascular causes than with other causes of death may reflect the function of education as an index of socioeconomic circumstances in early life, which appear to have a particular influence on the risk of cardiovascular disease.

Introduction

One of the most reproducible demographic findings, over time and within different countries, is the inverse association between socioeconomic position and mortality.[1-5] Several different indicators of socioeconomic position have been used in such studies,[6-11] including occupational social class, amount and type of education, employment grade, income, access to or ownership of various assets, and indices based on residential area characteristics. The choice of socioeconomic indicator often reflects which data are available, rather than any explicit theorisation of the possible effects of different dimensions of socioeconomic disadvantage. In the US, measures based on education have been widely used, because such information is the main socioeconomic indicator contained in various national datasets.[12] In

Britain occupational social class is the more usual measure and social class has been analysed with respect to mortality around each Census since 1911.[13-15] The various indicators of socioeconomic position are generally related in a similar manner to mortality, but only on a few occasions have different indicators within the same database been analysed with respect to mortality.[7-9,11,16-18] Different socioeconomic indicators show strong mutual associations[19-22] and sometimes appear to be treated as though they are interchangeable proxy measures of an underlying entity, 'socioeconomic status'. The associations between health and the different socioeconomic indicators may have different implications and causes, however. For example, the health effects of occupational hazards in unskilled manual jobs depend directly on work conditions, and reducing socioeconomic differentials consequent on such exposures requires changes to work environments.

Conversely, health differences according to level of education have been attributed to the direct effects of education, including the acquisition of knowledge regarding health-damaging behaviours, the ability to optimise use of health services, the development of time preferences favourable to health maintenance, an increasing willingness to invest in human capital, and the promotion of the psychological attributes of high self-esteem and self-efficacy.[21,23,24] If the influence of both occupational social class and education act through associated differentials in income and living conditions, similar interdependent associations with mortality risk would be expected. This study asks how different dimensions of socioeconomic position relate to health by analysing the association of education and occupational social class with health-related behaviours, physiological risk factors, health status, and mortality risk within a large cohort of working men followed up for 21 years after a screening examination and questionnaire survey carried out in the early 1970s. To our knowledge only one analysis relating mortality risk simultaneously to both occupational social class and education has not been performed with UK data before this study.[8]

Methods

This analysis is based on a cohort of men recruited from 27 workplaces in Glasgow, Grangemouth, and Clydebank (all in the west of Scotland) between 1970 and 1973. The workplaces included engineering, manufacturing, and petrochemical plants; a publishing house; civil service departments; administrative and professional divisions from British Rail; architectural institutes; legal and dental offices; and banking. Response rates were available for the workplaces from which 87% of the sample was recruited. For these sites, 70% of those invited completed the questionnaire and attended for examination. The achieved sample was 6,022 men and 1,006 women, from which 5,766 men aged 35-64 at the time of examination have been included in this report. The mortality experience of the women could not be analysed as only 176 deaths have occurred to date. The examinations used procedures which were developed for the series of MIDSPAN studies.[25-28] An extensive questionnaire, completed by the subject, was checked at the screening examination.

These examinations were conducted at clinics established for this purpose at, or near, the workplaces. The information collected at baseline examination included *sociodemographic data*: age, age at which the participant finished full-time education, occupational social class, whether a regular car driver; *health status measures*: angina, previous heart attack and intermittent claudication from the Rose questionnaire,[29] respiratory symptoms from the Medical Research Council questionnaire[30]; *health-related behaviours*: detailed smoking history; *physical examination*: height, weight, blood pressure (seated, taken with a London School of Hygiene and Tropical Medicine sphygmomanometer and with diastolic pressure being recorded at the disappearance of the fifth Korotkoff sound), lung function (with the Garthur Vitalograph), serum cholesterol and six lead electrocardiogram (leads I,II,III,aVR,aVL, and aVF).

Social class was coded according to the Registrar General's classification[31] and treated at six levels for analysis by social class alone and at four levels – I and II; III non-manual; III manual; IV and V – for analyses in which both social class and education were included. Age at leaving full-time education was categorised as 12-14; 15-16; 17-18, and 19+.

Persistent phlegm was defined as usually bringing up phlegm from the chest first thing in the morning on most days for as much as three months in winter each year. 'Infective phlegm' was defined as usually bringing up phlegm from the chest first thing in the morning in winter and having had a period of increased cough and phlegm lasting for three weeks or more in the past three years. Breathlessness was defined by responding positively to the question: 'Do you get short of breath walking with people of your own age on level ground?' Bronchitis was defined as having persistent and 'infective' phlegm and being breathless.[30]

Angina was considered present if chest pain or discomfort when walking uphill or hurrying was: sited in the sternum or the left chest and arm; caused the subject to stop or slow down; went away when the subject stopped or slowed down; and went away in 10 minutes or less.[29] For forced expiratory volume in one second (FEV_1), the best of two expirations was recorded. To estimate impairment, the expected FEV_1 was obtained from linear regression equations of age and height: Expected $FEV_1 = -278.06 + 4.33 \times$ height $- 3.06 \times$ age. Age is in years, height in cm, and the value is divided by 100 to give FEV_1 in litres. The coefficients were derived from a healthy subset of the population who never smoked and answered no to questions on phlegm, breathlessness, wheezy or whistling chest and if weather affected breathing. The adjusted FEV_1 was calculated by: Adjusted $FEV_1(\%) =$ (Actual FEV_1/Expected FEV_1) × 100. The ECG was coded according to the Minnesota system,[29] with any of the following codes, which encompass diagnoses of definite myocardial infarction, myocardial ischaemia, and left bundle branch block, being considered evidence of ischaemia: 1.1-1.3, 4.1-4.4, 5.1-5.3, 7.1. Data on social class and education were missing on nine and eight men respectively. These men were excluded from the present analyses, which are therefore based on 5,749 participants. Mortality over a 21-year follow-up period has been ascertained from flagging at the NHS Central Registry in Edinburgh, which also provides death certificates coded according to the Ninth Revision of the International Classification of Diseases (ICD-9).

Death rates have been calculated using a person years at risk based lifetable approach. These rates have been standardised for age by the direct method, using the total study population as the standard. Tests for trend for age-adjusted rates have been obtained through proportional hazards regression, using PROC PHREG in the SAS system, with age and the socioeconomic indicator (coded as a continuous variable) as covariates. Continuous variables have been age-standardised using PROC GLM, with tests for trend for age-adjusted means being obtained through PROC REG. Categorical variables have been age-standardised by the direct method and tests for trend performed in PROC LOGIST.

Proportional hazards coefficients and their standard errors were calculated using Cox's model.[32] Adjustment for age and other risk factors was performed by including terms for these in the proportional hazards models.

Exponentiated hazards coefficients are taken as indicators of relative rates of mortality. Stratification of the proportional hazards regression analysis was also performed, with social class or age at leaving full-time education as the stratification variable. This allows the baseline hazard to vary between strata, producing summary measures of the relative rates of mortality seen within the strata.

Relative index of inequality

To compare the magnitude of trends of current smoking and all-cause mortality with social class and with age at leaving full-time education, the relative index of inequality (RII)[5,14] has been calculated. Comparisons of ratio measures between social class or education groups suffer from the fact that the groups are of different size. It may be expected that the classification producing smaller groups at the margins would lead to larger ratios of, say, mortality, between the top and bottom categories, because finer discrimination of extremes of socioeconomic position is achieved. The RII is explicitly constructed to avoid this problem.

It requires classifications to be defined hierarchically – that is, social class being I and II, then IIIN, then IIIM, then IV and V; or age at leaving full-time education being 12-14, then 15-16, then 17-18, then 19+. Socioeconomic position of each group is assigned a value between 0 and 1, according to the proportion of participants with a higher position than the midpoint of each group within this hierarchy. This assignment is done separately within each five-year band for age at study entry, to allow production of an age-adjusted measure of inequality. If in a particular five-year age band 10% of men (that is, 0.1 as a proportion of the whole study population in this age band) is in the social class I and II category, this group is assigned a value of 0.05, which is the proportion of the population above its midpoint. If the next group, social class IIIN, contains an additional 12% of the men in this age band then the proportion of the population above the mid-point of this group is $0.1 + 0.12/2 = 0.16$. These indicators were created in a similar fashion for social class and age at leaving full-time education, in both cases using four levels. These numerical indicators of socioeconomic position (SEP) are then related to mortality through Poisson regression[5]: $\log (Dij) = \log (Pij) + \alpha_i + \beta*SEPj$, with D being the number of deaths and P the number of person-years at risk in the $_i$th five-year age group and $_j$th socioeconomic group.

Exponentiating β yields the RII, which is the relative risk of mortality comparing a socioeconomic position indicator of 1 to 0 – that is, the bottom to the top of the socioeconomic hierarchy. A similar logistic regression method, with D representing the number of smokers and P the number of study participants, was used to produce the RII for smoking, which in this case is the odds ratio for being a smoker at the bottom compared with the top of the socioeconomic hierarchy. The larger the RII, the greater the degree of inequality across a socioeconomic hierarchy.

Results

Characteristics of study participants

Table 1 gives the characteristics of the study population according to social class. On average, men in manual jobs were older, shorter, had higher blood pressure, lower serum cholesterol, poorer lung function, higher prevalences of angina and bronchitis, and were more likely to be current smokers but, if smokers, used less cigarettes per day.

Table I: Population characteristics according to social class (age-adjusted means and proportions)

	I	II	IIIN	IIIM	IV	V	Total	Trend
				Social class				
Number	762	1,102	1,036	1,648	993	208	5,749	
Age at screening[a]	47.7	47.9	47.7	48.1	49.0	51.5	48.2	p=0.0001
Systolic blood pressure (mm Hg)	131.1	131.2	133.1	136.4	136.3	133.0	134.0	p=0.0001
Diastolic blood pressure (mm Hg)	82.3	83.2	83.4	84.9	84.5	84.2	83.9	p=0.0001
Cholesterol (mmol/l)	6.4	6.1	6.0	5.7	5.6	5.6	5.9	p=0.0001
Height (cm)	176.3	175.0	173.2	171.2	170.6	170.4	172.8	p=0.0001
Body mass index (kg/m²)	24.9	25.3	25.1	25.3	25.1	25.3	25.2	p=0.15
FEV₁ score (%)	99.3	99.1	95.7	90.8	90.6	87.7	94.3	p=0.0001
Angina (%)	4.4	5.0	6.7	7.3	6.7	8.1	6.2	p=0.001
ECG ischaemia (%)	5.2	5.5	6.8	5.6	6.4	4.0	5.8	p=0.61
MRC bronchitis (%)	0.1	0.9	1.9	3.2	3.3	4.8	2.2	p=0.0001
Never smoked (%)	21.4	21.2	19.2	14.3	14.0	16.4	17.6	p=0.0001
Current cigarette smokers (%)	42.3	45.2	54.9	61.7	65.4	67.4	55.5	p=0.0001
Ex-smokers (%)	31.4	29.5	23.8	21.9	19.0	15.9	24.2	p=0.0001
Average number of cigarettes smoked per day[b]	20.2	19.4	18.3	19.2	18.6	17.4	19.0	p=0.004
Regular drivers (%)	75.4	72.1	42.6	47.8	34.7	18.4	51.8	p=0.0001
School leavers aged 16 or under (%)	24.2	65.6	84.8	98.3	98.7	99.1	79.8	p=0.0001

[a] Not age-adjusted.

[b] For current cigarette smokers only.

A strong association between social class and education was observed, and men in the manual classes were considerably less likely to be regular car drivers. Being a regular car driver is taken to be, in part, a marker for ownership of a car, which has been used in various studies as an indicator of available income.[8,11]

In Table 2 the data are presented according to age at leaving full-time education. The gradients by education are similar to those seen with respect to social class.

Smoking in relation to social class and education

Table 3 gives the age-adjusted prevalences of current smoking by social class and education. While there are few men in the manual social classes who had left school above the age of 16, the pattern of higher prevalence of smoking among the men in manual jobs within education strata seems clearer than the corresponding association between education and smoking within social class strata. The RIIs

Table 2: Population characteristics according to age at leaving full-time education (age-adjusted means and proportions)

| | Age at leaving full-time education | | | | |
	19+	17-18	15-16	12-14	Trend
Number	504	659	1,652	2934	
Age at screening[a]	47.1	47.7	46.3	49.7	p=0.0001
Systolic blood pressure (mm Hg)	131.4	131.3	134.1	134.9	p=0.0001
Diastolic blood pressure (mm Hg)	82.8	82.7	83.8	84.4	p=0.0001
Cholesterol (mmol/l)	6.4	6.2	5.9	5.7	p=0.0001
Height (cm)	176.7	175.4	173.4	171.3	p=0.0001
Body mass index (kg/m^2)	25.0	25.1	25.0	25.3	p=0.013
FEV$_1$ score (%)	101.2	99.4	95.1	91.5	p=0.0001
Angina (%)	3.5	5.9	5.2	6.8	p=0.002
ECG ischaemia (%)	4.7	5.8	6.4	5.6	p=0.75
MRC bronchitis (%)	0.5	0.3	1.4	3.2	p=0.0001
Never smoked (%)	20.5	21.0	19.4	15.5	p=0.0001
Current cigarette smokers (%)	41.7	47.6	53.2	60.4	p=0.0001
Ex-smokers (%)	33.1	27.5	24.8	22.2	p=0.0001
Average number of cigarettes smoked per day[b]	20.1	19.2	18.8	18.9	p=0.12
Regular drivers (%)	81.7	63.8	53.5	42.5	p=0.0001
Social class I or II (%)	95.6	72.2	37.1	11.8	p=0.0001

[a] Not age-adjusted
[b] For current cigarette smokers only.

Table 3: Age-adjusted prevalence (per 100) of current cigarette smoking (number in each category in parentheses)

| | Social class | | | | |
	I and II	IIIN	IIIM	IV and V	Test for trend
Age at leaving full-time education					
19+	39.5 (484)	60.0 (15)	100.0 (1)	100.0 (4)	p=0.010
17-18	45.2 (478)	53.2 (141)	53.7 (28)	50.0 (12)	p=0.13
15-16	45.4 (553)	54.4 (460)	58.2 (436)	64.5 (203)	p=0.0001
12-14	45.8 (349)	55.7 (420)	63.0 (1,183)	65.8 (982)	p=0.0001
Test for trend	p=0.066	p=0.69	p=0.021	p=0.63	

for current smoking are 2.66 (95% CI: 2.17–3.26) for education and 3.55 (2.93–4.30) for social class categorised at four levels. A test between these RIIs shows that they differ at a conventional level of significance (p=0.044). A logistic regression analysis, in which current smoking (yes/no) is the outcome, and linear terms for education and social class fitted together with age as independent variables, yielded odds ratios of 0.90 (0.84–0.96) for one education category and 0.77 (0.73–0.82) for one social class category, both at four levels. The logistic regression analysis thus supports the RII analysis in indicating that social class is more strongly related to smoking behaviour than is education.

Mortality according to social class and education

Mortality from all-causes and from broad cause of death groups show clear increases from the non-manual to the manual social classes (Table 4). Similar gradients are seen according to education (Table 5). The RIIs for all-cause mortality are 1.84 (1.54–2.19) for social class treated at four levels and 1.73 (1.42–2.10) for education. These do not differ significantly from each other (p=0.65). Proportional hazards models were also fitted containing age and linear terms for the socioeconomic measures. For a one category change in social class (treated at four levels), the age-adjusted relative rate of mortality is 1.17 (1.12–1.22). In analyses stratified by the four education groups, the relative rate for a one category change in social class is 1.12 (1.07–1.18). For a one category change in education, the age-adjusted relative rate of mortality is similar to that seen for social class: 1.19 (1.12–1.25). However, in this case stratifying by the four social class categories leads to greater attenuation of the relative rate of mortality according

Table 4: Age-adjusted 21-year death rates according to social class (per 10,000 person years)

	Social class						
	I	II	IIIN	IIIM	IV	V	Trend
All-cause							
Number of deaths	156	242	293	530	334	84	
Death rate	101.1	110.0	139.5	153.0	152.6	170.5	p=0.001
All CVD							
Number of deaths	65	138	155	273	172	38	
Death rate	48.0	66.8	79.8	86.4	87.7	78.7	p=0.0001
All cancer							
Number of deaths	64	68	91	166	109	25	
Death rate	41.7	35.4	52.7	57.4	57.8	60.1	p=0.005
Non CVD, noncancer							
Number of deaths	27	36	47	91	53	21	
Death rate	21.0	20.2	26.8	32.4	30.7	59.1	p=0.0001

Table 5: Age-adjusted 21-year death rates according to age at leaving full-time education (per 10,000 person years)

| | Age at leaving full-time education | | | | |
	19+	17-18	15-16	12-14	Trend
All-cause					
Number of deaths	96	150	397	996	
Death rate	100.8	112.8	129.3	148.5	p=0.0001
All CVD					
Number of deaths	40	81	212	508	
Death rate	47.5	66.7	75.0	83.9	p=0.0001
All cancer					
Number of deaths	36	47	125	315	
Death rate	38.9	39.6	47.4	54.4	p=0.004
Non CVD, noncancer					
Number of deaths	20	22	60	173	
Death rate	24.0	17.8	23.4	32.5	p=0.009

Table 6: Stratified and unstratified age-adjusted relative rates of mortality (and 95% CI) according to social class and age at leaving full-time education

	Social class	Social class (stratified by education)	Age at leaving full-time education	Age at leaving full-time education (stratified by social class)
All-cause	1.17	1.12	1.19	1.07
	(1.12-1.22)	(1.07-1.18)	(1.12-1.25)	(0.99-1.14)
All CVD	1.16	1.11	1.20	1.09
	(1.09-1.23)	(1.03-1.09)	(1.11-1.30)	(0.99-1.21)
All cancer	1.16	1.13	1.15	1.04
	(1.08-1.25)	(1.03-1.24)	(1.05-1.27)	(0.92-1.17)
Non-CVD, noncancer	1.22	1.18	1.20	1.03
	(1.10-1.35)	(1.04-1.34)	(1.05-1.37)	(0.87-1.23)

to education category, to 1.07 (0.99–1.14). Table 6 presents similar results for the major cause of death groups. Cardiovascular disease is the cause of death group most strongly associated with education, while the noncardiovascular noncancer category is the cause of death group most strongly associated with adulthood social class.

Mortality for different age groups

As average age at leaving full-time education changed over the period during which the men in this study were at school, mortality by age of leaving full-time education has been examined in two age bands (Table 7). Age at study entry correlates closely with relative age at the time of schooling, as the baseline screening period was short. Clear mortality differentials are seen for both age bands. Relative mortality differentials by both social class and education are greater in the younger age band (Table 8). Simultaneous analysis of education and social class within the age bands yields identical findings to those seen in the whole cohort. Differentials according to education are reduced to non-significance by stratification by social class, while differentials by social class are only moderately attenuated and remain significant on stratification by education (Table 8).

Discussion

British studies of the association between the socioeconomic position and mortality of individuals have generally used occupationally-based socioeconomic measures. Various versions of the Registrar General's social class classification have been used in the Decennial Supplements,[13-15] the major source of data on this subject. The

Table 7: Age-adjusted 21-year death rates according to age at study entry and age at leaving full-time education per 10,000 person years

	Age at leaving full-time education				
	19+	17-18	15-16	12-14	Trend
Age band 35-49					
Number of deaths	38	54	169	323	
Death rate	60.2	67.3	86.4	97.9	$p=0.0001$
Age band 50-64					
Number of deaths	58	154	228	673	
Death rate	151.8	169.9	183.4	212.0	$p=0.0001$

Table 8: Stratified and unstratified age-adjusted relative rates of mortality (and 95% CI) according to social class and age at leaving full-time education, according to age at study entry

Age band	Social class	Social class (stratified by education)	Age at leaving full-time education	Age at leaving full-time education (stratified by social class)
35-49	1.23	1.20	1.21	1.04
	(1.15-1.32)	(1.10-1.31)	(1.10-1.32)	(0.92-1.16)
50-64	1.14	1.09	1.17	1.07
	(1.08-1.20)	(1.02-1.16)	(1.09-1.25)	(0.98-1.17)

Longitudinal Study, involving the linkage of a 1% sample from the 1971 Census to death certification data, complements these reports by demonstrating large and increasing mortality differentials over the two decades of post-Census follow-up.[33]

Educational achievement, indicated by highest qualifications received, is also inversely associated with all-cause death rate in the Longitudinal Study.[7,8] The mortality differentials according to social class in this study are very similar to those for men of the same age group seen around 1981, the mid-point of the follow-up period, in Scotland. For men aged 55 to 64, social classes IV and V had death rates 66% higher than social classes I and II in the general Scottish population.[34] In this study population, social class IV and V men experienced an age-adjusted death rate 59% higher than that of social class I and II men. The general population data also show mortality differentials for the major cause of death groups similar in magnitude to those seen in this study. Our workplace sample thus appears a reasonable model for studying factors underlying socioeconomic differentials in mortality risk in the general population.

Age at leaving full-time education will be determined by several factors, including economic status of the family, aptitude of the child, employment opportunities at the time of reaching minimum school-leaving age, and legislation. It would be inappropriate to consider the effects of differences in age at leaving full-time education produced simply by legislative change, as this would merely reflect year of birth. The men included in this study were born between 1907 and 1938 and would have reached age 14 between 1921 and 1952. A minimum school-leaving age of 14 was introduced in 1904 in Scotland and was raised to 15 in 1947. However, enforcement was variable and many children left school at younger ages.[35,36] There were only 438 men in our study who, according to legislation, could not leave school at age 14 because of the 1947 legislative change. Excluding these men from the analyses did not materially change our findings. Analyses were also repeated in two age groups, to allow for any broad secular changes in the meaning and implications of age at leaving full-time education. Findings for the two age groups were very similar. Most studies that analyse education and adult socioeconomic measures separately in relation to mortality risk within the same dataset demonstrate associations in the expected direction.[7-9]

Analyses relating mortality risk to both occupational social class and education simultaneously have been performed only once with UK data before this study, to our knowledge.[8] We found that social class in adulthood seems to be the more important determinant of mortality. In the US, the National Longitudinal Mortality Study[9,18] has been analysed with respect to household income, years of education, and occupation. For working-age men, pronounced attenuation of the association between years of education and mortality occurs when other socioeconomic indices are taken into account.[18,37] In a US study, the National Longitudinal Survey of Older Men, years of education shows a strong inverse association with mortality risk. However, after adjustment for lifetime income and wealth this association essentially disappears.[38] In a collaborative study with centres in Kaunas (Lithuania) and Rotterdam (Netherlands) both occupational social class and education were related to mortality risk over a 10-year follow-up period. Adjustment for occupational level greatly reduced the association of mortality with education, while adjustment for education left a relatively substantial occupational effect.[39] Other studies have revealed contributions of both education and adult socioeconomic measures to mortality risk, although the analyses that have been presented do not allow for an adequate evaluation of the relative importance of these two factors.[40,41]

In this study, cigarette smoking was more strongly related to current occupational social class than age at leaving full-time education. This suggests that it is the social environment in adulthood that maintains, or initiates, smoking behaviour. Age at leaving full-time education is in this formulation mainly related to smoking behaviour through its determination of occupational level in adulthood. Similar findings, of more consistent differentials in smoking by occupation than by educational level, have come from Kaunas and Rotterdam.[39] A US study came to opposite conclusions, although the occupational classification used in this study and the manner in which it was statistically treated make the results hard to interpret.[21]

The pathways linking education and mortality have been discussed at some length.[23,24,42,43] Three basic positions can be distinguished. First, Fuchs and others have argued that people with different educational levels differ in unobservable ways, including having time preferences favourable to long-term investment in their future. Rather than good health being caused by education, underlying unobserved factors might lead to both good health and better education. Second, education may act through improving health-related knowledge, which allows the choice of healthier lifestyles, which in turn reduce mortality risk. Third, education may act through allowing for favourable employment opportunities with higher income levels and more favourable living conditions throughout adult life. Of health-related behaviours, smoking has probably been most investigated with respect to education.[43,44] When health-related knowledge is taken into account, strong associations between education and smoking remain.[43] This is consistent with the finding in this study that adulthood occupational social class is more strongly related to smoking behaviour than age at leaving full-time education and suggests that effects beyond those of knowledge are involved. Both the theory that unobservable differences in time preference and direct effects of education on health knowledge are responsible for the association between education and mortality risk would predict stronger associations with respect to education than occupational social class.

Our data suggest that both education and social class are serving as indices of lifecourse socioeconomic experience. In this sense, education is important for the opportunities it creates for improved material conditions of life that follow the completion of formal education, rather than for particular specific effects of education itself. The direct associations between socioeconomic position, either indexed by social class or by education, and serum cholesterol concentrations, are striking in this regard. Groups leaving school with more full-time education and those in the professional and managerial social classes have higher cholesterol values than those leaving school at minimum school-leaving age and those ending up in manual occupations. This suggests similar patterns with respect to dietary fat intake by socioeconomic position, however it is indexed, and no special effect of education on dietary practices in this regard. If education has its influence through an ability to assimilate health-related knowledge then an inverse gradient would have been expected, given that publicity relating animal fat intake to coronary heart disease risk was already circulating (albeit in limited form) in the early 1970s.

In this study, age at leaving full-time education was the only index of education available. We have no data regarding evening classes or day release schemes, which are important sources of post-school education. It may be that indices of educational achievement, rather than simply school leaving age, would show different associations with risk factors and mortality. There would, however, be a strong correlation between the two measures, with most people leaving at age 14 or under not obtaining the higher school qualifications that would have been achieved by those leaving at 17 or 18 and only those staying in full-time education to beyond the age of 19 obtaining college or university qualifications. Studies with detailed data on both amount of education and educational achievement, together with subsequent life trajectory, would be required to examine the hypothesis that underlying differences generate health differentials between those who do and do not obtain higher qualifications.

The main conclusion of this study is that age at leaving full-time education and occupational social class are both strongly related to risk factors and to mortality. There is no evidence that education plays a predominant role in this regard. Smoking behaviour seems more strongly related to the adulthood socioeconomic indicator, in keeping with the suggestion that it is social environment that maintains this behaviour.[45] Some differences in mortality associations for particular cause of death groups are seen in these data. In multivariable analysis, noncardiovascular disease noncancer mortality is considerably more strongly associated with occupational social class than with education. This could reflect direct occupational exposures that influence respiratory and digestive system disease, with such exposures being better indexed by social class than age at leaving full-time education. Cardiovascular disease mortality is the cause of death group most strongly associated with education, which may reflect the particular importance of socioeconomic circumstances in childhood (and factors related to this) with respect to risk of coronary heart disease and stroke.[46-48]

Single indicators of social economic position do not maximally discriminate between social groups at differing levels of mortality risk, with the use of cumulative or multiple indicators producing greater differentiation.[8,10,11,47] Future studies should collect measures of socioeconomic position across the lifecourse and use combined measures if they intend to show the full extent of socioeconomic differentiation or adequately control for possible confounding of associations between putative risk factors and disease risk by exposures which are socioeconomically patterned.

References

[1] Schellekens, J. (1989) 'Mortality and socioeconomic status in two eighteenth-century Dutch villages', *Population Studies*, vol 43, pp 391-404.

[2] Fox, J. (1989) *Health inequalities in European countries*, Aldershot: Gower.

[3] Davey Smith, G., Bartley, M. and Blane, D. (1990) 'The Black Report on socioeconomic inequalities in health 10 years on', *British Medical Journal*, vol 301, pp 373-7.

[4] **Davey Smith, G., Carroll, D. and Rankin, S. (1992) 'Socioeconomic differentials in mortality: evidence from Glasgow graveyards', *British Medical Journal*, vol 305, pp 1554-7.**

[5] Kunst, A.E. and Mackenbach, J.P. (1994) 'The size of mortality differences associated with educational level in nine industrialized countries', *American Journal of Public Health*, vol 84, pp 932-7.

[6] Liberatos, P., Link, B.G. and Kelsey, J.L. (1988) 'The measurement of social class in epidemiology', *Epidemiology Review*, vol 10, pp 87-121.

[7] Moser, K., Pugh, H. and Goldblatt, P. (1990) 'Mortality and the social classification of women', in P. Goldblatt (ed) *Longitudinal study: Mortality and social organisation*, London: HMSO, pp 145-62.

[8] Goldblatt, P. (1990) 'Mortality and alternative social classifications', in P. Goldblatt (ed) *Longitudinal study: Mortality and social organisation*, London: HMSO, pp 163-92.

[9] Rogot, E., Sorlie, P.D., Johnson, N.J. and Schmitt, C. (1993) *A mortality study of 1.3 million persons by demographic, social, and economic factors: 1979-1985 Follow-up*, US National Longitudinal Mortality Study, Washington, DC: NIH.

[10] Davey Smith, G., Blane, D. and Bartley, M. (1994) 'Explanations for socioeconomic differentials in mortality: evidence from Britain and elsewhere', *European Journal of Public Health*, vol 4, pp 131-44.

[11] **Davey Smith, G., Shipley, M.J. and Rose, G. (1990) 'The magnitude and causes of socioeconomic differentials in mortality: further evidence from the Whitehall Study',** *Journal of Epidemiology and Community Health*, **vol 44, pp 260-5.**

[12] Krieger, N. and Fee, E. (1994) 'Social class: the missing link in US health data', *International Journal of Health Services*, vol 24, pp 25-44.

[13] Stevenson, T.H.C. (1923) 'The social distribution of mortality from different causes in England and Wales, 1910-12', *Biometrika*, vol 15, pp 382-400.

[14] Pamuk, E.R. (1985) 'Social class inequality in mortality from 1921 to 1972 in England and Wales', *Population Studies*, vol 39, pp 17-31.

[15] Blane, D., Davey Smith, G. and Bartley, M. (1990) 'Social class differences in years of potential life lost: size, trends and principal causes', *British Medical Journal*, vol 301, pp 429-32.

[16] Hinkle, L.E., Whitney, H., Lehman, E.W. et al. (1968) 'Occupation, education and coronary heart disease', *Science*, vol 161, pp 238-46.

[17] Mare, R.D. (1990) 'Socioeconomic careers and differential mortality among older men in the US', in J. Vallin, S. D'Souza and A. Palloni (eds) *Measurement and analysis of mortality: New approaches*, Oxford: Clarendon Press, pp 362-87.

[18] Sorlie, P.D., Backlund, E. and Keller, J.B. (1995) 'US mortality by economic, demographic, and social characteristics: the National Longitudinal Mortality Study', *American Journal of Public Health*, vol 85, pp 949-56.

[19] Reid, I. (1989) *Social class differences in Britain: Life-chances and life-styles*, Glasgow: Fontana Press.

[20] OPCS (Office for Population Censuses and Surveys) (1990) *General Household Survey 1988*, London: DHSS.

[21] Winkleby, M.A., Jatulis, D.E., Frank, E. and Fortmann, S.P. (1992) 'Socioeconomic status and health: how education, income, and occupation contribute to risk factors for cardiovascular disease', *American Journal of Public Health*, vol 82, pp 816-20.

[22] Pekkanen, J., Tuomilehto, J., Uutela, A., Vartiainen, E. and Nissinen, A. (1995) 'Social class, health behaviour, and mortality among men and women in eastern Finland', *British Medical Journal*, vol 311, pp 589-93.

[23] Fuchs, V.R. (1979) 'Economics, health, and post-industrial society', *Milbank Memorial Fund Quarterly*, vol 57, pp 153-82.

[24] Pincus, T. and Callahan, L.F. (1994) 'Associations of low formal education level and poor health status: behavioural, in addition to demographic and medical, explanations?', *Journal of Clinical Epidemiology*, vol 47, pp 355-61.

[25] Hawthorne, V.M., Gillis, C.R., Lorimer, A.R., Calvert, F.R. and Walker, T.J. (1969) 'Blood pressure in a Scottish island community', *British Medical Journal*, vol 4, pp 651-4.

[26] Hawthorne, V.M., Gillis, C.R. and Maclean, D.S. (1972) 'Monitoring health in Scotland', *International Journal of Epidemiology*, vol 1, pp 369-74.

[27] Hawthorne, V.M. and Fry, J.S. (1978) 'Smoking and health: the association between smoking behaviour, total mortality, and cardiorespiratory disease in west central Scotland', *Journal of Epidemiology and Community Health*, vol 32, pp 260-6.

[28] Hawthorne, V.M., Watt, G.M.C., Hart, C.L., Hole, D.J., Davey Smith, G. and Gillis, C.R. (1995) 'Cardiorespiratory disease in men and women in urban Scotland: baseline characteristics of the Renfrew/Paisley (Midspan) study population', *Scottish Medical Journal*, vol 40, pp 102-7.

[29] Rose, G.A., Blackburn, H., Gillum, R.F. and Prineas, R.J. (1982) *Cardiovascular survey methods*, Geneva: WHO.

[30] Medical Research Council (1965) 'Definition and classification of chronic bronchitis for epidemiological purposes', *Lancet*, no I, pp 775-9.

[31] Office of Population Censuses and Surveys (1966) *Classification of occupations 1966*, London: HMSO.

[32] Cox, D.R. (1972) 'Regression models and life tables', *Journal of the Royal Statistical Society Series B – Statistical Methodology*, vol 34, pp 187-220.

[33] Harding, S. (1995) 'Social class differences in mortality of men: recent evidence from the OPCS Longitudinal Study', *Population Trends*, no 80, pp 31-7.

[34] Office of Population Censuses and Surveys (1986) *Occupational mortality 1979-1980, 1982-1983*, London: HMSO.

[35] Osborne, G.S. (1966) *Scottish and English schools*, London: Longman.

[36] Hunter, S.L. (1972) (2nd edn) *The Scottish educational system*, Oxford: Pergamon Press.

[37] Elo, I.T. and Preston, S.H. (1996) 'Educational differentials in mortality: US, 1979-85', *Social Science and Medicine*, vol 42, pp 47-57.

[38] Menchik, P.L. (1993) 'Economic status as a determinant of mortality among black and white older men: does poverty kill?', *Population Studies*, vol 47, pp 427-36.

[39] Bosma, H. (1994) *A cross-cultural comparison of the role of some psychosocial factors in the etiology of coronary heart disease*, Den Haag: CIP-DATA Koninklijke Bibliotheek.

[40] Seltzer, C.C. and Jablon, S. (1977) 'Army rank and subsequent mortality by cause: 23-year follow-up', *American Journal of Epidemiology*, vol 105, pp 559-66.

[41] Holme, I., Helgeland, A., Hjermann, I., Leren, P. and Lund-Larsen, P.G. (1980) 'Four-year mortality by some socioeconomic indicators: the Oslo Study', *Journal of Epidemiology and Community Health*, vol 34, pp 48-52.

[42] Leigh, J.P. (1983) 'Direct and indirect effects of education on health', *Social Science and Medicine*, vol 17, pp 227-34.

[43] Kenkel, D.S. (1991) 'Health behavior, health knowledge, and schooling', *Journal of Political Economy*, vol 99, pp 287-305.

[44] Farrell, P. and Fuchs, V.R. (1982) 'Schooling and health: the cigarette connection', *Journal of Health Economics*, vol 1, pp 217-30.

[45] Blane, D., Hart, C.L., Davey Smith, G., Gillis, C.R., Hole, D.J. and Hawthorne, V.M. (1996) 'Association of cardiovascular disease risk factors with socioeconomic position during childhood and during adulthood', *British Medical Journal*, vol 313, pp 1434-8.

[46] Barker, D.J.P. (1994) *Mothers, babies and disease in later life*, London: BMJ Publications.

[47] **Davey Smith, G., Hart, C., Blane, D., Gillis, C. and Hawthorne, V. (1997) 'Lifetime socioeconomic position and mortality: prospective observational study', *British Medical Journal*, vol 314, pp 547-52.**

[48] Davey Smith, G. and Ben-Shlomo, Y. (1997) 'Geographical and social class differentials in stroke mortality: the influence of early-life factors', *Journal of Epidemiology and Community Health*, vol 51, pp 134-7.

17

Adverse socioeconomic conditions in childhood and cause-specific adult mortality: prospective observational study

George Davey Smith, Carole Hart,
David Blane and David Hole

Abstract

Objective: To investigate the association between social circumstances in childhood and mortality from various causes of death in adulthood.

Design: Prospective observational study.

Setting: 27 workplaces in the west of Scotland.

Participants: 5,645 men aged 35-64 years at the time of examination.

Main outcome measure: Death from various causes.

Results: Men whose fathers had manual occupations when they were children were more likely as adults to have manual jobs and be living in deprived areas. Gradients in mortality from coronary heart disease, stroke, lung cancer, stomach cancer, and respiratory disease were seen (all $p<0.05$), generally increasing from men whose fathers had professional and managerial occupations (social classes I and II) to those whose fathers had semiskilled and unskilled manual occupations (social classes IV and V). Relative rates of mortality adjusted for age for men with fathers in manual versus non-manual occupations were 1.52 (95% CI: 1.24-1.87) for coronary heart disease, 1.83 (1.13-2.94) for stroke, 1.65 (1.12-2.43) for lung cancer, 2.06 (0.93-4.57) for stomach cancer, and 2.01 (1.17-3.48) for respiratory

British Medical Journal, 1998, vol 316, pp 1631-5

disease. Mortality from other cancers and accidental and violent death showed no association with fathers' social class. Adjustment for adult socioeconomic circumstances and risk factors did not alter results for mortality from stroke and stomach cancer, attenuated the increased risk of coronary heart disease and respiratory disease, and essentially eliminated the association with lung cancer.

Conclusions: Adverse socioeconomic circumstances in childhood have a specific influence on mortality from stroke and stomach cancer in adulthood, which is not due to the continuity of social disadvantage throughout life. Deprivation in childhood influences risk of mortality from coronary heart disease and respiratory disease in adulthood, although an additive influence of adulthood circumstances is seen in these cases. Mortality from lung cancer, other cancers, and accidents and violence is predominantly influenced by risk factors that are related to social circumstances in adulthood.

Introduction

The long-term influence of poor social circumstances in early life on risk of disease in adulthood has been recognised for many years.[1] Several studies relating socioeconomic position in childhood to adulthood morbidity and mortality have appeared,[2-4] and influences on mortality from all-causes and from cardiovascular disease have been observed.[4,5] A particular problem with such studies is that socioeconomic circumstances in childhood and adulthood are linked,[6] and the specific effects of socioeconomic conditions in early life, as opposed to the continuing effects of deprivation throughout life, have been difficult to isolate.

If the specific influence of socioeconomic environment in early life is to be investigated, studies with data on circumstances in early *and* later life are required. Associations can be investigated by examining different causes of morbidity and mortality as the processes initiated by socioeconomic deprivation in early life will have specific influences on particular diseases. Similarly, the expectation is that some causes of morbidity and mortality would be mainly influenced by circumstances in adulthood. We have investigated the association between socioeconomic position in early life and cause-specific mortality in the Collaborative Study, a large cohort of men in the west of Scotland, to identify the specific influences of socioeconomic environment in early life on later health.

Methods

This analysis is based on a cohort of 5,766 men aged 35-64 at the time of examination who were recruited from workplaces in the west of Scotland between 1970 and 1973. Full details regarding the present study population (the Collaborative Study) and the methods of data collection that were used have been presented previously.[7,8]

The information collected at baseline examination included:

- *Sociodemographic data:* age, father's occupation, subject's occupation at the time of screening (coded to social class), and whether he was a regular car driver.
- *Measures of health status:* angina from the Rose questionnaire and respiratory symptoms from the Medical Research Council questionnaire.
- *Health-related behaviours:* detailed smoking history.
- *Physical examination:* height, weight, blood pressure, lung function (forced expiratory volume in 1 second (FEV_1) expressed as a percentage of the expected value for age and height calculated from the subset of healthy participants[8]), serum cholesterol concentration, and electrocardiogram.

Data on social class of subjects' fathers or subjects' own social class were missing for 121 men. These were excluded from the present analyses, which are therefore based on 5,645 participants. The home address at the time of screening was retrospectively given a postcode, enabling an area-based deprivation category at the time of the 1981 Census to be ascertained.[8] Deprivation category varied from 1 (least deprived) to 7 (most deprived). In all analyses, fathers' social class was treated at four levels: social classes I and II (professional and managerial), IIIN (skilled non-manual), IIIM (skilled manual), and IV and V (semiskilled and unskilled manual). For the adjustments the subjects' own social class was treated at six levels.

Mortality over a 21-year follow-up period was ascertained by flagging at the NHS central registry in Edinburgh, which also provided death certificates coded according to the International Classification of Diseases, Ninth Revision (ICD-9).

Mortality rates were standardised for age by the direct method by using the total study population as the standard. Tests for trends of age-adjusted rates were obtained by proportional hazards regression with the PROC PHREG program in the SAS system, with age and social class (coded as a continuous variable) as covariates. Continuous variables were standardised for age with the PROC GLM program, with tests for trends in age-adjusted means obtained with the PROC REG program. Categorical variables were age-standardised by the direct method and tests for trends performed with the PROC LOGIST program. Proportional hazards coefficients and their standard errors were calculated with adjustment for age and other risk factors by including terms for these in the proportional hazards models. Exponentiated hazards coefficients were taken as indicators of relative rates of death.

Results

Data on demographic factors, morbidity, and cardiovascular risk factors according to fathers' occupational social class are presented in Table 1. Men with fathers in non-manual social classes (I, II and IIIN) were more likely to be in non-manual social classes themselves, to live in less deprived areas, to be taller, to be less likely to smoke, to report less angina or bronchitis, and to have lower diastolic blood pressure, higher FEV_1 scores, higher serum cholesterol concentrations, and lower body mass indices. Men with fathers in manual social classes (IIIM, IV and V) were less likely to be regular car drivers. Being a regular car driver was taken to be a marker for ownership of a car, which has been used in various studies as an indicator of available income.

Over the 21 years of follow-up, 1,602 cohort members died. Relative rates of mortality adjusted for age for all-causes, coronary heart disease, stroke, lung cancer, stomach cancer, other cancers, respiratory disease, and accidents and violence are presented in Table 2. The risks of all-cause mortality and the specific causes examined,

Table 1: Population characteristics according to father's social class (values are age-adjusted means or proportions unless stated otherwise)

| Characteristic | Father's social class | | | | |
	I and II (*n*=787)	IIIN (*n*=582)	IIIM (*n*=2,457)	IV and V (*n*=1,819)	*p* value for trend
Age (years)[a]	48.1	47.8	48.5	48.1	0.57
Current social class I and II (%)	72.2	54.4	27.6	15.0	0.0001
Regular drivers (%)	71.0	57.5	50.1	44.0	0.0001
Deprivation category 5-7 (%)	24.3	29.1	53.0	58.5	0.0001
Angina (%)	4.0	5.2	6.6	6.9	0.002
Ischaemia on electrocardiogram (%)	6.3	4.5	5.8	6.1	0.66
Bronchitis (%)	0.8	1.4	2.1	3.2	0.0001
Height (cm)	176.0	174.4	172.5	171.4	0.0001
FEV_1 score (%)	99.2	97.1	93.8	91.8	0.0001
Cholesterol (mmol/l)	6.18	6.05	5.85	5.75	0.0001
Body mass index (kg/m^2)	25.0	24.7	25.2	25.4	0.0001
Current cigarette smoker (%)	48.4	47.8	56.5	58.9	0.0001
Diastolic blood pressure (mm Hg)	82.5	83.1	84.1	84.3	0.0001

[a] Not age-adjusted.

Table 2: Relative rates of mortality (95% CI) adjusted for age and socioeconomic position in adulthood, with number of deaths

Cause of death and adjustment	Father's social class				p value for trend
	I and II	IIIN	IIIM	IV and V	
All-causes (n=1,602)					
Age	1	1.12 (0.89-1.40)	1.48 (1.25-1.75)	1.54 (1.29-1.82)	0.0001
Age and adult social class	1	1.06 (0.84-1.33)	1.28 (1.08-1.53)	1.26 (1.05-1.52)	0.011
Coronary heart disease (n=618)					
Age	1	0.96 (0.65-1.40)	1.47 (1.13-1.92)	1.53 (1.16-2.01)	0.0003
Age and adult social class	1	0.91 (0.62-1.33)	1.28 (0.96-1.69)	1.26 (0.93-1.70)	0.064
Stroke (n=130)					
Age	1	0.79 (0.31-1.97)	1.64 (0.91-2.98)	1.70 (0.92-3.15)	0.031
Age and adult social class	1	0.78 (0.31-1.96)	1.62 (0.87-3.02)	1.66 (0.86-3.24)	0.061
Lung cancer (n=185)					
Age	1	1.49 (0.74-3.02)	2.13 (1.24-3.68)	1.80 (1.02-3.17)	0.045
Age and adult social class	1	1.35 (0.67-2.74)	1.62 (0.92- 2.85)	1.24 (0.68-2.27)	0.75
Stomach cancer (n=50)					
Age	1	1.06 (0.24-4.74)	1.51 (0.51-4.46)	2.95 (1.03-8.47)	0.011
Age and adult social class	1	1.06 (0.24-4.77)	1.51 (0.49-4.65)	2.95 (0.95-9.16)	0.017
Other cancers (n=272)					
Age	1	1.49 (0.93-2.38)	1.27 (0.87-1.85)	1.05 (0.70-1.57)	0.78
Age and adult social class	1	1.45 (0.91-2.33)	1.18 (0.79-1.76)	0.95 (0.61-1.48)	0.46
Respiratory disease (n=105)					
Age	1	1.65 (0.60-4.55)	2.41 (1.09-5.31)	2.75 (1.23-6.14)	0.008
Age and adult social class	1	1.52 (0.55-4.22)	1.97 (0.87-4.47)	2.10 (0.90-4.90)	0.092
Accidents and violence (n=51)					
Age	1	0.52 (0.14-1.95)	0.84 (0.37-1.90)	1.15 (0.51-2.62)	0.47
Age and adult social class	1	0.43 (0.11-1.64)	0.50 (0.21-1.19)	0.58 (0.23-1.42)	0.42

with the exception of other cancer and accidents and violence, were higher among men whose fathers were in manual compared with non-manual occupations.

Relative mortalities adjusted for age and social class in adulthood are also presented in Table 2. The graded association between fathers' social class and mortality from lung cancer was essentially abolished by adjustment for subjects' social class in adulthood; for mortality from coronary heart disease and respiratory disease the association was attenuated but remained evident, while for mortality from stroke and stomach cancer there was essentially no attenuation of the association after adjustment for adult social class.

Table 3 presents relative mortalities adjusted for age, adult sociodemographic indicators, and other risk factors. The sociodemographic indicators adjusted for were adult social class,

Table 3: Relative rates of mortality for men with fathers of manual social class adjusted for socioeconomic indicators and other risk factors, with non-manual fathers' social class as baseline (p values for trend given for test across the four social class groupings used in Tables 1 and 2)

Cause of death and adjustment	Manual social class	p value for trend
All-causes		
Age	1.44*** (1.27-1.63)	0.0001
Age, adult social class, deprivation category, car	1.22** (1.06-1.39)	0.024
Age, adult social class, deprivation category, car, risk factors[a]	1.19** (1.04-1.37)	0.042
Coronary heart disease		
Age	1.52*** (1.24-1.87)	0.0003
Age, adult social class, deprivation category, car	1.28* (1.03-1.61)	0.11
Age, adult social class, deprivation category, car, risk factors[a]	1.26* (1.01-1.58)	0.12
Stroke		
Age	1.83** (1.13-2.94)	0.031
Age, adult social class, deprivation category, car	1.87* (1.12-3.12)	0.049
Age, adult social class, deprivation category, car, risk factors[a]	1.74* (1.05-2.90)	0.079
Lung cancer		
Age	1.65** (1.12-2.43)	0.045
Age, adult social class, deprivation category, car	1.23 (0.81-1.87)	0.89
Age, adult social class, deprivation category, car, risk factors[b]	1.23 (0.81-1.88)	0.84
Stomach cancer		
Age	2.06 (0.93-4.57)	0.011
Age, adult social class, deprivation category, car	2.03 (0.86-4.78)	0.014
Age, adult social class, deprivation category, car, risk factors[b]	2.03 (0.86-4.78)	0.012
Other cancer		
Age	0.98 (0.74-1.28)	0.78
Age, adult social class, deprivation category, car	0.92 (0.68-1.25)	0.48
Age, adult social class, deprivation category, car, risk factors[b]	0.90 (0.67-1.23)	0.43
Respiratory disease		
Age	2.01** (1.17-3.48)	0.008
Age, adult social class, deprivation category, car	1.53 (0.85-2.75)	0.13
Age, adult social class, deprivation category, car, risk factors[b]	1.60 (0.88-2.90)	0.12
Accidents and violence		
Age	1.22 (0.63-2.38)	0.47
Age, adult social class, deprivation category, car	0.68 (0.33-1.40)	0.34

* $p<0.05$; ** $p<0.01$; *** $p<0.001$.

[a] Adjusted for smoking, diastolic blood pressure, cholesterol, body mass index, and FEV_1 score.

[b] Adjusted for smoking, body mass index, and FEV_1 score.

deprivation category based on area of residence and car use. For mortality from all-causes, coronary heart disease and stroke, the risk factors adjusted for were smoking (number of cigarettes smoked, with an additional adjustment for being a former smoker), diastolic blood pressure, serum cholesterol concentration, body mass index, and adjusted FEV_1 score. These represent the available data on risk factors for cardiovascular disease, some of which are also important risk factors for other causes of death. For mortality from cancer and respiratory disease, the risk factors adjusted for were smoking, body mass index, and FEV_1 score as these factors have been identified as important predictors of death from these causes. After adjustment for the risk factors together with the adult sociodemographic indicators, the increased risk of mortality from stroke and stomach cancer, and to a lesser degree from coronary heart disease and respiratory disease, remained evident for men whose fathers were in manual occupations.

While adjustment for adult sociodemographic factors resulted in a non-significant trend across the four social class groupings for mortality from coronary heart disease, the increased risk among the men with fathers in manual occupations remained significant. For mortality from stroke the equivalent increased risk was more striking and remained after adjustment for adulthood social indicators.

To examine the hypothesis that deprivation in early life followed by later affluence is associated with an increased risk of mortality from cardiovascular disease, we examined mortality from coronary heart disease and stroke according to social class in childhood and adulthood (Table 4). The specific influence of socioeconomic position in childhood on risk of stroke was confirmed in these analyses.

There was no strong effect of upward social mobility on the risk of mortality from either coronary heart disease or stroke, with none of the tests of interaction between fathers' and participants' social class approaching significance.

Discussion

Studies of the association between socioeconomic circumstances and mortality have generally used assessments of socioeconomic position in adulthood. Attempts to explain the social distribution of all-cause mortality and death from specific causes have similarly focused on exposures such as health-related behaviours, unfavourable occupational factors, or inadequate healthcare acting during adult life.[9] The potential of adverse childhood circumstances to produce socioeconomic differentials in health in adulthood has, however, been recognised by some observers for many years.[1] Social position in adulthood is associated in similar fashion with many but not all[10] causes of death. Examining the association between childhood socioeconomic

Table 4: Mortality from coronary heart disease and stroke after 21 years follow-up according to social class at screening and fathers' social class (values are relative rates adjusted for socioeconomic factors and risk factor profiles)

Cause of death and adjustment	Participant non-manual at screening		Participant manual at screening	
	Non-manual father	Manual father	Non-manual father	Manual father
Coronary heart disease				
Age	1	1.51 (1.16-1.96)	1.68 (1.09-2.58)	1.82 (1.43-2.32)
Risk factors[a]	1	1.43 (1.10-1.86)	1.59 (1.02-2.48)	1.67 (1.27-2.18)
Stroke				
Age	1	1.84 (1.04-3.28)	1.12 (0.37-3.34)	1.88 (1.09-3.24)
Risk factors[a]	1	1.74 (0.97-3.12)	0.94 (0.30-2.91)	1.65 (0.90-3.03)

[a] Age, smoking, diastolic blood pressure, cholesterol, body mass index, FEV_1 score, deprivation category, and car.

circumstances and cause-specific mortality in adulthood, with adjustment for social conditions in adulthood, is one approach to determining which associations may reflect the specific influence of factors acting in early life. We have shown that stroke and stomach cancer, and to a lesser extent coronary heart disease and respiratory disease, seem to be influenced by childhood circumstances in a way that other causes of death, which are equally or more strongly socially patterned in adulthood, for example lung cancer and accidents and violence, are not.

Stroke and stomach cancer

Areas with high maternal and neonatal mortality earlier in the twentieth century have high current rates of death from stroke,[11] which could indicate that unfavourable environments in early life influence later risk of stroke. The inverse association between birth weight and stroke observed in one study,[12] together with extensive data demonstrating an inverse association between birth weight and later blood pressure,[11] provide more direct evidence of the potential early life origins of stroke, although such individually-based prospective studies remain susceptible to confounding by socioenvironmental factors in later life. Height in adulthood, in part an outcome of social environment in childhood, correlates negatively with mortality from stroke across the regions of England and Wales.[13]

Prospective studies also demonstrate an inverse association between height and risk of stroke.[14,15] By showing associations after adjustment for various indicators of socioeconomic position in adulthood and risk factor profiles our data suggest that current socioeconomic differentials in risk of stroke reflect socioeconomic differentials in childhood experiences which occurred earlier this century.

Stroke and stomach cancer share several epidemiological features: sizeable, continuing, and unexplained declines in mortality over the century and similar geographical distributions,[16] including unexpectedly low mortalities in the London area.[16] Migrant studies suggest that the risk of stomach cancer is in part determined during early life,[17] and current mortality correlates with markers of adverse socioeconomic circumstances earlier in the twentieth century.[18] Poor socioeconomic circumstances in childhood favour acquisition of *Helicobacter pylori*,[19] and such infection may be an important cause of stomach cancer.[20] Declining rates of *Helicobacter pylori* infection seem to have accompanied improving social conditions over the century[21] and thus may underlie the falling rates of death from stomach cancer. By allowing adjustment for socioeconomic position in adulthood, our study, the first prospective investigation of this issue to our knowledge, supports the notion that an early life factor, possibly *Helicobacter pylori* infection, strongly influences the socioeconomic distribution of stomach cancer in adulthood. Infections acquired in childhood have also been implicated in the risk of stroke, and this could be responsible for the common epidemiological features of stroke and stomach cancer.

Heart disease and respiratory disease

Most[2,4,5,22] but not all[23] studies investigating the association between socioeconomic circumstances in childhood and risk of coronary heart disease have found an association similar to that found in the present study, which is not purely due to the adverse social class destinations of those born into poor circumstances. Forsdahl hypothesised that deprivation in early life followed by later affluence combined to produce a high risk of mortality from coronary heart disease.[24] Our study, like several others that have examined this issue,[2,5,22] found no particular increase in risk of coronary heart disease among men born into families of manual social class who were themselves in non-manual jobs.

The influence of early life conditions on respiratory disease in adulthood has been studied for many years.[3] Respiratory infections in childhood have been related to poor respiratory health in later life, and environmental influences on childhood respiratory function such as damp housing, fumes from fuel burning, and air pollution could influence the risk of later respiratory disease.[25] In keeping with our findings that social circumstances in both childhood and adulthood influence mortality from respiratory disease, a cohort study from birth through to adulthood has shown that socially patterned exposures acting throughout life accumulate in their influence on adulthood respiratory health.[26]

Other causes of death

Deaths from lung cancer and accidents and violence are clearly influenced by exposures acting during adult life. Thus, adjustment for adulthood socioeconomic position and, in the case of lung cancer, cigarette smoking greatly attenuated (in the case of lung cancer) or reversed (in the case of accidents and violence) the association between fathers' social class and mortality. While the (non-significant) residual relation between mortality from lung cancer and social class in childhood is only moderately weaker than that between childhood social class and mortality from coronary heart disease, the important element is the change in relative risk after adjustment for confounders, rather than magnitude of the residual effect itself.[27]

Strengths and weaknesses of these methods

Information on social circumstances in childhood was based on recall in adulthood. Recall of childhood socioeconomic position on the basis of the occupational social class of the head of the household has been shown to be reliable in a middle-aged population in the US.[28] The question participants were asked in the present study related specifically to the main occupation of their father. In this cohort, for whom a change in socioeconomic circumstances during adult years would have been more likely than for their fathers, social mobility from labour market entry to middle age was low.[7] As there is little change in social class position after young adulthood, the type of employment the fathers of the participants were in for most of their lives would generally be the same or similar to that they were in when their children were young.[29]

A particular strength of the present study is the ability to use multiple measures of adult socioeconomic position in the analyses. It is likely that in previous investigations the measures used, such as social class in adulthood, have been inadequate as many studies show that the better the classification of socioeconomic position the greater the mortality differentials observed.[9] As there is likely to be more measurement error with respect to fathers' social class than participants' social class, we may be underestimating the influence of childhood social class in analyses that adjust for several well-indexed markers of adulthood socioeconomic position. Our analyses therefore represent a powerful test of the hypothesis that there are specific influences of childhood social circumstances on adult mortality risk that are not merely due to the continuity of disadvantage throughout life.

A second strength of our study is the ability to adjust statistically for several risk factors for cardiovascular disease. This may represent over-control as childhood social circumstances may act through these risk factors to influence cardiovascular disease in adulthood. This applies particularly to body mass index, for which exposures acting in childhood seem to be responsible for the higher levels among men with fathers of manual social class. The same considerations, but to a lesser degree, apply to blood pressure and lung function.[7]

Implications of our findings

There are several implications of our findings. Firstly, attempts to explain the social distribution of adult health and risk of mortality must consider the influence of socioeconomic circumstances acting across the entire lifecourse. Studies with data covering only one point in time, whether this is early life or adulthood, face serious limitations in their ability to advance understanding. Secondly, the contribution of social circumstances in early life varies greatly between causes of death. This highlights the inadequacies of models that consider socioeconomic differentials in health to reflect a heightened general susceptibility to all diseases among those in adverse social circumstances. Thirdly, current changes in mortality rates for certain causes, including reductions in rates of stomach cancer and stroke, will reflect social changes that occurred several decades ago. Finally, the increasing child poverty seen in Britain and elsewhere over the past 20 years may well herald unfavourable future trends in adult health.

References

[1] Kuh, D. and Davey Smith, G. (1993) 'When is mortality risk determined? Historical insights into a current debate', *Social History of Medicine*, vol 6, pp 101-23.

[2] Burr, M.L. and Sweetnam, P.M. (1980) 'Family size and paternal unemployment in relation to myocardial infarction', *Journal of Epidemiology and Community Health*, vol 34, pp 93-5.

[3] Elo, I.T. and Preston, S.H. (1992) 'Effects of early-life conditions on adult mortality: a review', *Population Index*, vol 58, pp 186-212.

[4] Vagero, D. and Leon, D. (1994) 'Effect of social class in childhood and adulthood on adult mortality', *Lancet*, vol 343, pp 1224-5.

5 Notkola, V., Punsar, S., Karvonen, M.J. and Haapakaski, J. (1985) 'Socioeconomic conditions in childhood and mortality and morbidity caused by coronary heart disease in adulthood in rural Finland', *Social Science and Medicine*, vol 21, pp 517-23.

6 Ben-Shlomo, Y. and Davey Smith, G. (1991) 'Deprivation in infancy or adult life: which is more important for mortality risk?', *Lancet*, vol 337, pp 530-4.

7 Blane, D., Hart, C.L., Davey Smith, G., Gillis, C.R., Hole, D.J. and Hawthorne, V.M. (1996) 'Association of cardiovascular disease risk factors with socioeconomic position during childhood and during adulthood', *British Medical Journal*, vol 313, pp 1434-8.

8 **Davey Smith, G., Hart, C., Blane, D., Gillis, C. and Hawthorne, V. (1997) 'Lifetime socioeconomic position and mortality: prospective observational study', *British Medical Journal*, vol 314, pp 547-52.**

9 Davey Smith, G., Bartley, M. and Blane, D. (1994) 'Explanations for socioeconomic differentials in mortality: evidence from Britain and elsewhere', *European Journal of Public Health*, vol 4, pp 131-44.

10 **Davey Smith, G., Neaton, J.D., Wentworth, D., Stamler, R. and Stamler, J. (1996) 'Socioeconomic differentials in mortality risk among men screened for the Multiple Risk Factor Intervention Trial: Part I – results for 300,685 white men', *American Journal of Public Health*, vol 86, pp 486-96.**

11 Barker, D.J.P. (1994) *Mothers, babies, and disease in later life*, London: BMJ Publishing.

12 Martyn, C.N., Barker, D.J.P. and Osmond, C. (1996) 'Mothers' pelvic size, fetal growth, and death from stroke and coronary heart disease in men in the UK', *Lancet*, vol 348, pp 1264-8.

13 Barker, D.J.P., Osmond, C. and Golding, J. (1990) 'Height and mortality in the countries of England and Wales', *Annals of Human Biology*, vol 17, pp 1-6.

14 Leon, D., Davey Smith, G., Shipley, M. and Strachan, D. (1995) 'Height and mortality in London: early life influences, socioeconomic confounding or shrinkage', *Journal of Epidemiology and Community Health*, vol 49, pp 5-9.

15 Watt, G.C.M., Hart, C.L., Hole, D.J., Davey Smith, G., Gillis, C.R. and Hawthorne, V.M. (1995) 'Risk factors for cardiorespiratory and all cause mortality in men and women in urban Scotland: 15 year follow up', *Scottish Medical Journal*, vol 40, pp 108-12.

16 Murray, M. (1962) 'The geography of death in England and Wales', *Annals of the Association of American Geography*, vol 52, pp 130-49.

17 Coggon, D., Osmond, C. and Barker, D.J.P. (1990) 'Stomach cancer and migration within England and Wales', *British Journal of Cancer*, vol 61, pp 573-4.

18 Barker, D.J.P., Coggon, D., Osmond, C. and Wickham, C. (1990) 'Poor housing in childhood and high rates of stomach cancer in England and Wales', *British Journal of Cancer*, vol 61, pp 575-8.

19 Mendall, M.A., Goggin, P.M., Molineaux, N., Levy, J., Toosy, T., Strachan, D. et al (1992) 'Childhood living conditions and *Helicobacter pylori* seropositivity in adult life', *Lancet*, vol 339, pp 896-7.

20 Forman, D., Newell, D.G., Fullerton, F., Yarnell, J.W.G., Stacey, A.R., Wald, N. et al (1991) 'Association between infection with *Helicobacter pylori* and risk of gastric cancer: evidence from a prospective investigation', *British Medical Journal*, vol 302, pp 1302-5

21 Banatvala, N., Mayo, K., Megraud, F., Jennings, R., Deeks, J.J. and Feldman, R.A. (1993) 'The cohort effect and *Helicobacter pylori*', *Journal of Infectious Diseases*, vol 168, pp 219-21.

22 Wannamethee, S.G., Whincup, P.H., Shaper, G. and Walker, M. (1996) 'Influence of fathers' social class on cardiovascular disease in middle-aged men', *Lancet*, vol 348, pp 1259-63.

23 Haste, H. (1990) 'Association between living conditions in childhood and myocardial infarction', *British Medical Journal*, vol 300, pp 289-98.

24 Forsdahl, A. (1977) 'Are poor living conditions in childhood and adolescence an important risk factor for arteriosclerotic heart disease?', *British Journal of Preventive Social Medicine*, vol 31, pp 91-5.

[25] Wu, J.M., Witorsch, R.J. and Witorsch, P. (1991) 'Respiratory effects of socioeconomic status, gas stove usage, and other factors in children: an analytical survey of the epidemiological literature', in L.D. Fechter (ed) *Proceedings of the fourth international conference on the combined effects of environmental factors*, Baltimore, MD: Johns Hopkins University.

[26] Mann, S.L., Wadsworth, M.E.J. and Colley, J.R.T. (1992) 'Accumulation of factors influencing respiratory illness in members of a national birth cohort and their offspring', *Journal of Epidemiology and Community Health*, vol 46, pp 256-92.

[27] Phillips, A. and Davey Smith, G. (1991) 'How independent are independent effects? Relative risk estimation when correlated exposures are measured imprecisely', *Journal of Clinical Epidemiology*, vol 44, pp 1223-31.

[28] Krieger, N., Okamoto, A. and Selby, J.V. (1998) 'Twins' recall of childhood social class and fathers' education: a validation study for public health research', *American Journal of Epidemiology*, vol 147, pp 704-8.

[29] Payne, G. (1987) *Employment and opportunity*, London: Macmillan.

18

Socioeconomic factors as determinants of mortality

George Davey Smith and Carole Hart

A recent study from the US[1] established that behavioural risk factors cannot account for the substantial socioeconomic differentials in mortality and found that income was a stronger determinant to mortality risk than education. These are crucial findings, as it is often asserted that education is the key socioeconomic variable with respect to health, particularly in the US literature.[2]

In Chapter Sixteen we reported on the association between education, occupational social class, and mortality in a large Scottish sample (n=5,749).[3] The indicator of adulthood social environments – in our case, occupational social class – was a more important determinant of overall mortality risk than education. In our study, extensive data on behavioural and physiological risk factors were available, and here we present data on the associations between social class, education, and mortality, with and without adjustment for risk factors (see Table 1). The socioeconomic differentials are shown to reflect a wider range of exposures than the behavioural and physiological characteristics often considered to underlie them.[2] In our analysis, we almost certainly are over-adjusting, in that many of the factors (such as lung function, body mass index, and even behaviours like smoking) should be viewed as outcomes of socioeconomic processes. They are therefore mediators rather than confounders of the association between social conditions and mortality.

Education and adulthood markers of socioeconomic position (such as income and occupational social class) should not be considered interchangeable measures that allow for more or less precise categorisation of some hypothetical underlying phenomena (sometimes referred to as 'socioeconomic status'). Education is strongly influenced by childhood socioeconomic circumstances, and exposures in childhood are important determinants of the social patterning of some causes of death, particularly stroke and stomach cancer.[4] Mortality due to coronary heart disease and respiratory disease is influenced by

Journal of the American Medical Association, 1998, vol 280, pp 1744-5

Table 1: Age-adjusted 21-year all-cause and cardiovascular disease (CVD) death rates according to social class and education (per 10,000 person years) and relative risks (RRs) adjusted for age and risk factors[a]

Mortality	I	II	IIIN	IIIM	IV	V
			Social class[c]			
All cause						
No of deaths	156	242	293	530	334	84
Death rate	101.1	110.0	139.5	153.0	152.6	170.5
Age-adjusted RR (95% CI)	1	1.07 (0.88-1.31)	1.45 (1.20-1.76)	1.65 (1.38-1.97)	1.63 (1.35-1.97)	1.74 (1.34-2.28)
Multivariate RR (95% CI)[b]	1	1.05 (0.86-1.29)	1.42 (1.17-1.73)	1.52 (1.26-1.83)	1.50 (1.23-1.83)	1.65 (1.26-2.17)
All CVD						
No of deaths	65	138	155	273	172	38
Death rate	48.0	66.8	79.8	86.4	87.7	78.7
Age-adjusted RR (95% CI)	1	1.47 (1.09-1.97)	1.84 (1.38-2.48)	2.03 (1.55-2.66)	2.00 (1.50-2.66)	1.86 (1.25-2.79)
Multivariate RR (95% CI)[b]	1	1.45 (1.08-1.95)	1.84 (1.38-2.47)	1.99 (1.51-2.63)	2.02 (1.50-2.71)	1.96 (1.30-2.95)

Mortality	19+	17-18	15-16	12-14
		Age at leaving full-time education (years)		
All cause				
No of deaths	96	150	397	996
Death rate	100.8	112.8	129.3	148.5
Age-adjusted RR (95% CI)	1	1.20 (0.93-1.55)	1.40 (1.12-1.75)	1.67 (1.35-2.06)
Multivariate RR (95% CI)[b]	1	1.23 (0.95-1.59)	1.37 (1.09-1.72)	1.56 (1.26-1.94)
All CVD				
No of deaths	40	81	212	508
Death rate	47.5	66.7	75.0	83.9
Age-adjusted RR (95% CI)	1	1.55 (1.06-2.26)	1.79 (1.28-2.51)	2.03 (1.47-2.80)
Multivariate RR (95% CI)[b]	1	1.67 (1.14-2.44)	1.88 (1.34-2.64)	2.07 (1.49-2.87)

[a] All comparisons, *p* trend <0.001.

[b] Adjusted for age, smoking, diastolic blood pressure, cholesterol level, body mass index, adjusted forced expiratory volume, angina, bronchitis, and electrocardiographic evidence of ischemia.

[c] Social class coded according to the Register General's schema: I, professional occupation; II, technical and managerial; IIIN, skilled non-manual occupations; IIIM, skilled manual occupations; IV, partly skilled occupations; V, unskilled occupations.

CI: confidence interval.

socially patterned exposures acting across the lifecourse,[5] whereas several other causes of death such as motor vehicle crashes, violence, and lung cancer are mainly influenced by socioeconomic factors during adulthood.[4] Therefore, the expectation is that education will be related more strongly to cardiovascular disease mortality than mortality due to other causes. This was not observed in the analyses by Lantz et al,[1] although their study lacked power. Based on three times as many deaths, we found that education is unrelated to cancer deaths and noncardiovascular, noncancer deaths after occupational social class was taken into account, but was associated with cardiovascular disease mortality.[3] Conversely, with respect to occupational social class, cancer mortality and noncardiovascular disease, noncancer mortality demonstrate the strongest independent associations after taking education into account. Education thus appears to act as an indicator of socioeconomic circumstances in early life.

References

[1] Lantz, P.M., House, J.S., Lepkowski, J.M., Williams, D.R., Mero, R.P. and Chen, J. (1998) 'Socioeconomic factors, health behaviours, and mortality: results from a nationally representative prospective study of US adults', *Journal of the American Medical Association*, vol 279, pp 1703-8.

[2] Pincus, T. and Callahan, L.F. (1994) 'Associations of low formal education level and poor health status: behavioural, in addition to demographic and medical, explanations?', *Journal of Clinical Epidemiology*, vol 47, pp 355-61.

[3] **Davey Smith, G., Hart, C., Hole, D., MacKinnon, P., Gillis, C., Watt, G., Blane, D. and Hawthorne, V. (1998) 'Education and occupational social class: which is the more important indicator of mortality risk?', *Journal of Epidemiology and Community Health*, vol 52, pp 153-60.**

[4] **Davey Smith, G., Hart, C., Blane, D. and Hole, D. (1998) 'Adverse socioeconomic conditions in childhood and cause-specific adult mortality: prospective observational study', *British Medical Journal*, vol 316, pp 1631-5.**

[5] Davey Smith, G. (1997) 'Socioeconomic differentials', in D. Kuh and Y. Ben Shlomo (eds) *A life course approach to chronic disease epidemiology*, Oxford: Oxford University Press, pp 242-73.

19

Lifecourse socioeconomic and behavioural influences on cardiovascular disease mortality: the Collaborative Study

George Davey Smith and Carole Hart

Abstract

Objectives: To demonstrate lifecourse influences on cardiovascular disease (CVD).

Methods: Prospective observational study.

Main outcome measure: Death from CVD.

Results: Combining four socioeconomic and behavioural risk indicators into a measure of lifecourse exposure produced five groups whose relative risk of CVD mortality ran from 1 for the group with the most favourable lifecourse exposures (baseline group) to 1.99, 2.60, 2.98 and finally 4.55 for the group with the most unfavourable lifecourse exposures. If the entire study population had the CVD mortality risk of the sub-sample with the most favourable lifecourse risk factor profile, around two thirds of cardiovascular deaths would not have occurred.

Conclusion: Cardiovascular disease risk is influenced in a cumulative fashion by socioeconomic and behavioural factors acting right across the lifecourse.

American Journal of Public Health, 2002, vol 92, pp 1295-8

Introduction

In 1941 Antonio Ciocco and colleagues concluded that the findings of their follow-up study of Maryland schoolchildren "reinforce the views held by many that disease in adulthood is often brought about by the cumulative effects over a long period of time of many pathological conditions, many incidents, some of which take place and are even perceived in infancy".[1] This lifecourse approach to chronic disease lost favour over the subsequent half-century, but has recently been revived.[2] This approach recognises that factors acting in early life accumulate and interact with factors acting in later life in the production of adulthood disease. Cardiovascular disease (CVD) is in many ways the paradigmatic adulthood health problem which illustrates the importance of a lifecourse perspective. Genomic and non-genomic intergenerational factors;[3,4] intrauterine environment;[5] growth, nutrition, health and social circumstances in childhood[6-9] and a variety of behavioural and socioeconomic factors in adulthood may all contribute to the development of CVD. Most studies to date have focused on only one stage of the lifecourse, on only one category of risk factor, or on cross-sectional measures of CVD risk factors or risk. Here we demonstrate the importance of lifecourse influences on CVD in a large cohort of men from the west of Scotland.

Methods

This analysis is based on a cohort of 5,766 men aged 35-64 at the time of examination, who were recruited from workplaces in the west of Scotland between 1970 and 1973. Full details regarding the present study population and the methods of data collection that were used have been presented previously.[9,10]

The data collected at baseline examination and included in this report were:

- *sociodemographic data:* age; father's occupation; age of leaving full-time education; participant's occupation at the time of screening.
- *health-related behaviours:* tobacco and alcohol use.

Alcohol consumption has been dichotomised as 15 units or more per week and less than 15 per week. This is the level of alcohol consumption above which we have previously reported that rates of cardiovascular disease mortality were increased in this cohort.[11]

The home address of the men at the time of screening was retrospectively postcoded, enabling the Carstairs index – an area-based deprivation category[12] – to be calculated, based on 1981 Census data. Deprivation category varied from 1 (least deprived) to 7 (most deprived); this has been dichotomised as 1-5 and 6-7.

Participants with missing data for any of the above variables were excluded from the present analyses, which are based on 5,628 participants.

Mortality over a 25-year follow-up period was ascertained by flagging at the NHS central registry in Edinburgh. CVD mortality (International Classification of Diseases, Ninth Revision [ICD-9] codes 390-459) is analysed in this report.

Age-adjusted odds ratios for associations between variables were calculated through logistic regression. Proportional hazards coefficients and their standard errors were calculated with adjustment for age. Exponentiated coefficients were taken as indicators of relative rates of death. Population attributable risk fractions were calculated using standard methods.[13]

Results

The social and behavioural exposures examined in this report are generally strongly interrelated (Table 1). People who are disadvantaged with respect to childhood social circumstances (as indexed by father's social class) are more likely to leave education early, have manual jobs in later adulthood, live in deprived areas as adults, be cigarette smokers and drink high quantities of alcohol.

Over the 25-year period 1,187 men died of CVD. Men whose fathers had manual occupations had a relative risk of CVD mortality of 1.61 (95% CI: 1.39-1.88) compared to men whose fathers had non-manual occupations. Table 2 presents relative rates of CVD mortality according to father's social class and later-life risk factors. Behavioural factors (smoking and heavy drinking), age at leaving

Table 1: Association between risk factors (age-adjusted odds ratios)

	Screening social class	Current smoking	Heavy alcohol consumption	Deprivation category	Education
Father's social class	8.26 (7.05-9.69)	1.45 (1.28-1.64)	1.82 (1.57-2.10)	3.36 (2.83-3.98)	8.44 (7.21-9.88)
Screening social class		1.89 (1.70-2.11)	2.78 (2.47-3.14)	4.15 (3.66-4.72)	9.27 (8.18-10.51)
Current smoking			1.95 (1.74-2.20)	1.64 (1.46-1.85)	1.60 (1.44-1.79)
Heavy alcohol consumption				1.99 (1.76-2.25)	2.17 (1.92-2.45)
Deprivation category					3.35 (2.95-3.81)

Note: Social class dichotomised as manual and non-manual; education dichotomised as leaving full-time education at 14 years of age or earlier and leaving full-time education at older than 14.

Table 2: Age-adjusted relative rates (and 95% CI) of CVD mortality by father's social class and later-life risk factors

Father's social class		Smoking	
		Other	Current cigarette
Non-manual	No (CVD deaths)	703 (75)	657 (133)
	Relative rate	1	2.20 (1.66-2.93)
Manual	No (CVD deaths)	1,811 (339)	2,457 (640)
	Relative rate	1.80 (1.40-2.31)	3.11 (2.45-3.95)
		Alcohol	
		<15 units/week	≥15 units /week
Non-manual	No (CVD deaths)	1,065 (158)	295 (50)
	Relative rate	1	1.28 (0.93-1.76)
Manual	No (CVD deaths)	2,847 (621)	1,421 (358)
	Relative rate	1.53 (1.28-1.82)	2.13 (1.77-2.57)
		Screening social class	
		Non-manual	Manual
Non-manual	No (CVD deaths)	1,148 (161)	212 (47)
	Relative rate	1	1.43 (1.03-1.97)
Manual	No (CVD deaths)	1,691 (354)	2,577 (625)
	Relative rate	1.56 (1.30-1.88)	1.85 (1.55-2.19)
		Deprivation category	
		1-5	6, 7
Non-manual	No (CVD deaths)	1,182 (175)	178 (33)
	Relative rate	1	1.17 (0.80-1.69)
Manual	No (CVD deaths)	2,831 (614)	1,437 (365)
	Relative rate	1.58 (1.34-1.87)	1.78 (1.49-2.14)
		Age at leaving full-time education	
		>14	≤14
Non-manual	No (CVD deaths)	1,126 (165)	234 (43)
	Relative rate	1	1.18 (0.84-1.65)
Manual	No (CVD deaths)	1,630 (299)	2,638 (680)
	Relative rate	1.48 (1.22-1.79)	1.77 (1.49-2.10)

full-time education and later life socioeconomic factors (social class, deprivation category) all provided additional discrimination of CVD mortality risk when combined with father's social class. In all cases the separate contribution of father's social class and the other risk indicator were significant at conventional ($p<0.05$) levels. In no cases were there substantial or conventionally significant interactions between father's social class and the later-life risk indicator.

We developed a strategy previously applied to analysis of this cohort, by producing a combined index of occasions in which people were disadvantaged with respect to a health risk indicator. Combining four risk indicators – father's and own social class, smoking and alcohol use – produced a strongly graded risk association (Table 3). This indicator ran from a score of 0 (unfavourable) (for those with a non-

Table 3: Cardiovascular mortality according to cumulative risk indicator (father's social class, screening social class, smoking, alcohol use)

	n	CVD deaths	Relative risk
4 favourable (0 unfavourable)	517	47	1
3 favourable (1 unfavourable)	1,299	227	1.99 (1.45-2.73)
2 favourable (2 unfavourable)	1,606	354	2.60 (1.92-3.52)
1 favourable (3 unfavourable)	1,448	339	2.98 (2.20-4.05)
0 favourable (4 unfavourable)	758	220	4.55 (3.32-6.24)

manual social class father, who had a non-manual job in adulthood and who were not current cigarette smokers nor heavy alcohol drinkers at the time of screening) through to 4 unfavourable (for those whose fathers were in manual jobs, who themselves had manual jobs in adulthood and who were smokers and heavy drinkers at the time of screening). The intermediate categories simply summed the number of occasions a man had an unfavourable risk indicator. Finally, all six socioeconomic and behavioural risk indicators included in these analyses were combined and a similar gradient of increasing risk was observed: relative risks running from the most favourable to least favourable exposure group: 1, 1.98 (1.39-2.82), 2.57 (1.82-3.64), 2.67 (1.89-3.77), 2.83 (2.01-3.98), 4.00 (2.84-5.63) and 4.48 (3.06-6.55). Population attributable risk fraction calculations indicate that if the entire cohort had the risk indicator profile of the most favourable group 63.4% of CVD deaths would be averted. This fraction is a little different to that produced by combining the four risk indicators utilised in Table 3 (62.6%).

Discussion

We have demonstrated that substantial differences in CVD mortality risk exist between groups defined by a small set of socioeconomic and behavioural risk factors. Previous reports have linked cumulative socioeconomic disadvantage with higher levels of CVD mortality,[9] morbidity[9,14] and risk factors.[14-16] Similar cumulative socioeconomic influences on all-cause mortality,[9,17-19] self-rated health,[20] and physical, psychological and cognitive functioning[21] have been demonstrated. Health-related behaviours have been utilised as control variables in our previous studies of cumulative social disadvantage with all-cause and CVD mortality risk, rather than as additional risk indicators. In such presentations the influence of smoking on socioeconomic gradients can be detected, but the additional contribution of smoking to health outcomes cannot be seen. A few previous studies have presented the joint effects of socioeconomic position in adulthood and smoking on mortality risk,[22,23] and one study has presented the joint effect of smoking and socioeconomic position on carotid intima-media thickness.[24]

An important issue relates to whether adulthood disease risk results from interactions between early-life and later-life risk indicators, or is more straightforwardly influenced by the accumulation of risk across the lifecourse. In the present cohort we have previously demonstrated that accumulation, rather than interaction, characterises the effects of childhood and adulthood social circumstances on CVD mortality risk.[7] In the present study we demonstrate that there are no important interactions between early-life socioeconomic circumstances and behavioural risk factors in adulthood, in keeping with evidence that there are no important interactions between smoking and adulthood social position.[22,23] Socioeconomic factors acting across the lifecourse seem to accumulate in their influence on CVD risk with two important health-related behaviours – smoking and heavy drinking – in adulthood.

We have previously demonstrated that in this cohort heavy drinking is associated with increased CVD – in particular stroke – risk.[11] Here we show that this is not dependent on socioeconomic confounding, either by childhood or adulthood social circumstances. In our cohort, alcohol consumption was probably of a binge drinking – rather than a sustained but low level – pattern, and this pattern has been associated with increased CVD risk in other studies.[25]

Favourable or adverse health-damaging exposures are not randomly distributed across individuals within society; they generally cluster within particular groups. People who are disadvantaged with respect to one exposure tend to be disadvantaged with respect to others, as demonstrated in Table 1. There are clear causal chains acting in this regard. Poor childhood social circumstances increase the risk of finishing education with few credentials, which in turn leads to an unfavourable occupational trajectory in adulthood and to membership of social groups which encourage the development and maintenance of certain patterns of health-damaging behaviours.[26-28] Interventions which simply select one item from this chain – almost invariably one of the health-related behaviours – and fail to recognise the societal basis for the distribution of risk are unlikely to be successful, as the failure of behavioural programmes targeted at individuals to reduce CVD risk attests.[29]

If our entire study population had the CVD mortality risk of the subsample with favourable profiles of lifecourse socioeconomic and behavioural factors, then nearly two thirds of cardiovascular deaths would not have occurred during the follow-up period. This was seen despite the loss of information entailed by dichotomising our exposure variables: if more categories had been used, an even greater proportion of cardiovascular deaths could be attributed to these simple indicators.

We have previously shown that health-related selection between childhood and adulthood social location does not account for CVD mortality differentials,[30] thus these risk indicators appear to be exogenous causes (at the distal level in the case of the socioeconomic measures) of increased cardiovascular mortality. Improving social circumstances and reducing harmful health behaviours in the population – all potentially possible – could lead to very substantial decreases in the population burden of CVD.

References

[1] Ciocco, A., Klein, H. and Palmer, C.E. (1941) 'Child health and the selective service physical standards', *Public Health Reports*, vol 56, pp 2365-75.

[2] Kuh, D. and Ben-Shlomo, Y. (1997) *A life course approach to chronic disease epidemiology*, Oxford: Oxford University Press.

[3] Austin, M.A. (1996) 'Genetic epidemiology of dyslipidaemia and atherosclerosis', *Annals of Medicine*, vol 28, pp 459-63.

[4] Davey Smith, G., Hart, C., Ferrell, C., Upton, M., Hole, D., Hawthorne, V. and Watt, G. (1997) 'Birth weight of offspring and mortality in the Renfrew and Paisley study: prospective observational study', *British Medical Journal*, vol 315, pp 1189-93.

[5] Barker, D.J.P. (1998) *Mothers, babies and health in later life*, Edinburgh: Churchill Livingstone.

[6] Gunnell, D.J., Davey Smith, G., Frankel, S., Nanchahal, K., Braddon, F.E.M., Pemberton, J. and Peters, T.J. (1998) 'Childhood leg length and adult mortality: follow up of the Carnegie (Boyd Orr) Survey of Diet and Health in Pre-war Britain', *Journal of Epidemiology and Community Health*, vol 52, pp 142-52.

[7] **Davey Smith, G., Hart, C., Blane, D. and Hole, D. (1998) 'Adverse socioeconomic conditions in childhood and cause-specific adult mortality: prospective observational study', *British Medical Journal*, vol 316, pp 1631-5.**

[8] Frankel, S., Davey Smith, G. and Gunnell, D. (1999) 'Childhood socioeconomic position and adult cardiovascular mortality: the Boyd Orr cohort', *American Journal of Epidemiology*, vol 150, pp 1081-4.

[9] Davey Smith, G., Hart, C., Blane, D., Gillis, C. and Hawthorne, V. (1997) 'Lifetime socioeconomic position and mortality: prospective observational study', *British Medical Journal*, vol 314, pp 547-52.

[10] Davey Smith, G., Hart, C., Hole, D., MacKinnon, P., Gillis, C., Watt, G., Blane, D. and Hawthorne, V. (1998) 'Education and occupational social class: which is the more important indicator of mortality risk?', *Journal of Epidemiology and Community Health*, vol 52, pp 153-60.

[11] Hart, C.L., Davey Smith, G., Hole, D.J. and Hawthorne, V.M. (1999) 'Alcohol consumption and mortality from all causes, coronary heart disease, and stroke: results from a prospective cohort study of Scottish men with 21 years of follow up', *British Medical Journal*, vol 318, pp 1725-9.

[12] Carstairs, V. and Morris, R. (1991) *Deprivation and health in Scotland*, Aberdeen: Aberdeen University Press.

[13] Hanley, J.A. (2001) 'A heuristic approach to the formulas for population attributable fraction', *Journal of Epidemiology and Community Health*, vol 55, pp 508-14.

[14] Wannamethee, S.G., Whincup, P.H., Shaper, G. and Walker, M. (1996) 'Influence of fathers' social class on cardiovascular disease in middle-aged men', *Lancet*, vol 348, pp 1259-63.

[15] Blane, D., Hart, C.L., Davey Smith, G., Gillis, C.R., Hole, D.J. and Hawthorne, V.M. (1996) 'The association of cardiovascular risk factors with socioeconomic position during childhood and adulthood', *British Medical Journal*, vol 313, pp 1434-8.

[16] Lynch, J.W. (2001) 'Socioeconomic factors in the behavioral and psychosocial epidemiology of cardiovascular disease', in N. Schneiderman, J. Gentry, J.M. da Silva, M. Speers and H. Tomes (eds) *Integrating behavioral and social sciences with public health*, Washington, DC: APA Press.

[17] Mare, R.D. (1990) 'Socioeconomic careers and differential mortality among older men in the US', in J. Vallin, S. D'Souza and A. Palloni (eds) *Measurement and analysis of mortality: New approaches*, Oxford: Clarendon Press, pp 362-87.

[18] Salhi, M., Caselli, G., Duchène, J., Egidi, V., Santini, A., Thiltgès, E. and Wunsch, G. (1995) 'Assessing mortality differentials using life histories: a method and applications', in A. Lopez, G. Caselli and T. Valkonen (eds) *Adult mortality in developed countries: From description to explanation*, Oxford: Clarendon Press.

[19] Wunsch, G., Duchène, J., Thiltgès, E. and Salhi, M. (1996) 'Socioeconomic differences in mortality: a life course approach', *European Journal of Population*, vol 12, pp 167-85.

[20] Power, C., Manor, O. and Matthews, S. (1999) 'The duration and timing of exposure: effects of socioeconomic environment on adult health', *American Journal of Public Health*, vol 89, pp 1059-65.

[21] Lynch, J.W., Kaplan, G.A. and Shema, S.J. (1997) 'Cumulative impact of sustained economic hardship on physical, cognitive, psychological and social functioning', *New England Journal of Medicine*, vol 337, pp 1889-95.

[22] **Davey Smith, G. and Shipley, M.J. (1991) 'Confounding of occupation and smoking: its magnitude and consequences', *Social Science and Medicine*, vol 32, pp 1297-300.**

[23] Marang-van de Mheen, P.J., Davey Smith, G. and Hart, C.L. (1999) 'The health impact of smoking in manual and non-manual social class men and women: a test of the Blaxter hypothesis', *Social Science and Medicine*, vol 49, pp 1851-6.

[24] Lamont, D., Parker, L., White, M., Unwin, N. et al (1999) 'Risk of cardiovascular disease measured by carotid intima-media thickness at age 49-51: life course study', *British Medical Journal*, vol 320, pp 273-8.

[25] Britton, A. and McKee, M. (2000) 'The relation between alcohol and cardiovascular disease in eastern Europe: explaining the paradox', *Journal of Epidemiology and Community Health*, vol 54, pp 328-32.

[26] Davey Smith, G., Bartley, M. and Blane, D. (1994) 'Explanations for socioeconomic differentials in mortality: evidence from Britain and elsewhere', *European Journal of Public Health*, vol 4, pp 131-44.

[27] Lynch, J.W., Kaplan, G.A. and Salonen, J.T. (1997) 'Why do poor people behave poorly? Variations in adult health behaviour and psychosocial characteristics, by stage of the socioeconomic life course', *Social Science and Medicine*, vol 44, pp 809-20.

[28] Davey Smith, G., Gunnell, D. and Ben-Shlomo, Y. (2001) 'Life-course approaches to socioeconomic differentials in cause-specific adult mortality', in D. Leon and G. Walt (eds) *Poverty, inequality and health*, Oxford: Oxford University Press.

[29] Ebrahim, S. and Davey Smith, G. (1997) 'Systematic review of randomised controlled trials of multiple risk factor interventions for preventing coronary heart disease', *British Medical Journal*, vol 314, pp 1666-74.

[30] Hart, C.L., Davey Smith, G. and Blane, D. (1998) 'Social mobility and 21 year mortality in a cohort of Scottish men', *Social Science and Medicine*, vol 47, pp 1121-30.

Section V
Further lifecourse
influences on health

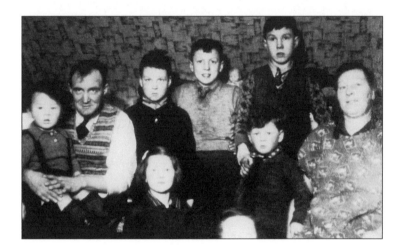

A family of nine living in a single attic room in Dundee, 1938.

20

Social circumstances in childhood and cardiovascular disease mortality: prospective observational study of Glasgow University students

George Davey Smith, Peter McCarron,
Mona Okasha and James McEwen

Background

Adverse socioeconomic circumstances in childhood have been related to increased cardiovascular disease (CVD) risk in adulthood in most, but not all, studies.[1] The findings of such studies can be difficult to interpret given the association of childhood social circumstances with social conditions and behavioural risk factors for CVD in adulthood. Statistical adjustment for these, however, generally indicates an important additional contribution of childhood socioeconomic background.[2] In this study we investigate the association between childhood circumstances and CVD mortality among male former students of Glasgow University, who will have experienced a relatively homogeneous and privileged adulthood social environment.

Methods and results

Students attending the University of Glasgow between 1948–68 were invited to participate in a medical examination carried out by the student health department.[3] Data collected included sociodemographic data, details of health behaviours and measured blood pressure. Participants were traced through the NHS Central Register. Full details are reported elsewhere.[3] The social class of the fathers of the students

Journal of Epidemiology and Community Health,
2001, vol 55, pp 340-1

was coded to the Registrar General's classification, with a combined social class III grouping being used since the distinction between III non-manual and III manual was not introduced until near the end of the recruitment period. Deaths up to 31 December 1998 were included in the analyses. Cox's proportional hazards models were used to estimate the association between fathers' social class and CVD, cancer and other (non-CVD, noncancer) mortality, adjusted for age and quintile of year of birth (to control for any cohort effect). Adjusted models for CVD included: smoking (no, 1-10, ≥11 cigarettes per day) and systolic blood pressure (mm Hg).

A total of 11,755 male students participated in the original examinations; the 3,576 female students were younger (as female intake increased over time) and provided too few deaths for analysis. We have traced 9,887 (84.1%) of the male students and social class was available for 8,856 of these (89.6%). Since age-adjusted results were similar for all individuals with social class data and for the 8,396 individuals with data available on smoking and blood pressure, we report only the latter here. There is a strong trend of increasing risk of all-cause and CVD mortality with lower paternal social class, with little trend evident for the other cause of death groups (Table 1). Adjustment for systolic blood pressure and smoking had little effect on the findings with respect to CVD mortality.

Table 1: Age-adjusted relative risks (with 95% CI) of mortality

Father's social class (n)	Cause of death (n)				
	All causes (n=866)	CVD (n=339)	Cancer (n=305)	Other (n=222)	CVD[a] (n=339)
I (1,686)	1.0	1.0	1.0	1.0	1.0
II (3,008)	1.13 (0.94-1.38)	1.51 (1.08-2.11)	1.11 (0.81-1.51)	0.81 (0.56-1.16)	1.46 (1.05-2.05)
III (3,085)	1.22 (1.00-1.47)	1.63 (1.17-2.27)	1.07 (0.78-1.46)	1.00 (0.70-1.42)	1.66 (1.19-2.32)
IV (492)	1.24 (0.90-1.70)	1.85 (1.12-3.07)	1.11 (0.65-1.91)	0.81 (0.42-1.57)	1.91 (1.15-3.17)
V (125)	1.32 (0.78-2.24)	2.36 (1.11-4.99)	0.47 (0.11-1.91)	1.34 (0.53-3.37)	2.31 (1.09-4.89)
p value for trend	0.038	0.002	0.90	0.74	0.001

[a] Adjusted for systolic blood pressure and smoking.

Note: All analyses adjusted for quintile of year of birth.

Discussion

We have demonstrated a strong and specific association between an indicator of childhood social circumstances and CVD mortality among male former Glasgow University students, in agreement with several other studies.[1] Our study has the advantage of having collected information on fathers' occupation at entry to further education (when most students would have been living at home), rather than relying on recall in middle age, which has been used in most studies of this issue. Furthermore, confounding by adulthood circumstances is unlikely to be as problematic as in most studies. Less than 5% of school leavers entered university over the period of this study[4] and those who did would generally have received educational credentials which placed them in a privileged social position in adult life. The association is specific for CVD mortality; other broad cause of death groups – which would be equally influenced by adulthood social circumstances and health-related behaviours – show no association with fathers' social class.

A range of factors – low birthweight, chronic infections acquired in childhood, and poor nutrition and growth in childhood – which are related to adverse socioeconomic circumstances in early life have been related to increased CVD risk in adulthood, and could account for the strong association observed here.[1] Blood pressure and smoking in early adulthood are related to subsequent CVD mortality in this cohort,[5,6] however, they are not strongly related to fathers' social class and thus do not confound the association reported here.

The existence of a socioeconomic gradient in CVD mortality among predominantly middle-class groups – such as civil servants in the Whitehall Study[1] – has been widely cited as evidence that psychological factors, generated by internalisation of position within social hierarchies, must be important, since there is a low prevalence of material deprivation in adulthood among these groups.[7] This study, however, indicates that childhood social circumstances strongly influence CVD mortality among an homogeneously affluent adulthood group. The socioeconomic gradient in CVD which is seen among middle-class adults could be generated by deprivation in childhood, which will have been almost entirely absent among the most privileged social groups (eg administrative level civil servants) but will have been experienced by a proportion of other middle-class groups in less favoured adulthood social locations.

References

[1] Davey Smith, G. (1997) 'Socioeconomic differentials', in D. Kuh and Y. Ben-Shlomo (eds) *A life course approach to chronic disease epidemiology*, Oxford: Oxford University Press, pp 242-73.

[2] **Davey Smith, G., Hart, C., Blane, D. and Hole, D. (1998) 'Adverse socioeconomic conditions in childhood and cause-specific adult mortality: prospective observational study', *British Medical Journal*, vol 316, pp 1631-5.**

[3] McCarron, P., Davey Smith, G., Okasha, M. and McEwen, J. (1999) 'Life course exposure and later disease: a follow-up study based on medical examinations carried out in Glasgow University (1948-68)', *Public Health*, vol 113, pp 265-71.

[4] *Higher education* (1963) Robbins Report, Cmnd 2154, London: HMSO.

[5] McCarron, P., Davey Smith, G., Okasha, M. et al (2000) 'Blood pressure in young adulthood and mortality from cardiovascular disease', *Lancet*, vol 355, pp 1430-1.

[6] McCarron, P., Davey Smith, G., Okasha, M. et al (in press) 'Smoking in adolescence and young adulthood and mortality in later life: prospective observational study', *Journal of Epidemiology and Community Health*.

[7] Syme, S.L. (1996) 'To prevent disease: the need for a new approach', in D. Blane, E. Brunner and R. Wilkinson (eds) *Health and social organisation*, London: Routledge.

21

Childhood socioeconomic position and adult cardiovascular mortality: the Boyd Orr cohort

Stephen Frankel, George Davey Smith and David Gunnell

Abstract

The relation between childhood socioeconomic position and adult cardiovascular mortality is examined in 3,750 individuals whose families took part in the Carnegie survey of family diet and health in England and Scotland between 1937 and 1939. The trend in coronary heart disease mortality across social position groups was not statistically significant at conventional levels ($p=0.12$), while a strong linear trend was seen for stroke mortality ($p=0.01$). Adjustment for the Townsend deprivation index of area of residence during adult life did not materially alter these findings, indicating that the effects of socioeconomic influences upon particular cardiovascular diseases differ according to the age at which they are experienced.

Introduction

Epidemiological interest has shifted over recent years from an almost exclusive interest in adult risk factors toward examining the extent to which adult disease may represent the outcome of processes occurring early in life. The relevance of this work to understanding mechanisms of disease and to guiding preventive strategies lies in determining the relative importance of early and later life influences and the interactions between them.[1,2] The broad impact of

American Journal of Epidemiology, 1999, vol 150, pp 1081-4

socioeconomic influences upon health is well known, but it is now becoming clear that these may have a cumulative effect over the lifecourse[3] and that different disease outcomes may be influenced by socioeconomic circumstances prevailing at different stages of life.[4] Here we investigate the extent to which cardiovascular disease may be associated with social position in childhood by means of a 60-year follow-up of a cohort of children studied in the 1930s.

Materials and methods

The methods used to establish the Boyd Orr cohort have been described elsewhere.[5,6] The material is drawn from the original records of the Carnegie survey of family diet and health in pre-war Britain, which was carried out on 1,352 families living in 16 urban and rural centres in England and Scotland between 1937 and 1939. The centres were chosen to reflect particular industrial and social conditions. The original purpose of the pre-war survey was to investigate the diets of families with children and, in particular, associations between diet, food expenditure, and the children's health. The researchers aimed to survey all families whose children attended particular schools, chosen on the advice of the local Medical Officer of Health.[7]

The NHS Central Register has been used to trace the 4,973 children whose families participated in the survey. Survey members who were alive and resident in Britain on 1 January 1948, are included in the mortality analyses that are based on deaths occurring up to 30 September 1997. Of this total population of 4,900, 767 were not traced, 293 individuals could not be assigned to social classes I-V, or identified as unemployed, and data were missing for date of death ($n=8$), and adult deprivation (Townsend) score ($n=87$); five subjects had missing data for more than one of these variables. The analyses presented here are therefore based on a total sample of 3,750.

The social position in childhood was classified according to the Registrar General's Decennial Supplement for 1931, and assignment was on the basis of the occupation of the male head of household. Social position was categorised into five groups: (1) I (professional and higher managerial) and II (intermediate); (2) III (skilled workers); (3) IV (semiskilled workers); (4) V (unskilled workers); and (5) unemployed. The proportion of subjects whose fathers were unemployed was high (33%). This was because the survey was carried out at a time of high unemployment (12% of the working population were unemployed),[8] and the survey sample was selectively drawn from families living in economically deprived areas. Weekly per capita household food expenditure was also assessed in the original pre-war survey, and we have used this to assess the validity of our measure of childhood social position. In the absence of information on the adult occupation of study members, an aggregate Census-based measure, the Townsend index, was used as a proxy measure of adult socioeconomic position. The Townsend index is constructed from Census data on levels of car ownership, unemployment, overcrowded housing, and housing tenure in the subject's health authority of residence.[9] Deaths due to coronary heart disease and stroke are those with International Classification of Diseases, Ninth Revision (ICD-9), codes 410-14 and 430-8, respectively.

Tests for trend for mean household expenditure and a Townsend deprivation score for the area of current residence or area of residence at the time of emigration or death were performed by linear regression of each continuous variable on childhood social position. Hazard ratios for the effects of childhood social position on mortality were calculated by entering the five social position groups into Cox's proportional hazards models as four dummy variables for each outcome of interest, adjusted for age, with social class III regarded as the reference category. These analyses were repeated with the Townsend deprivation score entered into the models to adjust for the level of adult deprivation for the area of current residence or area of residence at the time of emigration or death. Tests for trend for mortality rates across social position groups were performed by entering social position as a continuous variable into Cox proportional hazards models for each outcome of interest. We included the unemployed category of childhood social position in trend tests, as household food expenditure in the unemployed families was lower than in other families, as is the Townsend score for current area of residence (Table 1). To determine whether the associations between the Townsend score and mortality were consistent with a linear trend, we performed likelihood ratio

Table 1: Frequencies and mean age, household expenditure and Townsend score by childhood social position, Boyd Orr cohort, England and Scotland (1937-39)

Social position[a]	Number	%	Age at time of survey (years)	Mean household expenditure (£/week)	Townsend score
I and II	252	6.7	8.7 (4.9)[b]	0.51 (0.18)	−1.11 (2.69)[b]
III	721	19.2	6.9 (4.7)	0.37 (0.12)	−0.24 (4.02)
IV	888	23.7	7.1 (4.7)	0.36 (0.09)	−0.35 (2.93)
V	640	17.0	7.2 (4.9)	0.31 (0.09)	0.66 (5.2)
Unemployed	1,249	33.3	6.4 (4.7)	0.25 (0.07)	1.03 (4.75)
Trend test	−		−	p<0.001	p<0.001

[a] Social position groups: I, professional and higher managerial; II, intermediate; III, skilled workers; IV, semi-skilled workers; V, unskilled workers.

[b] Numbers in parentheses: standard deviation.

tests comparing models with quintiles of the Townsend score fitted as either four dummy variables or as a single linear term. Proportional hazards models were stratified for sex and district of residence at the time of the original survey. The analyses were repeated with interaction terms to test for interactions between sex and social position and between social position and adult the Townsend score. Analyses were performed using Stata software.[10]

Results

The mean household expenditure at the time of the survey shows a clear negative trend across childhood social position groups ($p<0.001$), with the children of families experiencing unemployment having approximately half the household expenditure of social classes I and II (Table 1). The Townsend score, reflecting levels of deprivation in the area of adult residence, shows a similar trend. The range of adult Townsend scores across the childhood social position groups was from –1.11 to 1.03 (a lower score implies relative affluence). The range of values across quintiles of Townsend scores was from –3.27 (standard deviation=0.51) to 7.58 (standard deviation=4.89). The correlation coefficients between childhood social class and Townsend score and between childhood household expenditure and Townsend deprivation score were 0.14 and –0.12 respectively.

An association between childhood social position and age-adjusted all-cause mortality was seen, with the hazard ratio rising from 0.84

Table 2: Hazard ratios and 95% CI for mortality (up to October 1997) in each childhood social position group (1937-39) adjusted for age and for age and adult Townsend score, stratified by sex and district, Boyd Orr cohort, England and Scotland

Social position[a]	All causes of death (n=776)		CHD[b] (n=189)		Stroke (n=50)		All-causes except CHD/stroke (n=537)	
	Age-adjusted	Age and Townsend adjusted	Age-adjusted	Age and Townsend adjusted	Age-adjusted	Age and Townsend adjusted	Age-adjusted	Age and Townsend adjusted
I and II	0.84	0.86 (0.61-1.22)	0.41	0.43 (0.19-0.98)	0.80	0.83 (0.16-4.37)	1.05	1.07 (0.71-1.60)
III	1.0	1.0	1.0	1.0	1.0	1.0	1.0	1.0
IV	1.16	1.17 (0.91-1.49)	0.88	0.89 (0.56-1.42)	1.53	1.55 (0.50-4.77)	1.27	1.27 (0.94-1.71)
V	1.20	1.19 (0.93-1.51)	1.14	1.12 (0.71-1.76)	1.43	1.40 (0.46-4.24)	1.21	1.20 (0.89-1.62)
Unemployed	1.28	1.28 (1.03-1.59)	1.04	1.04 (0.68-1.59)	2.89	3.00 (1.17-7.75)	1.28	1.28 (0.98-1.67)
Trend	$p=0.004$	$p=0.006$	$p=0.12$	$p=0.15$	$p=0.01$	$p=0.01$	$p=0.09$	$p=0.10$

[a] Social position groups: I, professional and higher managerial; II, intermediate; III, skilled workers; IV, semiskilled workers; V, unskilled workers.

[b] CHD, coronary heart disease.

for social classes I and II to 1.28 for unemployed people and with a clear trend across the social position groups (p=0.004) (Table 2). The hazard ratios for coronary heart disease mortality were raised in those from more deprived childhoods, with those in social classes I and II in childhood having lower mortality than the other more deprived childhood groups. The trend in coronary heart disease mortality across social position groups was not statistically significant at conventional levels (p=0.12). A strong trend across social position groups was seen for age-adjusted stroke mortality (p=0.01). The trend for causes of death other than coronary heart disease and stroke was small and non-significant. The reported hazard ratios were little affected by entering Townsend scores to adjust for adult socioeconomic circumstances. The likelihood ratio tests comparing models with the Townsend score as a categorical or linear term suggested the associations were consistent with a linear trend. The p values for the likelihood ratio tests comparing the two models were as follows: all-cause mortality (p=0.18); coronary heart disease (p=0.33); stroke (p=0.27); and deaths other than coronary heart disease and stroke (p=0.27). In the fully adjusted models including terms for age, Townsend score (as a linear variable), and social position, the hazard ratios for adult Townsend scores were the following: in relation to all-cause mortality (hazard ratio=1.02; 95% CI: 1.00-1.04; p=0.01); coronary heart disease mortality (hazard ratio= 1.04; 95% CI: 1.01-1.08; p=0.02); and stroke mortality (hazard ratio= 1.05; 95% CI: 0.98-1.12; p=0.2); and deaths other than coronary heart disease and stroke (hazard ratio=1.01; 95% CI: 0.99-1.04; p=0.2). No significant interactions between sex and social position or between childhood and adulthood socioeconomic measures were found in relation to all-cause, coronary heart disease, and stroke mortality.

Discussion

These findings indicate that the effects of socioeconomic influences on particular cardiovascular diseases differ according to the age at which they are experienced. The overall disadvantageous effects of deprivation in early life upon all-cause mortality are seen to correspond with a strong and graded trend in stroke mortality but a less marked trend in coronary heart disease.

Before this differential effect of socioeconomic circumstances upon these two forms of cardiovascular disease can be interpreted, the alternative explanation must be considered, that is, that social position in childhood is simply a marker for lifetime social circumstances. The finding that the associations between childhood social position and coronary heart disease, stroke, and other causes of death are different from those in relation to the adult Townsend score is an indication of a true difference between childhood and adult effects. In the absence of a direct measure of the participant's adult social class, this was the best proxy measure available to us, although we recognise that this ecological marker may not fully adjust for the effects of adult social class.

Social position in childhood does appear to be a robust marker for childhood living conditions, as is shown by the stepped differences in mean household food expenditure in the five social position groups. Unemployed people are the most deprived, as shown by their mean household food expenditure, and in line with contemporary evidence.[11] An association was found between childhood social position and adult living conditions, but this is not strong; the range of mean Townsend scores across childhood social position groups is small in comparison with the range across Townsend score fifths, and the correlations between Townsend score and both childhood social position and household expenditure were low. Finally, the trivial effects of entering the Townsend score into models of childhood social position on mortality indicate that these influences are operating through different pathways, and that childhood social position is not simply a proxy for adult living conditions. It therefore does appear that individuals carry throughout their lives a risk of stroke that is set in childhood and one more marked than the equivalent effect of childhood social circumstances upon the later risk of coronary heart disease.

This study closely replicates findings from the west of Scotland[4] and Norway, where height was negatively associated with stroke mortality; shorter stature can be regarded as a marker for those unfavourable conditions during early life that contribute to risk of stroke.[12] This effect did not emerge in a study of middle-aged US women,[13] and one other study showed no association between stroke and the father's social class, but this was a prevalence study of non-fatal stroke, and selective survival differences may have influenced the findings.[14]

The delineation of these differences in the timing of socioeconomic influences on these two forms of cardiovascular mortality is relevant to interpreting the epidemiology of coronary heart disease and stroke. It is striking that, while these conditions share so many adult risk factors, including hypertension, smoking, and obesity, the time trends and geographical patterns of the two diseases differ.[15] There is a clear relationship between stroke mortality and deprivation, but the complexity of this relation[16] may be explicable by the interaction between deprivation at an early age and later factors. Studies of this sort are consistent with patterns of disease arising from interactions between influences operating at different ages.[17] These findings strengthen the case that the origins of cardiovascular disease must be sought through investigation of factors operating throughout the lifecourse.

References

[1] Kuh, D. and Ben-Shlomo, Y. (eds) (1997) *A life course approach to chronic disease epidemiology*, Oxford: Oxford University Press.

[2] Barker, D.J.P. (1994) *Mothers, babies and disease in later life*, London: BMJ Publishing Group.

[3] **Davey Smith, G., Hart, C., Blane, D., Gillis, C. and Hawthorn, V. (1997) 'Lifetime socioeconomic position and mortality: prospective observational study', *British Medical Journal*, vol 314, pp 547-52.**

[4] **Davey Smith, G., Hart, C., Blane, D. and Hole, D. (1998) 'Adverse socioeconomic conditions in childhood and cause-specific adult mortality: the Collaborative Study', *British Medical Journal*, vol 316, pp 1631-5.**

[5] Gunnell, D.J., Frankel, S., Nanchahal, K. et al (1996) 'Life course exposure and later disease: a follow-up study based on a survey of family diet and health in pre-war Britain (1937-9)', *Public Health*, vol 110, pp 85-94.

[6] Frankel, S.J., Gunnell, D., Peters, T.J. et al (1998) 'Childhood energy intake and adult cancer – the Boyd Orr Cohort Study', *British Medical Journal*, vol 316, pp 499-504.

[7] Rowett Research Institute (1955) *Family diet and health in pre-war Britain*, Dunfermline: Carnegie UK Trust.

[8] Denman, J. and McDonald, P. (1996) 'Unemployment statistics from 1881 to the present day', *Labour Market Trends*, vol 104, pp 5-17.

[9] Phillimore, P., Beattie, A. and Townsend, P. (1994) 'Widening inequality of health in northern England, 1981-1991', *British Medical Journal*, vol 308, pp 1125-8.

[10] Stata Corporation (1996) *Stats statistical software: Release 5.0*, College Station, TX: Stata Corporation.

[11] Cole, G.D.H. and Cole, M.I. (1937) *The condition of Britain*, London: Victor Gollancz.

[12] Njølstad, I., Arnesen, E. and Lund-Larsen, P.G. (1996) 'Body height, cardiovascular risk factors, and risk of stroke in middle-aged men and women', *Stroke*, vol 94, pp 2877-82.

[13] Gliksman, M.D., Kawachi, I., Hunter, D. et al (1995) 'Childhood socioeconomic status and risk of cardiovasuclar disease in middle aged US women: a prospective study', *Journal of Epidemiology and Community Health*, vol 49, pp 10-15.

[14] Wannamethee, S.G., Whincup, P.H., Shaper, G. and Walker, M. (1996) 'Influence of fathers' social class on cardiovascular disease in middle-aged men', *Lancet*, vol 348, pp 1259-63.

[15] Davey Smith, G. and Ben-Shlomo, Y. (1997) 'Geographical and social class differentials in stroke mortality – the influence of early-life factors', *Journal of Epidemiology and Community Health*, vol 51, pp 134-7.

[16] Maheswaran, R., Elliott, P. and Strachan, D.P. (1997) 'Socioeconomic deprivation, ethnicity, and stroke mortality in Greater London and South East England', *Journal of Epidemiology and Community Health*, vol 51, pp 127-31.

[17] Frankel, S.J., Elwood, P., Sweetnam, P. et al (1996) 'Birthweight, body-mass index in middle age, and incident coronary heart disease', *Lancet*, vol 348, pp 1478-80.

22

Height and risk of death among men and women: aetiological implications of associations with cardiorespiratory disease and cancer mortality

George Davey Smith, Carole Hart,
Mark Upton, David Hole, Charles Gillis,
Graham Watt and Victor Hawthorne

Abstract

Objectives: Height is inversely associated with cardiovascular disease mortality risk and has shown variable associations with cancer incidence and mortality. The interpretation of findings from previous studies has been constrained by data limitations. Associations between height and specific causes of death were investigated in a large general population cohort of men and women from the West of Scotland.

Design: Prospective observational study.

Setting: Renfrew and Paisley, in the West of Scotland.

Participants: 7,052 men and 8,354 women aged 45-64 were recruited into a study in Renfrew and Paisley, in the West of Scotland, between 1972 and 1976. Detailed assessments of cardiovascular disease risk factors, morbidity and socioeconomic circumstances were made at baseline.

Main outcome measures: Deaths during 20 years' of follow-up classified into specific causes.

Journal of Epidemiology and Community Health,
2000, vol 54, pp 97-103

Results: Over the follow-up period, 3,347 men and 2,638 women died. Height is inversely associated with all-cause, coronary heart disease, stroke, and respiratory disease mortality among men and women. Adjustment for socioeconomic position and cardiovascular risk factors had little influence on these associations. Height is strongly associated with forced expiratory volume in one second (FEV_1) and adjustment for FEV_1 considerably attenuated the association between height and cardiorespiratory mortality. Smoking-related cancer mortality is not associated with height. The risk of deaths from cancer unrelated to smoking tended to increase with height, particularly for haematopoietic, colorectal and prostate cancers. Stomach cancer mortality was inversely associated with height. Adjustment for socioeconomic position had little influence on these associations.

Conclusion: Height serves partly as an indicator of socioeconomic circumstances and nutritional status in childhood and this may underlie the inverse associations between height and adulthood cardiorespiratory mortality. Much of the association between height and cardiorespiratory mortality was accounted for by lung function, which is also partly determined by exposures acting in childhood. The inverse association between height and stomach cancer mortality probably reflects *Helicobacter pylori* infection in childhood resulting in – or being associated with – shorter height. The positive associations between height and several cancers unrelated to smoking could reflect the influence of calorie intake during childhood on the risk of these cancers.

Introduction

The suggestion that stature is inversely related to the risk of disease and mortality dates back to the late 19th century.[1] Insurance industry data from the early decades of the 20th century demonstrated that taller people, on average, lived longer lives than shorter people.[2] More recently, height has been investigated in relation to coronary heart disease (CHD) risk, with case-control and prospective studies identifying inverse associations of height with the extent of atherosclerosis,[3] CHD incidence and CHD mortality.[4-7] A few studies have examined other illnesses and have generally,[7-10] but not always,[11] found inverse associations of height with stroke. Inverse associations have been found with respiratory disease risk,[7] and inconsistent results with respect to cancer.[6,7,10,12] Several mechanisms have been advanced to account for the associations that have been found. Firstly, height could serve as an indicator of growth, nutrition and social environment in earlier life. Poor foetal development[13] and poor growth during childhood[14] have been associated with increased cardiovascular disease risk in adulthood, as have indicators of unfavourable social circumstances in childhood.[15-17] Conversely, a high calorie intake in childhood may be related to an increased risk of cancer in later life.[18] Secondly, height is related to social class in adulthood and thus socially patterned exposures – including health-related behaviours, psychosocial influences, environmental factors and the physiological consequences of these – could account for the observed disease associations. Thirdly, the early stages of disease could lead to reductions in height and this process could generate the relation between height and mortality.[7] The studies of height and mortality that have been published to date have suffered from one or more of a series of limitations: they tend to be restricted to men; they have often used data sources in which information on socioeconomic position, cardiorespiratory disease risk factors and health-related behaviours have not been available; and they have generally involved small samples, so cause-specific mortality could not be examined. This study overcomes these limitations and presents a detailed analysis of height and mortality among a representative population sample of men and women from the west of Scotland.

Methods

The Renfrew/Paisley general population study was carried out between 1972 and 1976: the sampling frame was residents of the towns of Renfrew and Paisley aged 45-64 years, and a near 80% response rate was achieved. Full details of the study methodology have been reported previously.[19] A questionnaire was completed by each participant and this was checked when the participant attended a screening examination. The questionnaire recorded smoking habit, occupation, respiratory and cardiovascular symptoms. Social class was determined by regular occupation, according to the Registrar General's classification.[20] In the case of retired people, the last full-time occupation was taken. For housewives, husbands' or fathers' occupations were used. Participants were classified as non-manual if they were in social classes I, II or IIIN and manual if in social classes IIIM, IV or V. Blood pressure, height (to the nearest centimetre) and weight were measured and an electrocardiogram was recorded at the screening examination.

A non-fasting blood sample was also taken to measure plasma cholesterol concentration. Forced expiratory volume in one second (FEV_1) was measured and is treated both as a simple continuous variable and as an 'FEV score', expressed as a percentage of the expected FEV_1 for age and height, calculated from the subset of healthy never smoking participants.[21] The six lead electrocardiogram (ECG) (leads I, II, III, AVr, AVl and AVf) was taken with the subject sitting. Criteria for myocardial ischaemia on ECG were based on the Minnesota coding scheme. Any of the following codes were considered evidence of ischaemia, encompassing diagnoses of definite myocardial infarction, myocardial ischaemia and left bundle branch block: 1.1–1.3, 4.1–4.4, 5.1–5.3, 7.1. Angina was considered present if the definite or possible criteria of the Rose Angina Questionnaire were met.[22] Bronchitis was classified according to responses to the Medical Research Council questionnaire.[23] The home address at the time of screening was retrospectively postcoded, enabling an area-based deprivation category at the time of the 1981 Census to be ascertained.[24] Deprivation category varies from 1 (least deprived) to 7 (most deprived). Deprivation category and individual social class are related independently to mortality in the study population.[25] A total of 7,052 men and 8,354 women were included in the study. This differs slightly from numbers given in previous publications (7,058 men and 8,353 women) as 13 miscodings of sex and five people who attended twice were recently discovered. Height data were missing for three men and 10 women, who were excluded from all analyses. The analyses were therefore performed on 7,049 men and 8,344 women. For seven participants' addresses could not be postcoded and assigned a deprivation category and 423 participants had given insuffcient information on occupation to assign a social class. Dummy variables were created for these participants for inclusion in multivariable analyses. Participants were flagged at the NHS Central Register in Edinburgh and notification of deaths have been received for a 20-year follow-up period. Cause of deaths were coded to the International Classification of Diseases, Ninth Revision (ICD-9).[26] We classified the following as smoking related cancers; lip (ICD-9 140); tongue (141); mouth and pharynx (143–9); oesophagus (150); pancreas (157); respiratory tract (160–3) and urinary tract (188–9).[18] As height was measured to the nearest centimetre, the approximate quintile groups showed some variation in size. Analyses were conducted by height quintile and also according to a 10cm lower height, assuming a linear relation between height and outcome. Age-adjusted means for continuous variables were calculated using PROC GLM of the SAS system. Categorical variables were age-standardised by the direct method, using the male and female study populations as the standard. Age-adjusted mortality rates were calculated using a person-years at risk based lifetable approach and age standardisation was by the direct method. Trend tests were obtained through proportional hazards regression using PROC PHREG. Proportional hazards regression analyses of the whole cohort were stratified by sex within the PROC PHREG routine in SAS, except where sex-specific analyses have been reported. The exponentiated proportional hazards regression coefficients are referred to as relative rates.

Results

For men the mean height was 169.6 cm (standard deviation 6.8; first centile 154cm and 99th centile 185 cm). For women the mean height was 157.7cm (standard deviation 6.1cm; first centile 143cm and 99th

Table 1: Risk factors according to height quintiles (age-adjusted means or proportions)

	Height quintile (cm)					
	≤163	164-167	168-170	171-174	≥175	Trend[a]
Men						
Number	1,281	1,359	1,305	1,480	1,624	
Mean age at screening (years)[b]	55.2	54.7	54.2	53.8	53.1	p=0.0001
Mean diastolic BP (mm Hg)	85.8	85.5	86.4	85.5	86.9	p=0.019
Mean cholesterol (mmol/l)	5.87	5.85	5.87	5.85	5.87	p=0.60
Mean body mass index (kg/m²)	25.9	25.9	26.0	25.8	25.8	p=0.29
Mean FEV$_1$ (l)	2.18	2.37	2.49	2.63	2.82	p=0.0001
Mean-adjusted FEV$_1$ (%)	88.3	88.2	88.2	89.4	88.9	p=0.10
% never smoked	17.5	17.1	16.5	16.4	16.4	p=0.35
% current cigarette smokers	61.4	58.2	54.2	55.9	54.5	p=0.0003
% ex-smokers	19.5	22.2	27.0	25.7	27.6	p=0.0001
% deprivation category 5-7	68.2	62.6	59.6	53.1	49.7	p=0.0001
% social classes IV and V	37.7	31.2	28.6	25.6	22.4	p=0.0001
% angina (definite and possible)	21.6	18.9	17.5	15.2	15.3	p=0.0001
% bronchitis	7.6	6.4	6.4	4.4	4.5	p=0.0001
% ECG ischaemia	12.4	10.5	10.1	9.3	10.2	p=0.036
	≤152	153-155	156-158	159-162	≥163	Trend[a]
Women						
Number	1,638	1,378	1,606	2,003	1,719	
Mean age at screening (years)[b]	55.9	54.9	54.5	53.9	53.0	p=0.0001
Mean diastolic BP (mm Hg)	85.4	85.6	84.8	84.9	85.2	p=0.53
Mean cholesterol (mmol/l)	6.49	6.45	6.42	6.42	6.35	p=0.001
Mean body mass index (kg/m²)	26.5	26.2	25.8	25.8	25.0	p=0.0001
Mean FEV$_1$ (l)	1.55	1.66	1.78	1.84	2.00	p=0.0001
Mean-adjusted FEV$_1$ (%)	90.3	90.9	93.6	92.8	94.4	p=0.0001
% never smoked	45.8	46.6	46.2	44.9	45.3	p=0.11
% current cigarette smokers	48.5	47.7	45.6	47.2	45.0	p=0.29
% ex-smokers	5.5	5.7	8.2	7.8	9.6	p=0.0001
% deprivation category 5-7	66.9	60.6	58.5	56.7	50.9	p=0.0001
% social classes IV and V	48.3	42.3	39.8	35.0	29.2	p=0.0001
% angina (definite and possible)	20.9	17.0	17.2	15.9	13.9	p=0.0001
% bronchitis	6.5	3.8	4.2	3.1	3.2	p=0.0001
% ECG ischaemia	10.8	11.5	9.6	9.7	8.6	p=0.021

[a] Using height as a continuous variable.

[b] Not age-adjusted.

Table 2: Age-adjusted 20-year mortality (per 10,000 person years) in the Renfrew/Paisley study by height quintile

	Height quintile (cm)					RR[a] (95% CI)	RR[b] (95% CI)
	≤163	164-167	168-170	171-174	≥175		
Men (*n*=7,049)							
All-cause							
Number of deaths	685	704	600	661	697		
Death rate	257.5	255.5	234.7	232.5	233.1	1.13	1.10[c]
						(1.07-1.19)	(1.04-1.16)
CHD							
Number of deaths	278	248	238	251	266		
Death rate	132.6	115.1	111.6	105.3	107.5	1.14	1.12[c]
						(1.05-1.24)	(1.03-1.22)
Stroke							
Number of deaths	74	64	57	59	48		
Death rate	43.3	38.5	33.0	32.9	25.6	1.32	1.30[c]
						(1.11-1.57)	(1.10-1.55)
Respiratory disease							
Number of deaths	69	72	51	40	48		
Death rate	36.9	42.0	30.9	22.6	23.6	1.45	1.35[d]
						(1.21-1.72)	(1.12-1.61)
Smoking-related cancer							
Number of deaths	115	129	109	131	148		
Death rate	61.5	63.0	55.0	59.6	64.1	1.03	0.96[d]
						(0.91-1.15)	(0.86-1.09)
Smoking-unrelated cancer							
Number of deaths	60	81	64	70	90		
Death rate	35.2	43.7	35.2	35.9	40.5	0.92	0.88[e¶]
						(0.79-1.07)	(0.75-1.03)
Women (*n*=8,344)							
All cause							
Number of deaths	632	473	515	598	420		
Death rate	177.6	168.0	160.7	156.9	137.4	1.19	1.16[c]
						(1.11-1.26)	(1.08-1.23)
CHD							
Number of deaths	208	149	130	179	105		
Death rate	69.0	61.2	48.3	54.8	40.3	1.29	1.22[c]
						(1.15-1.45)	(1.08-1.37)
Stroke							
Number of deaths	101	78	75	75	57		
Death rate	35.2	34.9	30.5	27.7	25.9	1.23	1.20[c]
						(1.04-1.45)	(1.02-1.43)
Respiratory disease							
Number of deaths	54	43	36	32	23		
Death rate	19.1	19.6	15.2	10.5	9.6	1.75	1.77[d]
						(1.40-2.18)	(1.38-2.27)
Smoking related cancer							
Number of deaths	62	35	55	80	62		
Death rate	22.8	15.0	20.7	24.2	22.6	0.98	1.01[d]
						(0.81-1.18)	(0.83-1.23)
Smoking unrelated cancer							
Number of deaths	94	94	123	136	107		
Death rate	32.5	40.3	44.5	39.4	35.3	0.93	0.89[e]
						(0.81-1.07)	(0.77-1.02)

a Age-adjusted relative rate for 10cm lower height.
b Fully adjusted relative rate for 10cm lower height.
c Adjusted for social class, deprivation category, smoking, diastolic blood pressure, cholesterol, body mass index and FEV_1 score.
d Adjusted for social class, deprivation category, smoking, body mass index and FEV_1 score.
e Adjusted for social class, deprivation category, body mass index and FEV_1 score.

centile 172cm). The characteristics of the population according to height are presented in Table 1. For both men and women greater height was associated with younger age at screening, therefore data on all other factors were age adjusted. Taller participants were less likely to come from social class IV and V, less likely to live in deprived areas, less likely to report angina or bronchitis on a screening questionnaire, more likely to be ex-smokers, and less likely to have ischaemia detected on an ECG than shorter participants. Taller participants had higher FEV_1 than shorter participants and for women, but not men, this was also true for FEV_1 score. For men, but not women, taller participants had slightly higher blood pressure and were less likely to be current cigarette smokers than shorter participants. For women, but not men, taller participants had lower plasma cholesterol concentrations and lower body mass index than shorter participants.

Table 2 shows the mortality rates and relative rates associated with 10cm lower height. All-cause, coronary heart disease, stroke and respiratory disease mortality are inversely related to height. For both sexes, respiratory disease is the cause of death most strongly associated with height. For men, stroke is more strongly associated with height than coronary heart disease, while there is little difference for women. Adjustment for socioeconomic, behavioural and physiological risk factors had little influence on the association between height and mortality. In these adjustments the FEV_1 score was used as the measure of lung function. Raw FEV_1 is strongly correlated with height (r=0.38 for men and r=0.37 for women), and some studies have suggested that lung function accounts for the association of height with cardiovascular mortality and morbidity.[4] Including raw FEV_1 rather than FEV_1 score among the factors adjusted for resulted in considerable attenuation of the associations between height and cardiorespiratory mortality, with relative rates for 10cm lower height in men being 1.02 (95% CI: 0.93-1.11) for CHD; 1.19 (0.99-1.42) for stroke and 0.91 (0.75-1.09) for respiratory disease mortality in the fully adjusted models. For women the equivalent relative rates were 1.08 (0.95-1.22) for CHD 1.10 (0.92-1.31) for stroke and 1.28 (0.99-1.65) for respiratory disease mortality. We also examined the associations between raw FEV_1 and cardiorespiratory mortality (Table 3). The strong associations found were little influenced by adjustment for height.

Smoking-related cancer mortality is not associated with height (Table 2). Mortality from smoking unrelated cancers tended to be

Table 3: Age-adjusted relative rates (and 95% CI) for a 1 standard deviation lower FEV$_1$, with and without additional height adjustment

	CHD	Stroke	Respiratory disease
Men			
Age[a]	1.28 (1.21-1.36)	1.38 (1.22-1.55)	3.55 (3.14-4.01)
Age/height[b]	1.27 (1.20-1.36)	1.33 (1.17-1.51)	3.60 (3.18-4.07)
Women			
Age[a]	1.42 (1.31-1.53)	1.34 (1.20-1.49)	2.77 (2.39-3.20)
Age/height[b]	1.40 (1.29-1.51)	1.32 (1.17-1.48)	2.71 (2.32-3.17)

[a] Adjusted for age.
[b] Adjusted for age and height.

positively associated with height, although there was considerable heterogeneity within this category. Table 4 shows that stomach cancer is inversely associated with height. Mortality from haematopoietic cancers, colorectal cancer and prostate cancer tended to be directly related to height, while breast cancer was unrelated to height. The association between height and haematopoietic cancer was largely limited to lymphoma (ICD-9 200–3), with an age-adjusted combined relative rate of 0.44 (95% CI: 0.29-0.65) for 10cm lower height; for leukaemia (ICD-9 204–8) the equivalent relative rate was 0.89 (0.46-1.72). There were no significant interactions between height and sex in any of these analyses. For all-cause and cardiorespiratory disease

Table 4: Relative rates (and 95% CI) for 10cm lower height for cancers unrelated to smoking

	Number	Male RR[a]	Female RR[a]	Combined RR[a]	Combined RR[b]
All smoking unrelated cancers	919	0.92 (0.79-1.07)	0.93 (0.81-1.07)	0.92 (0.83-1.02)	0.89 (0.80-0.99)
Stomach (ICD-9 151)	103	1.43 (0.95-2.14)	1.54 (0.98-2.41)	1.47 (1.09-1.99)	1.33 (0.97-1.80)
Colorectal (ICD-9 153-4)	201	0.71 (0.53-0.96)	0.80 (0.58-1.10)	0.75 (0.60-0.94)	0.70 (0.56-0.88)
Breast (ICD-9 174)	147	–	1.13 (0.86-1.48)	–	–
Prostate (ICD-9 185)	59	0.77 (0.53-1.14)	–	–	–
Haematopoietic (ICD-9 200-8)	79	0.63 (0.39-1.03)	0.45 (0.28-0.73)	0.53 (0.38-0.75)	0.52 (0.36-0.73)
Other (remainder)	330	1.14 (0.87-1.49)	0.90 (0.72-1.13)	0.99 (0.83-1.18)	0.98 (0.82-1.17)

[a] Adjusted relative rate for age.

[b] Adjusted relative rate for age, social class and deprivation category.

mortality, associations were analysed separately for the first 10 years and second 10 years of follow-up. The only finding consistent between sexes was that the association between height and respiratory disease mortality was considerably stronger over the initial 10-year follow-up period than the later period. For men the relative rate for 10cm lower height over the first 10 years of follow up was 1.75 (1.32-2.33); over the second 10 years this was 1.28 (1.03-1.61). For women the equivalent relative rates were 2.20 (1.51-3.20) and 1.58 (1.21-2.07).

Discussion

Height in this large general population study is inversely associated with all-cause mortality among men and women over a 20-year follow-up period. The strength and direction of the association between height and mortality varies between broad cause of death groups, however. Among both men and women, respiratory disease mortality is most strongly associated with height, with inverse associations also being seen for cardiovascular disease mortality. Among men the association is stronger with respect to stroke than CHD, although among women there is little difference between these associations. Stomach cancer mortality is inversely associated with height, while smoking-related cancer mortality is not associated with height. Mortality from smoking-unrelated cancers, with the exception of stomach cancer, tends to be positively associated with height: taller people experience higher mortality rates.

General explanations of height–mortality associations

Two possible general explanations of inverse associations between height and mortality need to be considered. Firstly, height is associated with socioeconomic position: people in better socioeconomic circumstances are, on average, taller. This is shown in our own data with respect to occupational social class and area-based deprivation measures. Confounding by socioeconomic position would, then, be expected to produce inverse associations between height and mortality. If this explanation were the case then these associations should be seen for all causes of death that show strong socioeconomic gradients. Smoking-related cancers demonstrate some of the strongest associations with adverse socioeconomic circumstances,[27] however, they are not related to height. This argues against socioeconomic confounding as being key to the height–mortality associations, as does the robustness of the associations to adjustment for social class and area-based deprivation scores in the present data. Secondly, early stages of disease could lead to a loss of height.[7] This could either be real, because of disc space compression, or apparent, because of an inability to stretch during height measurement. In either case the lower measured height, on average, of the sick would produce inverse height-mortality associations.[7] This has been explored in a previous study by analysing mortality during earlier and later periods of mortality follow up. Such reverse causation should produce stronger inverse associations in the earlier period of follow-up, because as people with pre-existing disease die and are removed from the cohort they contribute less and less to the height–mortality associations. In an earlier study such attenuation over time was seen for both respiratory disease and CHD mortality.[7] In the present data such attenuation was only convincingly demonstrated for respiratory disease mortality. This suggests that such reverse causality is mainly an issue with respect to respiratory disease, a finding that is biologically plausible.

Height and cause-specific mortality

There are several factors, indexed by short stature, which could be responsible for the associations between height and mortality. Adult height is influenced by foetal development (indexed by birth weight), and growth during pregnancy and adolescence.[28] Factors that result in reduced birth weights – such as poor maternal nutrition and smoking – may, therefore, influence adult height. Genetic factors are also clearly of importance, although these could not be investigated in this study. Nutrition in infancy and adolescence are reflected in final adult height. Adverse social circumstances during childhood are also related to shorter stature in adulthood.[28] It is notable that, in this study, height is inversely associated with risk of stomach cancer, stroke, CHD and respiratory disease mortality. In a separate Scottish cohort we have demonstrated that adverse social circumstances in childhood – indexed by paternal occupational social class – are associated with high rates of mortality from these causes.[17] Early life determinants of stomach cancer mortality are implicated by ecological correlations between present day stomach cancer rates and indicators of adverse social circumstances, at the time when the cohorts who are currently developing stomach cancer were children.[29] *Helicobacter pylori* infection is generally acquired in childhood and this has been shown to be related to overcrowded housing and poor sanitary environments.[30] *H pylori* infection persisting from childhood is an important cause of stomach cancer[31] and is also associated with poorer growth and shorter attained height.[32,33] Thus the inverse association between height and stomach cancer mortality, also seen in a previous study,[34] could reflect chronic *H pylori* infection.

The higher stroke, CHD and respiratory disease mortality of people who experienced worse social circumstances in childhood is seen after socioeconomic position and cardiorespiratory risk factors in adulthood are taken into account.[17] Similarly, in the present data, adjusting for indicators of adulthood socioeconomic position, blood pressure, smoking, body mass index, cholesterol and FEV_1 score had little effect on the inverse association between height and cardiovascular mortality; a more substantial attenuation of the association between height and respiratory disease mortality was seen, although a substantial residual effect remained. Adjustment for raw FEV_1 greatly attenuated the associations between height and cardiorespiratory mortality, however. There has been considerable debate in the literature as to the appropriateness of adjusting for raw lung function measures when assessing the association between height and mortality.[4,35-39] Height is strongly correlated with raw FEV_1, in part simply because taller people have larger lungs. Thus adjusting for raw FEV_1 is adjusting for a proxy for height itself. In the present data, as in an earlier study,[35] it is noticeable that adjusting height–mortality associations for raw FEV_1 greatly attenuates the relative rates, while adjusting raw FEV_1-mortality associations for height has virtually no effect. If the problem was simply one of collinearity it should influence both sets of adjustments. The FEV_1 score is an index of lung health, while raw FEV_1 is an index of both lung health and lung capacity. In this simplified scheme, lung health includes a component attributable to airways geometry that is not proportional to height.[40] Raw FEV_1 is thus influenced both by body dimensions and by exposures acting across the lifecourse that influence lung function in adulthood. These factors include foetal development, childhood chest illnesses, smoking and occupational exposures in adulthood.[41] Adjustment for raw FEV_1 may, therefore, be equivalent to adjusting for a sensitive index of accumulating exposures acting across the lifecourse.[42]

The associations between adult height and cancer have been inconsistent across cancer sites, for cancer incidence or cancer mortality, and between studies,[7,10,12,43,44] although generally it is cancers unrelated to smoking that are found to be positively associated with height.[12,45] The positive associations we found between height and prostate cancer, colorectal cancer and lymphoma have been seen in most, but not all, previous studies.[7,11,43,44] In most previous studies, height has been positively associated with breast cancer risk,[46] although we did not find this. The interpretation of positive height–cancer associations has focused on caloric intake in early life as a determinant of both height and later cancer risk,[12,45] a suggestion that is strengthened by the recent demonstration of a direct association between energy intake in childhood and later risk of non-smoking related cancers.[18] Animal experiments have repeatedly demonstrated that caloric restriction from early age reduces the risk of cancer in later life.[47] Recent reports of positive associations between insulin-like growth factor-I (IGF-I) levels and prostate, colon and breast cancer provide a possible mechanism for the above associations.[48-50] Calorie restricted diets that decrease cancer risk in animals also decrease IGF–I levels.[51] Height may serve as an indicator of IGF–I levels during growth and developmental phases,[52] which has been proposed as the period during which IGF–I levels act to increase cancer risk in later life.[50]

Height may reflect other early life exposures, such as the absence or delay of childhood infections. Large sibships, which are associated with shorter height, have been associated with a reduced risk of Hodgkin's disease.[53] In another study in the west of Scotland[17] we have found an inverse association between number of siblings and risk of mortality from lymphoma (Davey Smith and Hart, unpublished observations).

Long-term secular trends in height have been associated with changing mortality rates in Britain and elsewhere.[54] In Britain for people born during the second quarter of the 19th century, height decreased with year of birth, then increased for people born after the mid-century.[54] This pattern is strikingly similar to mortality trends. All-cause mortality showed no improvement (and in some places even increased) over the second quarter of the century, and then from around 1850 mortality reductions were seen in a cohort-specific manner, first for children, then for young adults and then for older adults.[55,56] Both the height and mortality data suggest that childhood circumstances started to improve around the middle of the 19th century and that people who were young children during this period took with them, as their cohort aged, a reduced mortality risk. Our data on the cause-specific associations of mortality and height suggest that a similar co-dependency of height and mortality may be occurring presently. Height in Britain has continued to increase throughout the second half of the 20th century.[57] The causes of death that are inversely associated with height are those that tend to be decreasing, such as stroke, stomach cancer and respiratory disease mortality. The causes of death that show a positive association with height are those showing less favourable trends, such as prostate cancer, lymphoma and colorectal cancer. The factors that underlie the secular trend of increasing height in the population may also be influencing cause-specific mortality rates. Plausible underlying factors include increasing net energy balance (that is, energy intake minus that expended in physical activity, in keeping warm, etc) in childhood, and decreases and delays in infection in childhood.[58]

References

[1] British Association for the Advancement of Science (1883) *Final report of the Anthropometric Committee*, London: British Association for the Advancement of Science.

[2] Dublin, L.I., Lotka, A.J. and Spiegelman, M. (1949) *Length of life: A study of the life table*, New York, NY: The Ronald Press Company.

[3] Nwasokwa, O.N., Weiss, M., Gladstone, C. et al (1997) 'Higher prevalence and greater severity of coronary disease in short versus tall men referred for coronary arteriography', *American Heart Journal*, vol 133, pp 147-52.

[4] Walker, M., Shaper, A.G., Phillips, A.N. et al (1989) 'Short stature, lung function and risk of a heart attack', *International Journal of Epidemiology*, vol 18, pp 602-6.

[5] Palmer, J.R., Rosenberg, L. and Shapiro, S. (1990) 'Stature and the risk of myocardial infarction in women', *American Journal of Epidemiology*, vol 132, pp 27-32.

[6] Yarnell, J.G.W., Limb, E.S., Layzell, J.M. et al (1992) 'Height: a risk marker for ischaemic heart disease', *European Heart Journal*, vol 13, pp 1602-5.

[7] Leon, D., Davey Smith, G., Shipley, M. et al (1995) 'Adult height and mortality in London: early life, socioeconomic confounding or shrinkage?', *Journal of Epidemiology and Community Health*, vol 49, pp 5-9.

[8] Njolstad, I., Arnesen, E. and Lund-Larsen, P.G. (1996) 'Body height, cardiovascular risk factors, and risk of stroke in middle-aged men and women: a 14-year follow-up of the Finnmark Study', *Circulation*, vol 94, pp 2877-82.

[9] Walker, S.P., Rimm, E.B., Ascherio, A. et al (1996) 'Body size and fat distribution as predictors of stroke among US men', *American Journal of Epidemiology*, vol 144, pp 1143-50.

[10] Tverdal, A. (1989) *A mortality follow-up of persons invited to a cardiovascular disease study in five areas in Norway*, Oslo: National Health Screening Service.

[11] Wannamethee, S.G., Shaper, A.G., Whincup, P.H. et al (1998) 'Adult height, stroke and coronary heart disease', *American Journal of Epidemiology*, vol 148, pp 1069-76.

[12] Davey Smith, G., Shipley, M. and Leon, D. (1998) 'Height and cancer mortality among men: prospective observational study', *British Medical Journal*, vol 317, pp 1351-2.

[13] Barker, D.J.P. (1994) *Mothers, babies, and disease in later life*, London: BMJ Publishing Group.

[14] Gunnell, D.J., Davey Smith, G., Frankel, S.J. et al (1998) 'Childhood leg length and adult mortality: follow up of the Carnegie (Boyd Orr) survey of diet and health in pre-war Britain', *Journal of Epidemiology and Community Health*, vol 52, pp 142-52.

[15] **Davey Smith, G., Hart, C., Blane, D., Gillis, C. and Hawthorn, V. (1997) 'Lifetime socioeconomic position and mortality: prospective observational study', *British Medical Journal*, vol 314, pp 547-52.**

[16] Wannamethee, S.G., Whincup, P.H., Shaper, G. et al (1996) 'Influence of fathers' social class on cardiovascular disease in middle-aged men', *Lancet*, vol 348, pp 1259-63.

[17] **Davey Smith, G., Hart, C., Blane, D. and Hole, D. (1998) 'Adverse socioeconomic conditions in childhood and cause-specific adult mortality: prospective observational study', *British Medical Journal*, vol 316, pp 1631-5.**

[18] Frankel, S., Gunnell, D.J., Peters, T.J. et al (1998) 'Childhood energy intake and adult cancer – The Boyd Orr cohort study', *British Medical Journal*, vol 316, pp 499-504.

[19] Hawthorne, V.M., Watt, G.C.M., Hart, C.L. et al (1995) 'Cardiorespiratory disease in men and women in urban Scotland: baseline characteristics of the Renfrew/Paisley (Midspan) population study', *Scottish Medical Journal*, vol 40, pp 102-7.

[20] Anonymous (1966) *General Register Office classification of occupations*, London: HMSO.

[21] Hole, D.J., Watt, G.C.M., Davey Smith, G. et al (1996) 'Impaired lung function and mortality risk in men and women: findings from the Renfrew and Paisley prospective population study', *British Medical Journal*, vol 313, pp 711-15.

22 Rose, G.A., Blackburn, H., Gillum, R.F. et al (1982) *Cardiovascular survey methods*, Geneva: WHO.

23 Medical Research Council (1965) 'Definition and classification of chronic bronchitis for epidemiological purposes', *Lancet*, vol 1, pp 775-9.

24 Carstairs, V. and Morris, R. (1991) *Deprivation and health in Scotland*, Aberdeen: Aberdeen University Press.

25 **Davey Smith, G., Hart, C., Watt, G., Hole, D. and Hawthorn, V. (1998) 'Individual social class, area-based deprivation, cardiovascular disease risk-factors and mortality: the Renfrew and Paisley study', *Journal of Epidemiology and Community Health*, vol 52, pp 399-405.**

26 World Health Organisation (1977) *Manual of the international, statistical classification of diseases, injuries, and causes of death*, 9th revision, Geneva: WHO.

27 **Davey Smith, G., Leon, D., Shipley, M.J. and Rose, G. (1991) 'Socioeconomic differentials in cancer among men', *International Journal of Epidemiology*, vol 20, pp 339-45.**

28 Eveleth, P.B. and Tanner, J.M. (1990) *World-wide variation in human growth* (2nd edn), Cambridge: Cambridge University Press.

29 Barker, D.J.P., Coggon, D., Osmond, C. et al (1990) 'Poor housing in childhood and high rates of stomach cancer in England and Wales', *British Journal of Cancer*, vol 61, pp 575-8.

30 Malaty, H.M. and Graham, D.Y. (1994) 'Importance of childhood socioeconomic status on the current prevalence of *Helicobacter pylori* infection', *Gut*, vol 35, pp 742-5.

31 Forman, D., Newell, D.G., Fullerton, F. et al (1991) 'Association between infection with *Helicobacter pylori* and risk of gastric cancer: evidence from a prospective investigation', *British Medical Journal*, vol 302, pp 1302-5.

32 Patel, P., Mendall, M., Khulusi, S. et al (1994) '*Helicobacter pylori* infection in childhood: risk factors and effect on growth, *British Medical Journal*, vol 309, pp 1119-23.

33 Mendall, M., Molineaux, N., Levy, J. et al (1994) 'Association of *H pylori* with diminished adult height', *Gut*, vol 35, p S4.

[34] Hansson, L.-E., Baron, J., Nyrén, O. et al (1994) 'Early-life risk indicators of gastric cancer: a population-based case-control study in Sweden', *International Journal of Cancer*, vol 57, pp 32-7.

[35] Strachan, D.P. (1992) 'Ventilatory function, height, and mortality among lifelong non-smokers', *Journal of Epidemiology and Community Health*, vol 46, pp 66-70.

[36] Cook, N.R., Hebert, P.R., Satterfield, S. et al (1994) 'Height, lung function, and mortality from cardiovascular disease among the elderly', *American Journal of Epidemiology*, vol 139, pp 1066-76.

[37] Rich-Edwards, J.W., Manson, J.E., Stampfer, M.J. et al (1995) 'Height and the risk of cardiovascular disease in women', *American Journal of Epidemiology*, vol 142, pp 909-17.

[38] Walker, M., Phillips, A., Shaper, A.G. et al (1996) 'Re: Height and the risk of cardiovascular disease in women', Letter, *American Journal of Epidemiology*, vol 144, p 708.

[39] Rich-Edwards, J.W., Manson, J.E. and Hennekens, C.H. (1996) 'Re: Height and the risk of cardiovascular disease in women. Three authors reply', Letter, *American Journal of Epidemiology*, vol 144, pp 708-9.

[40] Martin, T.R., Feldman, H.A., Fredberg, J.J. et al (1988) 'Relationship between maximal expiratory flows and lung volumes in growing humans', *Journal of Applied Physiology*, vol 65, pp 822-8.

[41] Strachan, D.P. (1997) 'Respiratory and allergic diseases', in D. Kuh and Y. Ben-Shlomo (eds) *A life course approach to chronic disease epidemiology*, Oxford: Oxford University Press, pp 101-20.

[42] Mann, S.L., Wadsworth, M.E.J. and Colley, J.R.T. (1992) 'Accumulation of factors influencing respiratory illness in members of a national birth cohort and their offspring', *Journal of Epidemiology and Community Health*, vol 46, pp 286-92.

[43] La Vecchia, C., Negri, E., Parazzini, F. et al (1990) 'Height and cancer risk in a network of case-control studies from Northern Italy', *International Journal of Cancer*, vol 45, pp 275-9.

[44] Hebert, P.R., Ajani, U., Cook, N.R. et al (1997) 'Adult height and incidence of cancer in male physicians (US)', *Cancer Causes Control*, vol 8, pp 591-7.

45 Gunnell, D.J., Davey Smith, G., Holly, J.M.P. et al (1998) 'Leg length and cancer risk: indirect evidence of an aetiological role for growth factors in the Boyd Orr Cohort', *British Medical Journal*, vol 317, pp 1350-1.

46 Vatten, L.J. (1996) 'Body size and breast cancer risk', *The Breast*, vol 5, pp 5-9.

47 Shimokawa, I. and Higami, Y. (1994) 'Effect of dietary restriction on pathological processes', in B.P.Yu (ed) *Modulation of aging processes by dietary restriction*, London: CRC Press, pp 247-66.

48 Chan, J.M., Stampfer, M.J., Giovannucci, E. et al (1998) 'Plasma insulin-like growth factor-I and prostate cancer risk: a prospective study', *Science*, vol 279, pp 563-6.

49 Cats, A., Dullaart, R.P.F., Kleibeuker, J.H. et al (1996) 'Increased epithelial cell proliferation in the colon of patients with acromegaly', *Cancer Research*, vol 56, pp 523-6.

50 Hankinson, S.E., Willett, W.C., Colditz, G.A. et al (1998) 'Circulating concentrations of insulin-like growth factor-I and risk of breast cancer', *Lancet*, vol 351, pp 1393-6.

51 Ruggeri, B., Klurfeld, D., Kritchevsky, D. et al (1998) 'Calorie restriction and 7,12-dimethylben(a)anthracene-induced mammary tumor growth in rats: alterations in circulating insulin, insulin-like growth factors I and II, and epidermal growth factor', *Cancer Research*, vol 49, pp 4135-41.

52 Juul, A., Bang, P., Hertel, N.T. et al (1994) 'Serum insulin-like growth factor I in 1030 healthy children, adolescents, and adults: relation to age, sex, stage of puberty, testicular size, and body mass index', *Journal of Clinical Endocrinology and Metabolism*, vol 78, pp 744-52.

53 Bonelli, L., Vitale, V., Bistolfi, F. et al (1990) 'Hodgkin's disease in adults: association with social factors and age at tonsillectomy. A case-control study', *International Journal of Cancer*, vol 45, pp 423-7.

54 Floud, R., Wachter, K. and Gregory, A. (1990) *Height, health and history: Nutritional status in the UK, 1750-1980*, Cambridge: Cambridge University Press.

55 Kermack, W.O., McKendrick, A.G. and McKinlay, P.L. (1934) 'Death rates in Great Britain and Sweden: some general regularities and their significance', *Lancet*, vol 226, pp 698-703.

56 Kuh, D. and Davey Smith, G. (1993) 'When is mortality risk determined? Historical insights into a current debate', *Social History of Medicine*, vol 6, pp 101-23.

57 Kuh, D.L., Power, C. and Rodgers, B. (1991) 'Secular trends in social class and sex differences in adult height', *International Journal of Epidemiology*, vol 20, pp 1001-9.

58 Charlton, J. and Murphy, M. (1997) *The health of adult Britain 1841-1994*, London: The Stationery Office.

23

Leg length, insulin resistance, and coronary heart disease risk: the Caerphilly Study

George Davey Smith, Rosemary
Greenwood, David Gunnell,
Peter Sweetnam, John Yarnell
and Peter Elwood

Abstract

Background: Adult height has been inversely associated with coronary heart disease risk in several studies. The mechanism for this association is not well understood, however, and we have investigated this by examining components of stature, cardiovascular disease risk factors and subsequent coronary heart disease in a prospective study.

Methods: All men aged 45-59 years living in the town of Caerphilly, South Wales were approached, and 2,512 (89%) responded and underwent a detailed examination, which included measurement of height and sitting height (from which an estimate of leg length was derived). Participants were followed up through repeat examinations and the cumulative incidence of coronary heart disease – both fatal and non-fatal – over a 15-year follow-up period is the end-point in this report.

Results: Cross-sectional associations between cardiovascular risk factors and components of stature (total height, leg length and trunk length) demonstrated that factors related to the insulin resistance syndrome – the homoeostasis model assessment of insulin resistance, fasting triglyceride levels and total to HDL cholesterol ratio – were less favourable in men with shorter legs, while showing reverse or no associations with trunk

Journal of Epidemiology and Community Health,
2001, vol 55, pp 867-72

length. Fibrinogen levels were inversely associated with leg length and showed a weaker association with trunk length. Forced expiratory volume in one second was unrelated to leg length but strongly positively associated to trunk length. Other risk factors showed little association with components of stature. The risk of coronary heart disease was inversely related to leg length, but showed little association with trunk length.

Conclusion: Leg length is the component of stature related to insulin resistance and coronary heart disease risk. As leg length is unrelated to lung function measures it is unlikely that these can explain the association in this cohort. Factors which influence leg length in adulthood – including nutrition, other influences on growth in early life, genetic and epigenetic influences – merit further investigation in this regard. The reported associations suggest that pre-adult influences are important in the aetiology of coronary heart disease and insulin resistance.

Introduction

Height in adulthood has been found to be inversely related to coronary heart disease (CHD) risk in various cohort studies.[1-6] Since favourable socioeconomic circumstances are associated with greater height, the relationship between height and CHD incidence may be confounded by the effects of childhood and adulthood socioeconomic conditions. While this appears to be partly the case, associations persist after adjustment for socioeconomic circumstances during adult life,[6,7] childhood[3] and both simultaneously.[8] Birthweight, which is associated with both height[9] and CHD incidence[9,10] also fails to account for the relationship between adulthood height and CHD risk.[4,11]

Several mechanisms have been suggested for the association between height and CHD risk. These include: foetal growth[12] and childhood nutrition,[13] which influence achieved stature and also have long-term effects on CHD risk; genetic influences which determine height and health simultaneously;[2] the poorer lung function associated with shorter stature;[14] the lesser diameter of coronary vessels in people of shorter height;[15] and reverse causation, with poor health leading to both shrinkage and increased CHD risk in adulthood.[16]

While it is likely that several of these factors may contribute to the association between height and CHD risk, one approach to further elucidating the relationship is to analyse different components of height separately. It has been known for many years that the interruption of growth at any stage results in a relatively long torso and short legs.[17,18] If the rate of growth is sufficiently slowed down, for example by nutritional deficiency, the adult will have relatively short legs. Such proportions have been used as criteria for the study of nutrition and development in childhood, and have been investigated with respect to risk of cancer.[19,20] Recently, leg length measured in childhood has been shown to be the component of stature most sensitive to environmental influences[21] and to demonstrate a strong inverse association with risk of CHD mortality over a 50-year follow-up period.[13] In the present paper we relate components of adult stature to CHD risk in a prospective study, which also allows for the examination of a wide range of potential underlying, confounding or mediating factors.

Participants and methods

The Caerphilly Study is based on a 100% sample of men selected from the town of Caerphilly and five adjacent villages. The men were chosen by date of birth so that they were aged 45-59 years when examined between 1979 and 1983. A total of 2,512 men were seen – 89% of the 2,818 who were found to be eligible. Full details of screening and follow-up procedures have been reported elsewhere.[4,22-24] Measurements included blood pressure, total and HDL cholesterol, triglycerides, insulin, glucose, fibrinogen, forced expiratory volume in one second (FEV_1), own and father's occupational social class, father's unemployment, own employment and smoking behaviour. Lung function was indexed by FEV_1/height[25] and insulin resistance was estimated according to the homeostasis model assessment (HOMA)[26] as the product of fasting glucose and insulin, divided by the constant 22.5. The higher the value, the greater the level of insulin resistance. These HOMA scores are available for only 2,031 men because it was not assessed in diabetic men, those with a fasting blood glucose concentration ≥ 8 mmols per litre and participants with missing insulin or glucose measures.

Height was measured in millimetres using a Holtain stadiometer, with care being taken to ensure that the participant was standing upright with his back against the vertical stand, heels against the plate of the base and his chin down so that the middle of his ear was at the same horizontal level as his eyes. The participant was then asked to sit on a stool with his back against the vertical stand of the stadiometer and his sitting height was measured. For the purposes of these analyses, leg length has been calculated by subtracting sitting height from standing height. While this contains the stool height – which was the same for each man but was not measured – this will not influence the quintiles or standard deviation of the measure. Height or sitting height were missing on 82 men and one man was a double amputee. Therefore the base sample for the following analyses is 2,429 men.

Insulin resistance scores are available for only 2,031 of the men because the records of all men at the NHS Central Registry were flagged so that notification of death is automatic and a copy of the death certificate is received. Incident CHD was defined as in previous reports,[4,23,24] based on admission data to local hospitals, a questionnaire to men (whether still in the original area or having moved) regarding hospital admissions, hospital discharge letters from such admissions, and ECG recordings taken at follow-up clinics held at five-year intervals from the baseline measurements. The results recorded in the present study refer to mortality follow-up to the end of 1997 (between 14.25 and 18.25 years' follow-up) and for non-fatal CHD an average of 13.75 years' follow-up.

Statistical methods

Pearson's correlation coefficients were calculated between the anthropometric variables. To illustrate the direction and shape of any associations between the three height variables – leg length, trunk length and total height – and other variables, quartiles were used. Age-standardised means and prevalence of risk factors were determined for these quartiles. Age standardisation of prevalence was by the direct method in five three-year age bands, 45-47, 48-50, 51-53, 54-56, and 57-59. Age standardisation of means was carried out with general linear modelling in the SAS procedure GLM. Statistical testing of possible associations was carried out using multiple regression, and using the continuous stature variables. Serum triglyceride and HOMA scores were found to be log normal, the geometric means have been quoted, and the natural log of the variables used in the regression models. Multiple logistic regression was used to explore the effects of other risk factors on the association between CHD and the height variables.

Results

Interrelationships between the various anthropometric measures are presented in Table 1. Several of these associations are consequences of variable construction – for example, the sizeable correlations between height and both leg and trunk length reflect the fact that the latter are constituents of the former; while body mass index is a measure explicitly computed because of its lack of association with height. However, the relatively low correlation between leg length and trunk length reflect the importance of considering these components separately. Short legs are associated with higher body mass index, while the reverse is the case for trunk length. Men with a high leg to

Table 1: Pearson's correlation coefficients (and partial correlation coefficients controlling for age) for the correlations between, height, trunk, leg length, leg length/trunk ratio and body mass index (BMI)

	Height	Trunk length	Leg length	Leg:trunk ratio	BMI
Height	1.00				
Trunk length	0.78 (0.78)	1.00			
Leg length	0.88 (0.88)	0.40 (0.39)	1.00		
Leg:trunk ratio	0.72 (0.73)	0.13 (0.13)	0.96 (0.96)	1.00	
BMI	−0.013 (−0.017)[a]	0.17 (0.16)	−0.14 (−0.15)	−0.20 (−0.20)	1.00

Note: All correlations $p<0.0001$ except [a], direct correlation $p=0.53$; partial correlation $p=0.40$.

trunk length ratio have a lower body mass index than men with a low ratio.

Total mortality, CHD mortality and cumulative fatal and non-fatal incident CHD are displayed according to the anthropometric measures divided into quarters of their distributions in Table 2. Longer legs are associated with lower CHD risk. Height and trunk length are not related to either fatal or total CHD rates after adjusting for age.

Cardiovascular disease risk factors and demographic data are presented according to quartiles of the anthropometric measures in Table 3. Blood pressure is not strongly related to any anthropometric measure while total cholesterol levels are inversely related to all the anthropometric measures. Lung function is positively related to both overall height and to trunk length, but not to leg length. Factors related to the insulin resistance syndrome – HOMA scores, triglyceride levels and total/HDL cholesterol ratio – are associated in opposite directions with leg and trunk length. Men with shorter legs are more liable to have high HOMA scores and high triglyceride levels, while associations in the opposite direction are seen with trunk length. Height, on the other hand, tends to be unrelated to these measures.

All anthropometric measures are related to the occupational social class of the men, the occupational social class of the father of the men and whether their father had been unemployed at any time during their childhood. Indicators of childhood socioeconomic circumstances were particularly strongly related to leg length. All anthropometric measures were positively related to the men being in employment. Smoking behaviour was unrelated to any of the anthropometric measures.

Risk of incident CHD in relation to the anthropometric measures, both before and after various adjustments for potential confounding or mediating factors, is detailed in Table 4. Leg length and leg length to trunk ratio were both inversely associated with CHD risk. Adjustment for various potential confounding or intermediary factors had little influence on the effect estimates, although the level of significance was attenuated.

Table 2: Fifteen year age-adjusted mortality and cumulative incidence of CHD per 100 men, according to different leg length, trunk length, height and leg/trunk length ratio quartiles, with standard errors

	Leg length				
	1 – lowest quartile	2	3	4 – highest quartile	*p* value
All deaths (639)	27.7 (1.8)	26.9 (1.8)	25.7 (1.8)	24.2 (1.7)	0.18
CHD deaths (263)	11.3 (1.3)	12.0 (1.3)	11.5 (1.3)	8.2 (1.1)	0.17
All incident CHD (435)	19.1 (1.6)	19.7 (1.6)	18.6 (1.6)	14.3 (1.4)	0.05

	Trunk length				
	1 – lowest quartile	2	3	4 – highest quartile	*p* value
All deaths (639)	25.8 (1.7)	28.9 (1.8)	25.8 (1.7)	24.7 (1.8)	0.82
CHD deaths (263)	9.9 (1.2)	12.0 (1.3)	11.2 (1.3)	10.3 (1.3)	0.49
All incident CHD (435)	16.6 (1.6)	19.9 (1.6)	18.2 (1.5)	17.2 (1.6)	0.40

	Height				
	1 – lowest quartile	2	3	4 – highest quartile	*p* value
All deaths (639)	26.0 (1.7)	28.4 (1.8)	25.2 (1.7)	24.9 (1.8)	0.30
CHD deaths (263)	10.1 (1.2)	12.4(1.3)	11.4 (1.3)	9.1 (1.2)	0.55
All incident CHD (435)	17.3 (1.5)	20.4 (1.6)	19.0 (1.5)	15.1 (1.5)	0.36

	Leg length/trunk length ratio				
	1 – lowest quartile	2	3	4 – highest quartile	*p* value
All deaths (639)	28.0 (1.7)	26.3 (1.7)	25.9 (1.8)	24.6 (1.7)	0.18
CHD deaths (263)	11.7 (1.3)	10.3 (1.2)	12.1 (1.3)	8.8 (1.2)	0.10
All incident CHD (435)	19.8 (1.6)	17.7 (1.6)	18.7 (1.5)	15.0 (1.5)	0.02

Note: p values based on continuous variables for stature, not quartiles.
Standard errors in parenthesis.

Table 3: Mean or prevalence and standard error (SE) of the mean or prevalence of age-adjusted risk factors in men by leg length, sitting height, height and leg: trunk ratio quartiles

Variable	1 – lowest quartile Mean or prevalence (SE)	2 Mean or prevalence (SE)	3 Mean or prevalence (SE)	4 – highest quartile Mean or prevalence (SE)	p value for trend
Leg length					
Age	52.5 (0.2)	52.5 (0.2)	51.9 (0.2)	51.4 (0.2)	0.0001
Systolic blood pressure (mm Hg)	141.8 (0.8)	139.9 (0.8)	140.8 (0.8)	140.6 (0.8)	0.43
Diastolic blood pressure (mm Hg)	90.0 (0.5)	88.0 (0.5)	88.4 (0.5)	88.3 (0.5)	0.19
Total cholesterol (mmol/l)	5.79 (0.05)	5.74 (0.05)	5.64 (0.05)	5.66 (0.05)	0.037
HDL cholesterol (mmol/l)	1.10 (0.01)	1.15 (0.01)	1.12 (0.01)	1.12 (0.01)	0.56
Total/HDL cholesterol	5.70 (0.08)	5.44 (0.08)	5.47 (0.08)	5.41 (0.08)	0.063
Triglyceride (mmol/l)[a]	1.82 (0.02)	1.66 (0.02)	1.65 (0.02)	1.62 (0.02)	0.0008
Fibrinogen (g/l)	3.81 (0.04)	3.81 (0.04)	3.76 (0.04)	3.69 (0.03)	0.004
FEV_1/height^2 (cl/m^2)	89.1 (1.0)	91.0 (1.0)	90.2 (1.0)	91.3 (0.9)	0.11
Insulin resistance[a] (HOMA)	1.43 (0.04)	1.24 (0.04)	1.26 (0.04)	1.22 (0.04)	0.013
Non-manual social class (%)	20.2 (1.7)	28.8 (1.9)	36.1 (2.0)	42.7 (2.0)	0.0001
Father in non-manual social class (%)	8.8 (1.2)	8.9 (1.2)	12.7 (1.4)	18.8 (1.6)	0.0001
Father unemployed (%)	50.4 (2.3)	49.5 (2.3)	46.4 (2.3)	36.2 (2.2)	0.0001
Subject employed at baseline (%)	75.2 (1.7)	78.9 (1.7)	81.3 (1.6)	85.9 (1.4)	0.0001
Ever smoker (%)	84.0 (1.5)	84.8 (1.5)	85.0 (1.4)	82.7 (1.5)	0.90
Trunk length					
Age	53.1 (0.2)	52.5 (0.2)	51.8 (0.2)	51.0 (0.2)	0.0001
Systolic blood pressure (mm Hg)	140.7 (0.8)	140.0 (0.8)	140.5 (0.8)	141.4 (0.8)	0.34
Diastolic blood pressure (mm Hg)	88.6 (0.5)	88.1 (0.5)	88.3 (0.5)	89.5 (0.5)	0.24
Total cholesterol (mmol/l)	5.75 (0.05)	5.80 (0.05)	5.67 (0.05)	5.64 (0.05)	0.016
HDL cholesterol (mmol/l)	1.16 (0.01)	1.13 (0.01)	1.12 (0.01)	1.08 (0.01)	0.0001
Total/HDL cholesterol	5.40 (0.09)	5.56 (0.08)	5.45 (0.08)	5.61 (0.09)	0.062
Triglyceride (mmol/l)[a]	1.66 (0.02)	1.69 (0.02)	1.65 (0.02)	1.76 (0.02)	0.055
Fibrinogen (g/l)	3.82 (0.04)	3.76 (0.04)	3.76 (0.03)	3.73 (0.04)	0.093
FEV_1/height^2 (cl/m^2)	86.2 (1.0)	90.1 (0.9)	91.4 (0.9)	93.5 (1.0)	0.0001
Insulin resistance[a] (HOMA)	1.23 (0.04)	1.24 (0.04)	1.26 (0.04)	1.45 (0.04)	0.0025
Non-manual social class (%)	24.3 (1.8)	29.5 (1.9)	31.7 (1.9)	43.7 (2.1)	0.0001
Father in non-manual social class (%)	11.0 (1.4)	11.4 (1.4)	13.1 (1.4)	14.4 (1.5)	0.006
Father unemployed (%)	47.8 (2.4)	47.8 (2.3)	43.9 (2.2)	42.1 (2.3)	0.0001
Subject employed at baseline (%)	76.5 (1.8)	79.5 (1.6)	81.3 (1.6)	82.8 (1.6)	0.012
Ever smoker (%)	85.9 (1.5)	84.1 (1.5)	82.5 (1.5)	84.3 (1.5)	0.22

(continued)

Table 3: contd.../

Variable	1 – lowest quartile Mean or prevalence (SE)	2 Mean or prevalence (SE)	3 Mean or prevalence (SE)	4 – highest quartile Mean or prevalence (SE)	*p* value for trend
Height					
Age	53.0 (0.2)	52.6 (0.2)	51.6 (0.2)	51.2 (0.2)	0.0001
Systolic blood pressure (mm Hg)	141.6 (0.8)	140.0 (0.8)	140.0 (0.8)	141.3 (0.8)	0.96
Diastolic blood pressure (mm Hg)	89.6 (0.5)	88.1 (0.5)	87.9 (0.5)	89.0 (0.5)	0.76
Total cholesterol (mmol/l)	5.74 (0.05)	5.78 (0.05)	5.69 (0.05)	5.64 (0.05)	0.008
HDL cholesterol (mmol/l)	1.14 (0.01)	1.13 (0.01)	1.11 (0.01)	1.11 (0.01)	0.047
Total/HDL cholesterol	5.47 (0.09)	5.55 (0.08)	5.57 (0.08)	5.45 (0.08)	0.75
Triglyceride (mmol/l)[a]	1.70 (0.02)	1.73 (0.02)	1.68 (0.02)	1.65 (0.02)	0.19
Fibrinogen (g/l)	3.77 (0.04)	3.81 (0.04)	3.79 (0.03)	3.69 (0.03)	0.005
FEV_1/height^2 (cl/m^2)	88.2 (1.0)	89.2 (1.0)	92.2 (1.0)	91.8 (0.9)	0.0001
Insulin resistance[a] (HOMA)	1.35 (0.04)	1.23 (0.04)	1.30 (0.04)	1.27 (0.04)	0.89
Non-manual social class (%)	20.1 (1.7)	28.9 (1.9)	35.8 (2.0)	43.1 (2.1)	0.0001
Father in non-manual social class (%)	7.7 (1.2)	11.9 (1.4)	13.8 (1.5)	16.0 (1.6)	0.0001
Father unemployed (%)	49.7 (2.4)	49.7 (2.3)	42.4 (2.3)	39.2 (2.2)	0.0001
Subject employed at baseline (%)	75.2 (1.8)	79.9 (1.6)	80.8 (1.6)	85.3 (1.5)	0.0001
Ever smoker (%)	82.7 (1.6)	85.7 (1.5)	83.9 (1.5)	83.7 (1.5)	0.47
Leg length/trunk length ratio					
Age	52.3 (0.2)	52.4 (0.2)	51.9 (0.2)	51.7 (0.2)	0.011
Systolic blood pressure (mm Hg)	141.7 (0.8)	140.3 (0.8)	141.0 (0.8)	140.2 (0.8)	0.27
Diastolic blood pressure (mm Hg)	90.1 (0.5)	88.0 (0.5)	88.3 (0.5)	88.2 (0.5)	0.074
Total cholesterol (mmol/l)	5.78 (0.05)	5.72 (0.05)	5.69 (0.05)	5.64 (0.05)	0.13
HDL cholesterol (mmol/l)	1.09 (0.01)	1.13 (0.01)	1.14 (0.01)	1.13 (0.01)	0.047
Total/HDL cholesterol	5.74 (0.08)	5.43 (0.08)	5.46 (0.08)	5.38 (0.08)	0.013
Triglyceride (mmol/l)[a]	1.83 (0.02)	1.66 (0.02)	1.64 (0.02)	1.60 (0.02)	0.0001
Fibrinogen (g/l)	3.80 (0.03)	3.79 (0.03)	3.76 (0.03)	3.70 (0.04)	0.012
FEV_1/height^2 (cl/m^2)	90.2 (1.0)	90.6 (1.0)	90.4 (1.0)	90.2 (1.0)	0.89
Insulin resistance[a] (HOMA)	1.47 (0.04)	1.25 (0.04)	1.21 (0.04)	1.21 (0.04)	0.0004
Non-manual social class (%)	22.2 (1.7)	28.0 (1.8)	37.3 (2.0)	40.7 (2.0)	0.0001
Father in non-manual social class (%)	8.4 (1.2)	10.7 (1.3)	11.7 (1.4)	18.5 (1.7)	0.0001
Father unemployed (%)	48.9 (2.3)	52.4 (2.3)	44.5 (2.3)	36.0 (2.2)	0.0001
Subject employed at baseline (%)	75.6 (1.7)	78.0 (1.7)	82.8 (1.5)	85.0 (1.5)	0.0001
Ever smoker (%)	82.5 (1.5)	86.3 (1.4)	84.1 (1.5)	83.5 (1.5)	0.82

[a] geometric means, standard errors refer to logged data.

Note: Age is the only variable not age-adjusted.

Table 4: Odds ratios for CHD incidence for increase in 1 standard deviation of leg length, trunk length, height and leg length/trunk length ratio

Variables in model	Number of men with full data on variables considered	Unadjusted odds ratio for increase of one standard deviation[a]	95% CI	Adjusted odds ratio for increase of one standard deviation[a]	95% CI
		Leg length			
Anthropometric variables[b]	2,427	0.90	(0.81-1.00)	0.90	(0.80-1.07)
CHD risk factors[c]	2,152	0.89	(0.79-1.00)	0.94	(0.84-1.06)
Insulin resistance[d]	1,904	0.88	(0.78-0.99)	0.89	(0.79-1.00)
Socioeconomic position[e]	2,370	0.90	(0.81-1.00)	0.91	(0.82-1.02)
All listed variables[f]	1,771	0.87	(0.76-0.99)	0.88	(0.76-1.02)
		Trunk length			
Anthropometric variables[b]	2,427	1.05	(0.94-1.16)	1.07	(0.95-1.20)
CHD risk factors[c]	2,152	1.04	(0.93-1.17)	1.08	(0.96-1.22)
Insulin resistance[d]	1,904	1.01	(0.89-1.14)	0.98	(0.86-1.10)
Socioeconomic position[e]	2,370	1.06	(0.95-1.18)	1.08	(0.96-1.20)
All listed variables[f]	1,771	1.03	(0.91-1.17)	1.12	(0.97-1.30)
		Height			
Anthropometric variables[b]	2,427	0.95	(0.86-1.06)	1.05	(0.89, 1.23)
CHD risk factors[c]	2,152	0.94	(0.84-1.06)	1.00	(0.88, 1.12)
Insulin resistance[d]	1,904	0.92	(0.81-1.04)	0.91	(0.80, 1.03)
Socioeconomic position[e]	2,370	0.96	(0.86-1.07)	0.98	(0.87, 1.09)
All listed variables[f]	1,771	0.92	(0.81-1.05)	1.12	(0.91, 1.36)
		Leg length/trunk length ratio			
Anthropometric variables[b]	2,427	0.88	(0.80-0.98)	0.88	(0.75-1.03)
CHD risk factors[c]	2,152	0.87	(0.77-0.98)	0.92	(0.81-1.03)
Insulin resistance[d]	1,904	0.87	(0.77-0.98)	0.89	(0.79-1.01)
Socioeconomic position[e]	2,370	0.88	(0.79-0.98)	0.89	(0.80-1.00)
All listed variables[f]	1,771	0.86	(0.75-0.97)	0.83	(0.68-1.01)

[a] Age-adjusted odds ratio for increase in leg length of one standard deviation (4.4 cm), sitting height of one standard deviation (3.3 cm), height of one standard deviation (6.5 cm) and leg length/trunk length ratios of one standard deviation (3.3 cm).

[b] Anthropometric variables in the model.

[c] CHD risk factors in the model: body mass index, FEV_1/H^2, cholesterol, fibrinogen, diastolic blood pressure, ever smoked, currently smoke.

[d] Insulin resistance factors in the model: HOMA, log triglycerides, HDL cholesterol

[e] Indicators of socioeconomic position in the model: own social class, father's social class (including a category for not known), father unemployed (including a category for not known).

[f] All variables from all four categories entered in the model.

Discussion

Height has been inversely related to CHD risk in many studies [1-6,11,12,14,16,27] and a higher prevalence and greater severity of coronary atherosclerosis found at arteriography has also been reported among shorter men.[28] The weak and non-significant inverse association between overall height and incident CHD seen in this longer follow-up of the Caerphilly Study represents an attenuation of the stronger inverse association seen over a five-year follow-up.[4] A similar decrease in the magnitude of the inverse association between height and CHD mortality with longer follow-up has been seen in the Whitehall Study[16] and it was there postulated that this may reflect some of the height–CHD association being due to greater reductions in height occurring with ageing among ill people. As the group of already sick individuals decreases in size due to selective mortality, this group will have increasingly less influence on height–CHD incidence associations and the attenuation with follow-up that is seen would be expected. While this may contribute to the association between overall height and CHD being weaker at this longer follow-up in the Caerphilly Study, it is unlikely to account for an inverse association between leg length and CHD incidence. Longitudinal studies examining reductions in height with age suggest that this occurs preferentially in the trunk rather than leg component of total height, probably due both to shrinkage in the vertebral column and scoliosis.[29] Thus, associations between leg length, which is less affected by ageing, and CHD incidence are unlikely to be confounded by adult disease processes leading to shrinkage in those with ill health.[15]

The specific association of leg length and CHD incidence has implications for other potential mechanisms linking height and CHD risk. In the present study we see that trunk length, rather than leg length, is positively associated with lung function. This is the expectation which follows from simple mechanical considerations. If the association between height and CHD risk were mediated through lung function, as has been suggested,[14] it would be expected that trunk length, rather than leg length, would be the important component of total height. The fact that the reverse is the case suggests that the lung function hypothesis cannot provide a full explanation of the association between height and CHD risk. Inhibited foetal development, reflected in lower height in adulthood, has been advanced to explain the association between height and CHD. The hypothesis here is that it is poor foetal development which is the fundamental causal factor, and height serves as a marker of this. However, the correlations between birthweight, the indicator of foetal development used in many of the prospective studies investigating the foetal origins of CHD, and the two components of height are similar, $r=0.17$ for trunk length and $r=0.12$ for leg length in the present study. Data from other studies also demonstrate similar correlations of birthweight (and birthweight adjusted for birth length) with trunk length and leg length.[30] If impaired foetal development underlays the height–CHD associations it would be expected that both components of height would have similar associations with CHD. Again this is counter to the results we obtained.

Leg length appears to serve as an indicator of nutritional status in childhood.[31] It is the component of overall height that grows proportionately more in the years up to puberty,[32] as shown by changes in the sitting height: height ratio from birth to adulthood from around 0.66 to around 0.52,[33] and secular increases in height are thought to be largely due to leg length increases.[34] Thus, in the observed relationships between leg length and CHD mortality, leg length may be acting as a sensitive marker for environmental exposures in childhood leading both to growth retardation and later predisposition to CHD.

Other explanations for the height–CHD relationship may be classified under two headings – confounding and mechanical. Height–CHD relationships may be confounded by adult risk factors. For example children exposed to environmental factors that retard growth may be more likely to become adult smokers;[35] similarly taller children are more likely to experience upward social mobility[36] and adults in upper socioeconomic groups are at reduced CHD risk. Adjustment for both adult risk factors and social class partially attenuated the hazard ratios seen in our analyses. Attenuation with respect to adult risk factors may be because alterations of these are the mechanism through which childhood exposures affect adult CHD risk. Thus, rather than adjusting for a confounding factor, one is adjusting for a risk factor lying on the causal pathway of the observed associations, thereby diminishing 'true' effects. Mechanical explanations suggest that reduced stature is associated with diminished coronary artery lumen diameter, and thereby with greater risk of occlusion.[15] If this explanation were valid, one might expect to see stronger relationships with trunk length, as this may more directly relate to body mass and hence heart and coronary size. This was not found in our analyses.

Height in adulthood has been inversely associated with the risk of adult-onset diabetes and impaired glucose tolerance in some[37-39] but not all[40] previous studies. This association could reflect common genetic factors influencing both height and later glucose tolerance; intrauterine development and its associations with adulthood height and later glucose tolerance; or childhood circumstances, which influence final attained height and later glucose tolerance. Evidence that the inverse association between height and glucose tolerance is independent of birth weight has been interpreted as indicating that the association does not simply reflect the influence of intrauterine environment. In our analyses we demonstrate clearly that the association between stature and insulin resistance – together with other components of the metabolic syndrome, including triglyceride levels and obesity – are linked specifically to leg length. Since birth weight is similarly associated with height, with leg length and with trunk length, the specific associations between leg length and components of the metabolic syndrome are unlikely to reflect the common influence of intrauterine development, which is reflected by birthweight. However, the relevance of insulin resistance[41] and the components of the metabolic syndrome for subsequent development of CHD have been questioned among non-diabetics.[42] Statistical adjustment for components of the insulin resistance syndrome did not greatly attenuate the association between leg length and incident CHD. Thus it appears that additional mechanisms link leg length to risk of CHD.

Adverse social circumstances in childhood are related to increased risk of CHD mortality,[43] and to components of the metabolic syndrome.[44] Leg length and leg length to trunk length ratio, both in childhood and in adulthood, may reflect the influence of growth patterns, which, in turn, influence later disease risk. In both the present study and in the Boyd Orr cohort[13] – in which leg length was measured in childhood – the association between components of stature and adult disease risk were statistically independent of socioeconomic indicators in both childhood and in adulthood. Thus the leg length association with adulthood disease does not appear to simply reflect confounding by social circumstances.

Leg length and leg length to trunk length ratio in adulthood appear to be influenced by factors constraining early childhood growth (poorer socioeconomic circumstances result in shorter legs and a lower leg length to trunk length ratio), however, later puberty (which may also reflect adverse circumstances) results in greater leg length to trunk length ratios.[45] Thus leg length and leg to trunk length ratio in adulthood will be a less useful indicator of childhood circumstances than leg length measured in childhood. This may explain why the associations with CHD were of greater magnitude in the Boyd Orr cohort, in which anthropometric measurements were taken in childhood, than in the present study.[13]

Conclusions

Leg length is inversely associated with the risk of CHD and with components of the insulin resistance syndrome among adults. This provides supportive evidence for the hypothesis that impaired growth during childhood increases the risk of these conditions. The finding should, however, be considered in the light of evidence suggesting that high calorie intake in childhood, longer legs in childhood and greater final achieved stature are associated with an increased risk of non-smoking-related cancers.[6,16,19,20] Further research is required to delineate the overall influence of encouraged growth in childhood on adult health.

References

[1] Greig, M., Pemberton, J., Hay, I. and MacKenzie, G. (1980) 'A prospective study of the development of coronary heart disease in a group of 1202 middle-aged men', *Journal of Epidemiology and Community Health*, vol 34, pp 23-30.

[2] Waaler, H.T. (1984) 'Height, weight and mortality', *Acta Medica Scandinavica Supplementum*, vol 679, suppl.

[3] Notkola, V., Punsar, S., Karvonen, M.J. and Haapakoski, J. (1985) 'Socioeconomic conditions in childhood and mortality and morbidity caused by coronary heart disease in adulthood in rural Finland', *Social Science and Medicine*, vol 21, pp 517-23.

[4] Yarnell, J.W.G., Limb, E.S., Layzell, J.M. and Baker, I.A. (1992) 'Height: a risk marker for ischaemic heart disease: prospective results from the Caerphilly and Speedwell heart disease studies', *European Heart Journal*, vol 13, pp 1602-5.

[5] Hebert, P.R., Rich-Edwards, J.W., Manson, J.E., Ridker, P.M., Cook, N.R., O'Connor, G.T., Buring, J.E. and Hennekens, C.H. (1993) 'Height and incidence of cardiovascular disease in male physicians', *Circulation*, vol 88, pp 1437-43.

[6] **Davey Smith, G., Hart, C., Upton, M., Hole, D., Gillis, C., Watt, G. and Hawthorne, V. (2000) 'Height and risk of death among men and women: aetiological implications of associations with cardiorespiratory disease and cancer mortality',** ***Journal of Epidemiology and Community Health*, vol 54, pp 97-103.**

[7] **Davey Smith, G., Shipley, M.J. and Rose, G. (1990) 'The magnitude and causes of socioeconomic differentials in mortality: further evidence from the Whitehall Study',** ***Journal of Epidemiology and Community Health*, vol 44, pp 265-70.**

[8] Peck, A.N.M. and Vågerö, D. (1989) 'Adult body height, self perceived health and mortality in the Swedish population', *Journal of Epidemiology and Community Health*, vol 43, pp 380-4.

[9] Frankel, S., Elwood, P., Sweetnam, P., Yarnell, J. and Davey Smith, G. (1996) 'Birthweight, adult risk factors and incident coronary heart disease: the Caerphilly Study, *Public Health*, vol 110, pp 139-43.

[10] Barker, D.J.P. (1994) *Mothers, babies, and disease in later life*, London: BMJ Publishing Group.

[11] Rich-Edwards, J.W., Manson, J.E., Stampfer, M.J., Colditz, G.A., Willett, W.C. et al (1995) 'Height and risk of cardiovascular disease in women', *American Journal of Epidemiology*, vol 142, pp 909-17.

[12] Barker, D.J.P., Osmond, C. and Golding, J. (1990) 'Height and mortality in the counties of England and Wales', *Annals of Human Biology*, vol 17, pp 1-6.

[13] Gunnell, D., Davey Smith, G., Frankel, S., Nanchahal, K., Braddon, F.E.M., Pemberton, J. and Peters, T.J. (1998) 'Childhood leg length and adult mortality: follow up of the Carnegie (Boyd Orr) Survey of diet and health in pre-war Britain', *Journal of Epidemiology and Community Health*, vol 52, pp 142-52.

[14] Walker, M., Shaper, A.G., Phillips, A.N. and Cook, D.G. (1989) 'Short stature, lung function and the risk of a heart attack', *International Journal of Epidemiology*, vol 18, p 602-6.

[15] Palmer, J.R., Rosenberg, L. and Shapiro, S. (1990) 'Stature and the risk of myocardial infarction in women', *American Journal of Epidemiology*, vol 132, pp 27-32.

[16] Leon, D.A., Davey Smith, G., Shipley, M. and Strachan, D. (1995) 'Adult height and mortality in London: early life, socioeconomic confounding, or shrinkage?', *Journal of Epidemiology and Community Health*, vol 49, pp 5-9.

[17] Leitch, I. (1951) 'Growth and health', *British Journal of Nutrition*, vol 5, pp 142-51.

[18] Mitchell, H.S. (1962) 'Nutrition in relation to stature', *Journal of American Dietetic Association*, vol 40, pp 521-4.

[19] Gunnell, D.J., Davey Smith, G., Holly, J.M.P. and Frankel, S. (1998) 'Leg length and risk of cancer in the Boyd Orr cohort', *British Medical Journal*, vol 317, pp 1350-1.

[20] Albanes, D., Jones, D.Y., Schatzhin, A., Micozzi, M.S. and Taylor, P.R. (1988) 'Adult stature and risk of cancer', *Cancer Research*, vol 48, pp 1658-62.

[21] Gunnell, D.J., Davey Smith, G., Frankel, S.J., Kemp, M. and Peters, T.J. (1998) 'Socioeconomic and dietary influences on leg length and trunk length in childhood: a reanalysis of the Carnegie (Boyd Orr) survey of diet and health in pre-war Britain (1937-39)', *Paediatric and Perinatal Epidemiology*, vol 12, suppl 1, pp 96-113.

[22] The Caerphilly and Speedwell Collaborative Group (1984) 'Caerphilly and Speedwell collaborative heart disease studies', *Journal of Epidemiology and Community Health*, vol 38, pp 259-62.

[23] Yarnell, J.W.G., Sweetnam, P.M., Marks, V., Teale, J.D. and Bolton, C.H. (1994) 'Insulin in ischaemic heart disease: are associations explained by triglyceride concentrations? The Caerphilly prospective study', *British Heart Journal*, vol 71, pp 293-6.

[24] Yarnell, J.W.G., Baker, I.A., Sweetnam, P.M., Bainton, D., O'Brien, J.R., Whitehead, P.J. and Elwood, P.C. (1991) 'Fibrinogen, viscosity and white blood cell count are major risk factors for ischaemic heart disease: the Caerphilly and Speedwell collaborative heart disease studies', *Circulation*, vol 83, pp 836-44.

[25] Cole, T.J. (1975) 'Linear and proportional regression models in the prediction of ventilatory function', *Journal of the Royal Statistical Society*, vol 138, pp 297-338.

[26] Matthews, D.R., Hosker, J.P., Rudenski, A.S., Naylor, B.A., Treacher, D.F. and Turner, R.C. (1985) 'Homoeostasis model assessment: insulin resistance and beta-cell function from fasting plasma glucose and insulin concentrations in man', *Diabetologia*, vol 28, pp 412-19.

[27] Williams, S.R.P., Jones, E., Bell, W., Davies, B. and Bourne, M.W. (1997) 'Body habitus and coronary heart disease in men', *European Heart Journal*, vol 18, pp 376-93.

[28] Nwasokwa, O.N., Weiss, M., Gladstone, C. and Bodenheimer, M.M. (1997) 'Higher prevalence and greater severity of coronary disease in short versus tall men referred for coronary arteriography', *American Heart Journal*, vol 133, pp 147-52.

[29] Friedlaender, J.S., Costa, P.T., Bosse, R., Ellis, E., Rhoads, J.G. and Stoudt, H.W. (1977) 'Longitudinal physique changes among healthy white veterans in Boston', *Human Biology*, vol 49, pp 541-58.

[30] Gunnell, D., Davey Smith, G., McConnachie, A., Greenwood, R., Upton, M. and Frankel, S. (1999) 'Separating in-utero and postnatal influences on later disease', *Lancet*, vol 354, pp 1526-7.

[31] Gunnell, D. (2001) 'Commentary: early insights into height, leg length, proportionate growth and health', *International Journal of Epidemiology*, vol 30, pp 221-2.

[32] Martorell, R., Malina, R.M., Castillo, R.O., Mendoza, F.S. and Pawson, I.G. (1988) 'Body proportion in three ethnic groups: children and youths 2-17 years in NHANES II and HHANES', *Human Biology*, vol 60, pp 205-22.

[33] Gerver, W.J.M. and Bruin, R.D. (1995) 'Relationship between height, sitting height and subischial leg length in Dutch children: presentation of normal values', *Acta Paediatrica*, vol 84, pp 532-5.

[34] Tanner, J.M., Hayashi, T., Preece, M.A. and Cameron, N. (1982) 'Increase in length of leg relative to trunk in Japanese children and adults from 1957 to 1977: comparison with British and with Japanese Americans', *Annals of Human Biology*, vol 9, pp 411-23.

[35] Kandel, D.B., Wu, P. and Davies, M. (1994) 'Maternal smoking during pregnancy and smoking by adolescent daughters', *American Journal of Public Health*, vol 84, pp 1407-13.

[36] Power, C., Fogelman, K. and Fox, A.J. (1986) 'Health and social mobility during the early years of life', *Quarterly Journal of Social Affairs*, vol 2, pp 397-413.

[37] Brown, D.C., Byrne, C.D., Clark, P.M.S. et al (1991) 'Height and glucose tolerance in adult subjects', *Diabetologia*, vol 34, pp 531-3.

[38] Njølstad, I., Arnesen, E. and Lund-Larsen, P.G. (1998) 'Sex differences in risk factors for clinical diabetes mellitus in a general population: a 12-year follow-up of the Finnmark Study', *American Journal of Epidemiology*, vol 147, pp 49-58.

[39] Sayeed, M.A., Banu, A., Khan, A.R. et al (1995) 'Prevalence of diabetes and hypertension in a rural population of Bangladesh', *Diabetes Care*, vol 18, pp 555-8.

[40] Colditz, G.A., Willett, W.C., Stampfer, M.J. et al (1990) 'Weight as a risk factor for clinical diabetes in women', *American Journal of Epidemiology*, vol 132, pp 501-13.

[41] Yarnell, J.W.G., Patterson, C.C. and Sweetnam, P.M. (1995) 'Simple measure of insulin resistance', *Lancet*, vol 346, pp 1108-9.

[42] Yarnell, J.W.G., Patterson, C.C., Bainton, D. and Sweetnam, P.M. (1998) 'Is Metabolic Syndrome a discrete entity in the general population? Evidence from the Caerphilly and Speedwell population studies', *Heart*, vol 79, pp 248-52.

[43] **Davey Smith, G., Hart, C., Blane, D. and Hole, D. (1998) 'Adverse socioeconomic conditions in childhood and cause-specific adult mortality: prospective observational study', *British Medical Journal*, vol 316, pp 1631-5.**

[44] Davey Smith, G. and Hart, C. (1997) 'Insulin resistance syndrome and childhood social conditions', *Lancet*, vol 349, pp 284-5.

[45] Buckler, J.M.H. (1998) 'Growth at adolescence', in C.J.H. Kelnar, M.O. Savage, H.F. Sterling and P. Saenger, *Growth disorders*, London: Chapman and Hall.

Section VI
Ethnicity and health inequalities

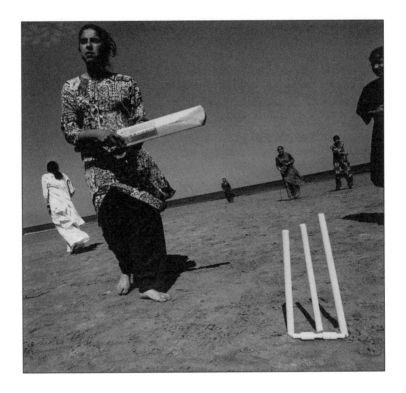

Humber, from 'The shipping forecast'. Photograph by
Mark Power. Reproduced with permission of Mark Power.

24

Ethnic inequalities in health: a review of UK epidemiological evidence

George Davey Smith, Nish Chaturvedi, Seeromanie Harding, James Nazroo and Rory Williams

Introduction

Associations between ethnicity and health status have been noted from the time when quantitative health data were first recorded. Thus in 1845 Frederich Engels noted the poor health and mortality record of the Irish living in England.[1] Engels also drew attention to the miserable social and environmental circumstances in which the majority of the Irish population lived and it is clear that he considered these to underlie their poor health. Similarly, in a 1916 report from the US, John W. Trask concluded that the lower death rates among white people than black people reflected more favourable socioeconomic circumstances, rather than any inherent ethnic differences.[2] Since then the complex interrelationships between ethnicity, social position and health have remained a central concern of studies in this area, as the material presented in this chapter indicates.

The approach we have taken is an epidemiological one. Descriptive epidemiology provides data on how disease, disability and death are distributed between and within populations. Analytical epidemiology aims at uncovering the causes of disease and thus the reasons for the distribution of disease that are seen. Epidemiological studies concerned with ethnicity have taken both descriptive and analytical approaches. There are now extensive data demonstrating differentials in health status between ethnic groups and a growing body of literature analysing the contribution of socioenvironmental factors to this. There are also some attempts at investigating the specific factors involved in the

Critical Public Health, 2000, vol 10, pp 375-408

high or low rates of certain conditions seen among particular ethnic groups – the investigation of high rates of coronary heart disease and low rates of colon cancer among South Asians and high hypertension prevalence among African Caribbeans are examples of this. We will provide descriptive data on ethnic health differentials in the UK initially and then proceed to investigate the contribution of socioeconomic factors to these differentials.

We will conclude with a discussion of the different approaches that have been taken to understanding differentials in health status between ethnic groups. The main test of these approaches is their capacity to point to modifiable causes of inequality, rather than to novel aetiological hypotheses.[3]

Ethnicity and health: illustrative data

Adult mortality by country of birth

Mortality data according to ethnic group come from various sources, all of which have their limitations. Here we concentrate on data for England and Wales for the years around the 1991 Census. Deaths around this Census year have been classified according to country of birth, as given on the death certificate, and the population was classified according to country of birth in the 1991 Census. This allows the calculation of mortality rates for country of birth groups. The country of birth groupings used in these analyses are those born in the Caribbean commonwealth, West and South Africa, the East African commonwealth, the Indian subcontinent (India, Pakistan, Bangladesh, Sri Lanka), Scotland, and Ireland (both Northern Ireland and Republic of Ireland). The disaggregation of the African grouping is carried out because the majority of East Africans are of Indian origin while those from West/South Africa are of 'Black African' origin. Data are presented separately for those born in India, Pakistan and Bangladesh when numbers of deaths are high enough to allow disaggregation. Tables 1 and 2 present standardised mortality ratios (SMRs) for deaths from all-causes and from various specific causes, according to country of birth groups for men and women of working age. All-cause mortality is markedly higher for men and women born in West/South Africa, East Africa, Scotland and Ireland.

Ischaemic heart disease and lung cancer are major causes of death, regardless of ethnic group. Ischaemic heart disease mortality is particularly high for men and women born in the Indian subcontinent, but low in people born in the Caribbean. Stroke mortality is elevated for all of the country of birth groups examined. Lung cancer mortality is lower for men and women born in all countries examined except Scotland and Ireland, who show high rates. Deaths from accidents

Table 1: SMRs for men aged 20-64 years, by country of birth, England and Wales (1991-93)[4]

	All causes	Ischaemic heart disease	Stroke	Lung cancer	Other cancer	Accidents and injuries	Suicide
Total	100	100	100	100	100	100	100
Caribbean	89*	60*	169*	59*	89	121	59*
West/South Africa	126*	83	315*	71	133*	75	59*
East Africa	123*	160*	113	37*	77	86	75*
Indian subcontinent	107*	150*	163*	48*	65*	80*	73*
India	106*	140*	140*	43*	64*	97	109
Pakistan	102	163*	148*	45*	62*	68*	34*
Bangladesh	133*	184*	324*	92	74*	40*	27*
Scotland	129*	117*	111	146*	114*	177*	149*
Ireland	135*	121*	130*	157*	120*	189*	135*

Note: *p<0.05, compared to overall rate.

Table 2: SMRs for women aged 20-64 years, by country of birth, England and Wales (1991-93)[4]

	All causes	Ischaemic heart disease	Stroke	Lung cancer	Other cancer	Accidents and injuries	Suicide
Total	100	100	100	100	100	100	100
Caribbean	104	100	178*	32*	87	103	49*
West/South Africa	142*	69	215*	69	120	a	102
East Africa	127*	130	110	29*	98	a	129
Indian subcontinent	99	175*	132*	34*	68	93	115
Scotland	127*	127*	131*	164*	106	201*	153*
Ireland	115*	129*	118*	143*	98	160*	144*

[a] Too few deaths.
Note: *p<0.05, compared to overall rate.

and injuries are high for men and women born in Scotland and Ireland, as is suicide. Suicide is low among men and women born in the Caribbean.[4]

Routine data for Britain only allow mortality to be related to country of birth, although the 1991 Census was the first to collect information on ethnicity. Ethnicity may also become available on death certificates in time, allowing for the direct examination of mortality in relation to ethnicity. The 1971 Census included a question on country of birth of parents and this information has been used in the longitudinal study – a follow-up of a 1% sample of the population of England and Wales – to demonstrate that second generation Irish people living in England and Wales experience high mortality rates, particularly the younger adults (Table 3).[5,6] The elevated all-cause mortality for second generation Irish people is strongly influenced by a high lung cancer death rate among younger men. The numbers

Table 3: SMRs of second generation Irish people living in England and Wales (1971-92)[5]

Age at death (years)	SMR	Age at death (years)	SMR
Men		*Women*	
15-44	147	15-44	153
45-64	120	45-64	121*
65-74	114	65-74	107
≥75	97	≥75	110
≥15	109	≥15	112

Note: *p<0.05.

of deaths are relatively small, but there also appears to be a high rate of ovarian, cervical and prostate cancers, and accidental and violent death.

Mortality in men of patrilineal Irish decent in the west of Scotland has been shown to be elevated for overall mortality, coronary heart disease mortality and accidental and violent death.[7] Original immigration of the ancestors of these men would have been in the 19th century in many cases. This demonstrates that differential mortality experience need not disappear rapidly following immigration and can persist across several generations.

Child and infant mortality by country of birth

Mortality in the first year of life (infant mortality) shows distinctive patterns in relation to ethnic group. In Table 4 perinatal mortality rates are higher among infants of mothers born outside the UK for all the groups considered. Neonatal mortality is high for the offspring of mothers born in Pakistan and the Caribbean, but shows only small or no elevations for the offspring of mothers born in India. Post-neonatal mortality is low for the offspring of mothers born in East Africa, India or Bangladesh and elevated for the other groups considered. Infant deaths and stillbirths from congenital anomalies

Table 4: Mortality in the first year of life per 1,000 births by mother's country of birth, England and Wales (1996)[10]

	UK	East Africa	Bangladesh	India	Caribbean	Pakistan
Perinatal mortality	8.2	12.4	9.5	11.3	11.5	15.8
Neonatal mortality	3.9	4.1	4.2	3.9	4.7	6.5
Postneonatal mortality	1.9	2.0	2.2	1.5	3.6	3.6
Infant mortality	5.8	6.1	6.3	5.4	8.4	10.1

are markedly elevated for the offspring of mothers born in Pakistan, moderately elevated in mothers born in other parts of the Indian subcontinent and lower for the offspring of mothers born in West Africa than for the offspring of mothers born in the UK. Sudden Infant Death Syndrome, which accounts for around 40% of all post-neonatal deaths of infants in England and Wales, has been a less frequent cause of death among offspring of mothers born in Africa or the Indian subcontinent.[8] It has been suggested that sleeping positions (on their backs)[9] for infants may be responsible for the low rates of Sudden Infant Death Syndrome among the offspring of mothers born in Africa or the Indian subcontinent. The recent fall in rates of sudden infant death syndrome is making this difference less obvious, however.

The analysis of mortality in childhood is rendered problematic by the small numbers of deaths on which analyses can be based. Overall there is evidence for higher mortality among 1–4 and 5–14 year olds born in the Indian subcontinent and in the African commonwealth.[10]

Morbidity in adulthood

Representative data on morbidity among minority ethnic groups have, until recently, been sparse. Data from the 1991 Census show higher rates of longstanding illness reported to limit activities among all of the ethnic minority groups compared to white people, apart from Chinese people. While there have been several local studies and disease-specific investigations limited to particular ethnic groups, the inclusion of a detailed health component in the Fourth National Survey of Ethnic Minorities[34] has allowed a considerably more detailed analysis of morbidity differentials than has been carried out previously. We therefore concentrate on data from this source in this chapter, cross-referencing other studies where appropriate.

Table 5 presents age and gender-standardised prevalence rates of various health problems according to ethnic group membership. Self-assessed general health is particularly poor among Pakistani/ Bangladeshi and Caribbean people. The longstanding illness data in the Fourth National Survey show lower rates among Chinese people, in line with the Census data, but also lower rates among South Asian groups, which are the reverse of the Census. This may reflect the fact that the Census question asked about limiting longstanding illness rather than longstanding illness alone. Data from other sources have suggested that there is a higher threshold for reporting ill health as constituting longstanding illness among ethnic minority groups. Table 6 presents data from a relatively small study of health among ethnic minorities in Bristol[11] which demonstrates that a high percentage of respondents answer 'No' to a question regarding longstanding illness,

Table 5: Age and gender-standardised prevalence rates (per 100) of reported health problems according to ethnicity[34]

	White	All ethnic minorities	Caribbean	All South Asians	Indian or African Asian	Pakistani or Bangladeshi	Chinese
Fair or poor health	27	32	34	32	27	39	26
A longstanding illness	27	21	27	18	17	21	15
Long-standing illness limiting work	11	12	13	12	11	13	7
Diagnosed angina or heart attack	4.2	4.0	3.7	4.2	3.3	6.0	3.0
Hypertension	12	11	17	9	8	11	5
Diabetes	1.7	5.7	5.3	6.2	4.7	8.9	3.0
Accidents resulting in hospital treatment	13	6	9	4	4	5	8

Table 6: Respondents with a particular condition which has been treated by a doctor who responded 'No' when asked if they had a 'long-standing illness, disability or infirmity'[11]

Condition	Number of respondents	Answered 'No' to longstanding illness
Diabetes	53	27
Asthma	79	60
Cancer	4	3
Epilepsy/fits	6	3

disability or infirmity who are receiving, or have received, treatment by a doctor for several important forms of morbidity.

Within the Fourth National Survey adding a question regarding whether ability to work was limited by the illness produced a pattern across ethnic groups that was more similar to those from the Census (Table 5). Table 7 shows the specific activities limited by health and it can be seen that Chinese people tend to have the lowest rates of limitation – lower than the majority ethnic group in most cases – while other ethnic minority groups, in particular Bangladeshi and Pakistani people, have higher rates of limitation.

Taking the definitions of coronary heart disease used in the Fourth National Survey, Pakistani/Bangladeshi people had considerably higher rates than white people, although the prevalence rates for Indian and African Asian people were very similar to those for the majority ethnic group (Table 5). This is not in line with the mortality data presented above, nor with the results of some other studies.[12] This may reflect the self-reported nature of the data in the Fourth National Survey. The prevalence rates of hypertension also need to be treated with

Table 7: Age and gender-standardised prevalence rates (per 100) for specific activities limited by health problems according to ethnicity: Fourth National Survey of Ethnic Minorities[34]

	White	All ethnic minorities	Caribbean	All South Asians	Indian or African Asian	Pakistani or Bangladeshi	Chinese
Several flights of stairs	12	15	13	16	13	22	6
One flight of stairs	4	6	5	8	5	13	1
Walking more than one mile	7	13	9	16	11	23	8
Walking half a mile	4	9	5	10	7	17	6
Walking 100 yards	2	4	3	5	4	8	1
Carrying groceries	8	11	10	12	10	16	6
Bending, kneeling or stooping	9	10	12	10	8	13	4
Bathing or dressing	3	4	3	5	4	6	2

caution, since they are based on self-reports. The picture of a higher rate of hypertension among Caribbean people is consistent with the findings from surveys in which blood pressure is measured (see later). The higher prevalence rates of diabetes among all the ethnic minority groups for whom data could be analysed in the Fourth National Survey are also in keeping with several specific studies of this issue.[13-15] All the ethnic minority groups studied except Caribbeans had considerably lower prevalences of respiratory symptoms than white people. A lower prevalence of respiratory symptoms among children of families originating from the Indian subcontinent has been found elsewhere,[16] although not all studies agree on this.[17] Similarly, some studies of respiratory symptoms in adults have found similar rates for South Asian groups to the majority ethnic population.[18,19]

The lower risk of having an accident resulting in hospital treatment for all the ethnic minority groups is consistent with the mortality data for the Indian subcontinent groups, although not for Caribbean people. It may be that there are differences in the propensity to attend hospital following accidents between the groups.

Relative differences in cardiovascular disease and diabetes morbidity by ethnic group reflect the differences in mortality. Thus, mean blood pressure is greater in South Asian,[20] and African Caribbean people than the general population (Table 8). These differences are particularly

Table 8: Mean systolic blood pressure (mmHg) by ethnicity

Ethnic group	Age group	Men	Women
Europeans	40-64	121	120
South Asians	40-64	126	126
African Caribbeans	40-64	128	135
Chinese	25-64	123	121

striking for African Caribbean women, where over a third of those in middle age are hypertensive. In contrast, blood pressure in Chinese people is similar to that of the general population.[21] Assessing the burden of heart disease is difficult, as there may be ethnic differences in the proportion of people with heart disease being given this diagnosis by a doctor, and differences in interpretation of standard angina questionnaires. Changes consistent with ischaemic heart disease on an electrocardiogram are less prone to an ethnic bias. Numbers of women with these changes are too small in existing studies, but in men it appears that while South Asian people have twice the prevalence of heart disease compared with the general population,[13] African Caribbean and Chinese people have rates which are about a quarter of that of the general population (Table 9).[14,21] The prevalence of adult diabetes is three and five times greater in African Caribbean and South Asian people respectively compared with the general population (Table 10).[14,20] Current data suggest that diabetes prevalence is not different in Chinese people compared with the general population.[15]

Table 9: Prevalence of major Q waves (indicative of coronary artery disease) on an electrocardiograph (men only)

Ethnic group	Age group	Prevalence (%)
Europeans	40-64	2.3
South Asians	40-64	4.0
African Caribbeans	40-64	0.5
Chinese	25-64	0.6

Table 10: Prevalence (%) of non-insulin dependent diabetes in different ethnic groups[a]

Ethnic group	Age group	Men	Women	Total	Relative risk[b]
Europeans	40-64	5	2	4	1.0
South Asians	40-64	20	16	19	4.8
African Caribbeans	40-64	13	18	16	3.2
Chinese	45-64	–	–	8	1.3

[a] Includes people with previously diagnosed diabetes and that found on screening with oral glucose tolerance test and the WHO criteria.

[b] Relative risk compared to the European comparator used in the study from which the data have been taken.

Childhood morbidity

Low birthweight is a risk factor for infant (in particular perinatal) mortality and recent evidence suggests that low birthweight may also be a risk factor for diseases in later life, including coronary heart disease, stroke, diabetes and respiratory illness. The birthweight distribution according to mother's country of birth is such that a higher percentage of births are of low weight (under 2,500g) and there is, indeed, a shift of the whole distribution of birthweights downwards, with a higher percentage of deliveries also being in the next two lowest categories (2,500g-2,999g and 3,000g-3,499g) for the offspring of mothers born on the Indian subcontinent, East Africa, West/South Africa and the Caribbean.[10]

There are very limited data on morbidity in childhood according to ethnic group. In the absence of data on general morbidity there has been particular attention to issues such as congenital anomalies, vitamin D deficiency (producing rickets) and haemoglobinopathies such as sickle cell trait, seen among as many as 1 in 10 African Caribbean babies, and thalassaemia minor seen among 1 in 10 to 1 in 20 offspring of mothers born in the Indian subcontinent.[10] These conditions are not in themselves generally causes of serious morbidity although sickle cell disease and thalassaemia major, which occur if both parents carry these traits, lead to serious ill health. However, the concentration of studies on conditions which are considered to be of particular relevance to minority ethnic populations may, in fact, ignore differences in causes of ill health which affect more people.

A study from Glasgow looked at the prevalence of morbidity and health-related behaviours among 14- to 15-year-olds of British Asian

Table 11: Glasgow 14- to 15-year-olds: ethnic differences in self-reported health (%) [19, 22]

	Male		Female	
Self-reported health	**British Asian**	**Other origin**	**British Asian**	**Other origin**
Health fairly/not good in last 12 months	45	40**	49	57**
Health fair/poor versus others own age	22	22**	36	29
Fitness moderate/not very good	23	23**	46	42**
Long-standing illness or disability	19	26	16	23
Limiting long-standing illness	12	16	7	15*
Indications of chronic phlegm	9	10	2	11**
Accidents/injuries in last three years	27	41**	17	23
Lost 1+ second teeth	20	30*	18	29*
Report 6+ symptoms in last month	40	29*	44	45

Note: British Asian versus other origin within sexes.

* $p<0.05$; ** $p<0.01$; *** $p<0.001$.

and other ethnic origin (Tables 11 and 12).[19,22] At age 14-15, compared with non-Asian counterparts, fewer British Asian girls reported limiting illness or chronic phlegm, fewer boys reported accidents, and fewer of both sexes had lost second teeth; more of both sexes reported not smoking, drinking alcohol, or using drugs; and fewer reported frequent exercise.

Table 12: Glasgow 14- to 15-year-olds: ethnic differences in reported health behaviour[19, 22]

	Male		Female	
Reported health behaviour	**British Asian**	**Other origin**	**British Asian**	**Other origin**
Age 14				
Drinking alcohol				
– never	88	27	87	18
– tried once or twice	6	21	4	18
– used to but gave up	0	2	0	4
– on special occasions	6	37	4	39
– regularly	0	13***	5	21***
Smoking				
– never	72	53	65	41
– tried once or twice	16	20	27	25
– used to but gave up	10	4	3	12
– occasionally	2	5	4	8
– regularly	0	18**	1	14***
Drugs				
– tried (soft or hard)	4	27***	1	21***
Age 15				
Drinking alcohol				
– never	80	25	89	11
– tried once or twice	10	20	4	21
– used to but gave up	2	6	1	4
– on special occasions	4	33	4	40
– regularly	4	16***	2	24***
Smoking				
– never	70	51	84	36
– tried once or twice	16	22	9	27
– used to but gave up	3	10	1	8
– occasionally	7	8	5	9
– regularly	4	9**	1	20***
Drugs				
– tried (soft or hard)	10	26**	3	25***
Age 14-15				
Physical exercise for 20 minutes				
– daily	26	40	16	20
– 4-6 times per week	27	30	15	26
– 2-3 times per week	29	22	53	39
– once a week or less	18	8**	16	15*

Note: British Asian versus other origin. * $p<0.05$; ** $p<0.01$; *** $p<0.001$.

Ethnicity and health: the role of socioeconomic position

The contribution of socioeconomic factors to ethnic differences in mortality – especially to the higher mortality among black people than white people in the US – has been discussed and investigated for many years.[23-25] In the UK less attention has been paid to this issue, partly because of data limitations. While health data are often analysed according to socioeconomic position, or according to ethnic group, there have been relatively few analyses of socioeconomic differentials in health within minority ethnic groups. Recent analyses of data from around the 1991 Census have demonstrated social class differences in mortality of men of working age among most ethnic groups which are similar to those of the majority population. For Caribbean men the social class gradient was weak and inconsistent, while there was no gradient at all for West/South Africans (Table 13). The numbers of deaths in the categories stratified by social class and ethnicity are small, making it difficult to analyse cause-of-death specific social class gradients among minority ethnic groups. For ischaemic heart disease, manual rates were substantially higher than non-manual rates for men born in East Africa, the Indian subcontinent, Scotland and Ireland, but not for men born in the Caribbean or West/South Africa. Stroke was higher among manual men in all of the above-mentioned groups, although the difference among men from West/South Africa was small.[4]

In the Fourth National Survey, morbidity was analysed according to ethnicity and social class. Households were divided into those that were manual and non-manual with a third group of respondents coming from households containing no full-time worker. Table 14 presents morbidity according to household social class and ethnic group membership. Social class differences are seen within the majority and minority populations for most of the causes of ill health and health-related behaviours examined, although differences are also seen between ethnic groups within social class strata. People living in households in which there is no full-time worker were, for many causes of morbidity, in worse health than those living in households with a full-time worker. In some cases this could be because the respondent to the survey who would normally work was out of employment because of ill health.

Table 13: SMRs for men aged 20-64, all-causes, by social class and country of birth[4]

			Country of birth							
Social class	All countries	Caribbean	West/ South Africa	East Africa	Indian subcontinent	Scotland	Ireland (all parts)	India	Pakistan	Bangladesh
I/II	71[b]	83[b]	136[b]	104	96	82[b]	95	94	101	132[b]
IIIN	100	84[b]	103	138[b]	112[b]	121[b]	127[b]	105	120	159[b]
IIIM	117[b]	105	177[b]	150[b]	120[b]	169[b]	166[b]	124[b]	104	148[b]
IV/V	135[b]	99	112	120[b]	158[b]	186[b]	173[b]	146[b]	147	233[b]
Non-manual	77[b]	83[b]	128[b]	113[b]	100	89[b]	102	96	106	144[b]
Manual	124[b]	102	137[b]	136[b]	140[b]	176[b]	169[b]	135[b]	128[b]	201[b]
All[a]	100	89[b]	126[b]	123[b]	107[b]	129[b]	135[b]	106[b]	102[b]	137[b]

[a] includes unclassified
[b] SMR significantly different from 100, p<0.05.

Table 14: Age and gender-standardised prevalences per 100: Fourth National Survey of Ethnic Minorities[34]

	White	All ethnic minorities	Caribbean	Indian or African Asian	Pakistani or Bangladeshi
Reported fair or poor health					
Non-manual	21	24	25	20	30
Manual	23	30	29	27	35
No full-time worker in household	37	38	38	34	44
Respiratory symptoms					
(coughing up phlegm or a wheeze)					
Non-manual	23	14	16	13	13
Manual	23	17	28	13	12
No full-time worker in household	35	21	26	17	20
Diabetes					
Non-manual	1.1	4.1	4.1	2.8	6.4
Manual	1.1	4.5	3.2	3.5	8.3
No full-time worker in household	2.1	6.3	4.5	7.1	7.6
Hypertension					
Non-manual	8	8	15	5	6
Manual	12	11	15	9	10
No full-time worker in household	11	12	18	8	11
Angina or heart attack by tenure					
Owner-occupier	3.0	3.2	2.7	2.5	5.2
Tenant	4.1	4.0	3.8	3.5	5.2
No full-time worker in household	3.9	4.5	4.0	4.3	5.4
Regular current smoking					
Non-manual	21	16	24	9	16
Manual	33	18	30	8	18
No full-time worker in household	46	25	39	19	18
Ever drinks alcohol					
Non-manual	95	49	81	45	7
Manual	91	46	83	39	5
No full-time worker in household	84	46	84	41	2

The contribution of socioeconomic position to health differentials

In an analysis around the 1971 Census, occupational social class was found to explain little or none of the mortality differentials between ethnic groups.[26] We present more recent data from around the 1991 Census in Table 15. SMRs adjusted for age are presented in the top line of each row in the table, with SMRs following adjustment for social class as well as age being shown below these. Thus the SMR of 89 for all-cause mortality for Caribbean men is further reduced, to 82, after adjustment for social class. This is seen because Caribbean men are more likely to be in manual social class groups, which generally have higher mortality than non-manual social class groups. Thus the

Table 15: SMRs for men aged 20-64, before and after adjustment for social class[4]

	All causes	Ischaemic heart disease	Stroke	Lung cancer	Accidents and injuries	Suicide
Total	100	100	100	100	100	100
Caribbean						
Age	89*	60*	169*	59*	121	59*
Age/social class	82*	55*	146*	49*	109*	57*
West/South Africa						
Age	126*	83	315*	a	a	a
Age/social class	135*	79*	372*			
East Africa						
Age	123*	160*	113	a	86	75*
Age/social class	137*	188*	128*		104*	75*
Indian subcontinent						
Age	107*	150*	163*	48*	80*	73*
Age/social class	117*	165*	175*	52*	87*	76*
Scotland						
Age	129*	117*	111	146*	117*	149*
Age/social class	132*	121*	112*	151*	184*	160*
Ireland						
Age	135*	121*	130*	157*	189*	135*
Age/social class	129*	115*	124*	145*	169*	134*

[a] Numbers too small.

* p<0.05, compared to overall rate.

Note: The SMRs which are just age-adjusted are sometimes a little different from the equivalent age-adjusted SMRs in Table 1. This is because the analyses only included the men on whom social class data were available on death certificates.

expectation would be that Caribbean men would have high, rather than low, mortality and taking social class into account in the statistical adjustments makes this discrepancy between what is seen and what would be expected more apparent.

In studies of second and later generation Irish people living in the UK it has been possible to adjust for a range of socioeconomic factors.[5] Among second generation Irish men of working ages the SMR of 126 is little changed by adjustment for social class (it becomes 132) or for housing tenure and car access, which serve as indices of socioeconomic position (it becomes 124). Similarly, for women, the age-adjusted SMR of 129 becomes 130 on adjustment for social class and 126 on adjustment for housing tenure and car access. Among men of patrilineal Irish descent in the west of Scotland, adjustment for indicators of socioeconomic position over the lifecourse – including father's social class, own social class in adulthood and car access – reduced the elevation in all-cause mortality from 26% to 17%, and in the case of cardiovascular disease from 50% to 40%.[27]

There is a clear social class gradient in perinatal, neonatal, post-neonatal and infant mortality for all countries of birth, with those born in the lowest social classes generally having the highest mortality rate.[10] However, the lower occupational social class of many people from minority ethnic groups cannot account for the overall ethnic differences in mortality. Within each social class, for example, infant mortality rates were about twice as high in Pakistani children as in those born in England and Wales, except for those in social class I (possibly due to the small number of deaths observed in this group). Perinatal, post-neonatal and infant mortality is thus highest in children born to Pakistani parents, even when social class is taken into account. Conversely, when social class is taken into account, infants born to parents from Bangladesh, East and West Africa have lower post-neonatal mortality rates than those born to parents from the UK, and similarly, infant mortality rates are also lower in Bangladeshi children.

In the Fourth National Survey the role of socioeconomic factors in accounting for the differences in morbidity and health-related behaviours according to ethnic group membership was studied in detail).[34] As shown in Table 14, while the usual social class differences in morbidity are seen within each ethnic group, differences between ethnic groups are also seen within each social class stratum. A standard of living index was also constructed within this study, putting together various markers of socioeconomic position. Information on overcrowding of accommodation, the presence of basic household amenities, the ownership of consumer durables and access to cars was used for this purpose. This, as is discussed later, was considered to be a more discriminatory marker of socioeconomic position than social class. Differences in morbidity were then adjusted for social class, for housing tenure (a commonly used indicator of socioeconomic

285

position in UK studies) and the standard of living index. Table 16 presents data on reporting health as fair or poor according to ethnic group after adjustments for socioeconomic measures. A relative risk of 1.25, for example, indicates a 25% higher chance of reporting fair or poor health among Caribbean people than the majority ethnic community. When this is reduced to 1.15 on adjustment for social class (as well as age and gender) this indicates that after taking social class into account there is only a 15% higher risk of reporting fair or poor health among Caribbean people. For Pakistani and Bangladeshi people it can be seen that adjustment for the standard of living index produces considerably greater attenuation of the degree to which their reported health is worse than the majority ethnic community than does adjustment for social class or housing tenure. Tables 17, 18 and 19 report equivalent data for diabetes, respiratory symptoms and diagnosed heart disease. As can be seen, the elevated risk of diabetes among all the ethnic minority groups considered is largely independent of current socioeconomic position.

Table 16: Relative risk compared with the ethnic majority community of reported fair or poor health, standardised for socioeconomic factors: Fourth National Survey of Ethnic Minorities[34]

	Caribbean	Indian and African Asian	Pakistani and Bangladeshi	All ethnic minorities[a]
Age and gender	1.25	0.99	1.45	1.17
	(1.1-1.4)	(0.9-1.1)	(1.3-1.6)	(1.1-1.3)
Class, age and gender	1.15	1.00	1.36	1.14
	(1.03-1.3)	(0.9-1.1)	(1.2-1.5)	(1.1-1.2)
Tenure, age and gender	1.17	1.04	1.45	1.18
	(1.04-1.3)	(0.9-1.2)	(1.3-1.6)	(1.1-1.3)
Standard of living, age and gender	1.15	0.94	1.24	1.08
	(1.03-1.3)	(0.9-1.04)	(1.1-1.4)	(0.99-1.2)

[a] Includes the displayed groups plus Chinese people.

Table 17: Relative risk of diabetes compared with the ethnic majority community, standardised for socioeconomic factors: Fourth National Survey of Ethnic Minorities[34]

	Caribbean	Indian and African Asian	Pakistani and Bangladeshi	All ethnic minorities[a]
Age and gender	2.6	2.6	4.9	3.0
	(1.6-4.0)	(1.7-3.9)	(3.3-7.2)	(2.1-4.3)
Class, age and gender	2.8	3.1	5.2	3.5
	(1.8-4.3)	(2.0-4.6)	(3.4-7.8)	(2.4-5.0)
Tenure, age and gender	2.3	2.7	4.8	3.1
	(1.4-3.6)	(1.8-4.1)	(3.3-6.9)	(2.2-4.4)
Standard of living, age and gender	2.2	2.4	4.1	2.8
	(1.4-3.4)	(1.6-3.6)	(2.9-6.0)	(2.0-3.9)

[a] Includes the displayed groups plus Chinese people.

Table 18: Relative risk of respiratory symptoms compared with the ethnic majority community, standardised for socioeconomic factors: Fourth National Survey of Ethnic Minorities[34]

	Caribbean	Indian and African Asian	Pakistani and Bangladeshi	All ethnic minorities[a]
Age and gender	0.89	0.53	0.65	0.66
	(0.7-1.05)	(0.4-0.6)	(0.6-0.8)	(0.6-0.7)
Class, age and gender	0.86	0.53	0.55	0.64
	(0.7-1.01)	(0.4-0.6)	(0.5-0.7)	(0.6-0.7)
Tenure, age and gender	0.85	0.58	0.65	0.68
	(0.7-1.01)	(0.5-0.7)	(0.6-0.8)	(0.6-0.8)
Standard of living, age and gender	0.83	0.50	0.50	0.61
	(0.7-0.98)	(0.4-0.6)	(0.4-0.6)	(0.5-0.7)

[a] Includes the displayed groups plus Chinese people.

Table 19: Relative risk of diagnosed heart disease compared with the ethnic majority community, standardised for socioeconomic factors: Fourth National Survey of Ethnic Minorities[34]

	Caribbean	Indian and African Asian	Pakistani and Bangladeshi	All ethnic minorities[a]
Age and gender	0.95	0.77	1.50	0.97
	(0.6-1.4)	(0.5-1.1)	(1.1-2.0)	(0.7-1.3)
Class, age and gender	1.05	0.92	1.49	1.10
	(0.7-1.6)	(0.6-1.3)	(1.1-2.1)	(0.8-1.5)
Tenure, age and gender	0.93	0.85	1.57	1.05
	(0.6-1.4)	(0.6-1.2)	(1.2-2.1)	(0.8-1.4)
Standard of living, age and gender	1.02	0.67	1.24	0.92
	(0.7-1.5)	(0.5-0.96)	(0.9-1.7)	(0.7-1.2)

[a] Includes the displayed groups plus Chinese people.

Similarly the reduced risk of respiratory symptoms is, as would be expected, not a reflection of socioeconomic differences, since in general socioeconomic indicators are less favourable for the ethnic minority people and in all groups people in worse socioeconomic circumstances report higher levels of respiratory symptoms. An elevated risk of diagnosed heart disease is only seen for Pakistani and Bangladeshi people after standardisation for socioeconomic factors, age and gender. The apparent reduced risk among Indian and African Asian people for diagnosed heart disease after such standardisation stands in contrast to other research on this issue[4,12] and should be treated with caution.

Several studies have examined blood pressure and glucose intolerance (an indicator of diabetes risk) according to both ethnicity and social class. As can be seen in Table 20 while mean blood pressure was higher in people from manual occupations compared to those from

Table 20: Blood pressure and glucose intolerance by social class in African Caribbeans and Europeans

	European		African Caribbean	
	Men	Women	Men	Women
Mean systolic pressure (mm Hg)				
Non-manual	122	116	126	131
Manual	123	119	129	136
Prevalence of glucose intolerance (%)				
Non-manual	8	12	33	32
Manual	21	13	27	33

non-manual occupations, in African Caribbean and European men and women these differences were relatively modest, and occupational social class could not account for the large observed ethnic difference in blood pressure. The prevalence of glucose intolerance (combining those at high risk of diabetes and those with frank diabetes), was only markedly higher in European men from manual occupations compared to non-manual. In the other groups, no such differences could be found.

Ethnicity and health: approaches to understanding the relationship

When considering differentials in health status between ethnic groups it is useful to categorise models of explanation. This is not intended to suggest that one explanatory category is adequate to account for the health differentials and it is likely that most, if not all, categories make some contribution to the pattern which is observed.

Categories of explanation for sociodemographic differences in health have been developed and refined over many years[28] and have been modified and expanded for application specifically to health differentials between ethnic groups.[29]

Artefact

Artefact explanations suggest that the relationships between ethnicity and health could be produced by the processes of data collection and analysis. For example, if country of birth is reported differently on death certificates than at the Census, using these two sources to estimate mortality rates could be seriously misleading. The measurement of health status could also differ across groups. Self-reported health has been used in several studies discussed above and it could be that members of different ethnic groups have different propensities for reporting ill-health at a given level of objective morbidity, although there is evidence against this.[30] For other health outcomes ethnicity could also influence classification of illness status. For example it has been suggested that the apparently higher prevalence of schizophrenia among young African Caribbean men than young men of the majority ethnic population is due to a greater propensity to diagnose schizophrenia among them, rather than any real difference in disease prevalence. While it is always important to consider the degree to which the processes of measurement and data analysis may generate apparent health differentials when no such differentials exist, it is likely that the overall contribution of artefact explanations to understanding the association between ethnic group and health is limited, although in particular circumstances it could be an important factor.

Migration

A history of migration is often the root factor in the formation of self-conscious ethnic minorities and majorities, and is often a key issue in explaining patterns of health. The migration may have been of the current minority (eg South Asian or African Caribbean people in Europe, or Irish people in Britain, US and Australasia) or of the current majority (eg the white populations among Maori or Aborigine or native American peoples in Australasia and North America). Among the migrants, this means that there is always biographical experience of at least two economic systems, one current and one in the past, and of at least two cultures. Among their descendants, likewise, there is a continuing consciousness of this dual experience. Hence all the factors enumerated below are complicated by this duality, for example, material factors in both economic systems may have shaped migrants' health, and the culture of migrants is not straightforwardly that of the country of origin, but will have been affected almost immediately by experiences in the receiving country.

Factors associated with the period immediately surrounding the migration also frequently present specific explanations for the health of ethnic minorities or, more often, alternative explanations which need to be ruled out in analysis or guarded against in the design of studies. Migrants tend to be selected by health characteristics from the population of origin – usually having better health if they are long-distance migrants.[26] These health characteristics are present at the time of decision to migrate and will be reflected in the health of migrants in their place of destination. However, over time such differentials 'wear off' and the health of migrants will tend to revert to the mean standard of the population of origin, particularly when the next generation is considered.

In the case of long-distance migrants, the 'wearing off' of the protection produced by the tendency of migrants to be a healthy subgroup of their source population may mean a relative decline in the health of migrants, compared to health in the country of destination, over time.

An alternative health selection aspect of migration is the possibility that returning to one's birthplace when sick or through the desire to die in one's original home could lead to the selective return of those with high mortality risk. This phenomenon – which has been called the 'Salmon Bias'[31] phenomenon – would therefore artificially reduce the mortality rate of migrant populations. This would occur whether or not there was complete recording of the return migrants leaving the UK. If recording is complete – and therefore denominators can be adjusted for those leaving the UK – then it is still the case that the remaining people born in a particular country and living within the UK would be a selected healthy group with low mortality. In addition, if there is incomplete recording of people who leave the country then they will erroneously remain part of the denominator for calculating mortality rates and artificially reduced rates of death will be generated. While the 'Salmon Bias' has been investigated in US studies with regard to the low levels of mortality among Latino populations (and has been found not to explain the low levels of adult mortality of these groups) there has been little equivalent investigation in the UK. Williams and Ecob showed that among English residents in the 1971 Longitudinal Study, those born in the Republic of Ireland have higher proportions not present at the next Census and lower proportions recorded as dying, suggesting return migration of those who will die, as well as over-estimation of the denominator population.[32] Similarly the low mortality for those of post-retirement age among the Irish-born or second generation Irish people compared to the elevated mortality at younger ages suggests there may be an issue relating to the return of ill people at elevated mortality risk.[32]

A second factor associated with the migration period is stress of various kinds.[33] This would normally lead to worse health, but as it is a transitional phenomenon it should be followed by improvement over time, if other things are equal. The elevated risk seen long after migration and among second generation migrants cannot be due to the acute stress of migration.

Socioeconomic factors

Given that there is such a strong relationship between socioeconomic factors and health, and there are important differences in the

Table 21: Socioeconomic position by ethnic group: Fourth National Survey of Ethnic Minorities[34]

	White	Caribbean	Indian	African Asian	Pakistani	Bangladeshi	Chinese
Registrar General's social class							
I/II	35	22	30	35	20	11	40
IIn	15	18	19	23	15	18	26
IIIm	31	30	21	23	32	32	20
IV/V	20	30	30	19	33	40	13
Economically active unemployed (%)	11	24	16	13	38	42	7
Lacking one or more basic housing amenities (%)[a]	16	17	19	10	39	32	19

[a] That is, exclusive use of: bath or shower, bathroom, inside toilet, kitchen, hot water from a tap, and central heating.

distribution of socioeconomic circumstances of different ethnic groups (summarised in Table 21)[34] it would seem to make sense to explore how far ethnic variations in health remain once socioeconomic differences between ethnic groups have been controlled. This was the strategy adopted by Marmot et al,[26] but they found that once they had standardised for class differences in the immigrant mortality data they used, ethnic variations in health remained more or less unchanged. In addition, they found that class had a variable relationship with mortality rates for the different migrant groups. A more consistent picture, with social class differentials among minority ethnic groups being in the same direction as the general population, has emerged in the 1990s,[4] but, as Table 15 shows, conventional adjustment for occupational social class still accounts for little if any of the differences in mortality risk between members of different ethnic groups.

However, there are two key reasons why class effects might be suppressed in immigrant mortality data. First, such data use occupation as recorded on death certificates to define social class. The inflating of occupational status on death certificates (where, according to Townsend and Davidson,[35] occupation is recorded as the 'skilled' job held for most of the individual's life rather than the 'unskilled' job held in the last few years of life) will be particularly significant for immigrant mortality data if migration to Britain was associated with downward social mobility for members of ethnic minority groups, a process that has been clearly documented.[36,37] So, the occupation recorded on the death certificates of migrants may well be an inaccurate reflection of their experience in Britain prior to death. In addition, given the socioeconomic profile of ethnic minority groups in Britain, this inflation of occupational level would only need to happen in relatively few cases for the figures representing the small population in higher classes to be distorted upwards.

Second, there has been an increasing recognition of the limitations of traditional class groupings, which are far from internally homogeneous. A number of studies have drawn attention to variations in income levels and death rates among occupations that comprise particular social classes.[38] Within an occupational group, it is certainly likely that, as a result of the racialisation of disadvantage, ethnic minorities will be more likely to be found in lower or less prestigious occupational grades, to have poorer job security, to endure more stressful working conditions and to be more likely to work unsocial hours (eg see the account of the situation in nursing).[39] Evidence from the Fourth National Survey illustrates this point clearly.[34] Table 22 shows that ethnic minority people had a lower income than white people in the same class, that unemployed ethnic minority people had been unemployed for longer than equivalent white people, and that some ethnic minority groups had poorer quality housing than

Table 22: Variations within socioeconomic bands by ethnic group: Fourth National Survey of Ethnic Minorities[34]

	White	Caribbean	Indian and African Asian	Pakistani and Bangladeshi
Mean income by Registrar General's social class (£)[a]				
I/II	250	210	210	125
IIIn	185	145	135	95
IIIm	160	145	120	70
IV/V	130	120	110	65
Median duration of unemployment (months)	7	21	12	24
Lacking one or more basic housing amenities (%)[b]				
Owner-occupiers	11	12	14	38
Renters	27	23	28	37

[a] Based on bands of equivalised household income. The mean point of each band is used to make this calculation, which is rounded to the nearest £5.

[b] That is, exclusive use of: bath or shower, bathroom, inside toilet, kitchen, hot water from a tap, and central heating.

white people regardless of tenure. Similar findings have been reported from elsewhere in the UK and in the US.[40-42]

The conclusion to be drawn is that, while standard indicators of socioeconomic position have some use for making comparisons *within* ethnic groups, they are of little use for 'controlling out' the impact of socioeconomic differences.

Another problem with using data that have been standardised for socioeconomic position is worth highlighting. Such an approach to analysis and interpretation regards socioeconomic position as a confounding factor that needs to be 'controlled out' to reveal the 'true' relationship between ethnicity and health.[43] This results in the importance of socioeconomic factors becoming obscured and their explanatory role lost. The presentation of 'standardised' data leaves both the author and reader to assume that all that is left is an 'ethnicity' effect, be that cultural or biological. This gives the impression that different types of explanation operate for ethnic minority groups compared with the general population. While for the latter, factors relating to socioeconomic position are shown to be crucial, for the former they are not visible, so differences are assumed to be related to some aspect of ethnicity or 'race', even though socioeconomic factors are important determinants of health for all groups. Theories based on apparent 'pure' ethnic characteristics can in this way be used to explain the residual effects in models that claim to, but, as described above, cannot, take full account of socioeconomic factors.

Culture, beliefs, behaviour

Culture is usually assumed to affect health through such factors as health-related behaviours and beliefs (eg smoking, drinking alcohol, diet, exercise, sexual behaviour, concepts of health, images of the body, lay theories of illness etc), or the organisation of family and kinship (affecting childrearing, gender roles and patterns of social support), or language and communication (mainly affecting health service use).

Health-related behaviours are the best-documented of these factors. Smoking is generally at lower levels among black and South Asian groups than in the general population, especially among the women,[44] although smoking levels of African Caribbean and Pakistani men are approaching similar levels to the general population, and higher levels have been recorded for Bangladeshi men.[45] Alcohol consumption, even more than smoking, is at low levels among black and South Asian groups, again particularly among the women.[44] However, aggregated data may conceal high levels of alcohol consumption among Sikhs, and levels approaching those of the general population among Hindus.[46] By contrast with this picture, among Caribbean and South Asian groups, both smoking and drinking levels have been reported to be high among Irish people.[47] Smoking and drinking patterns have been reported to persist into the second generation,[48] but data on a longer-established Irish community in Britain suggest that differences are slight or non-existent, and rates of smoking and drinking in Ireland are generally similar to those in Britain.[49]

Patterns of diet are more difficult to summarise, and have recently been reviewed.[50] Concern has been expressed that dietary control may be needed to reduce coronary risk factor (especially abdominal obesity) among South Asian groups, and to reduce risk of hypertension and stroke (and excess weight for height) among African Caribbeans. Among largely vegetarian groups such as Gujaratis, saturated fat intakes are not an issue, but total fat intake may be. In addition, low vitamin D and iron intakes in vegetarian groups have been connected with tuberculosis and childhood growth problems. Among meat-eating groups such as Punjabis, intakes of saturated and total fat may be an issue.

The other side of excess weight problems is exercise: low levels of exercise have been found among black and South Asian groups, with the exception of young African Caribbean men.[45] Short stature among South Asian groups, and among people of Irish descent in Britain, suggests the possibility of a more general nutritional deficit, or a greater exposure to infections, in childhood. The stature of Irish people in Ireland is not shorter than that of the general population in Britain.[7]

The organisation of family and kinship is another complex subject. There are some recent statistical overviews,[51] although the area has not been reviewed in relation to health. South Asians groups have larger average household sizes, both in number of adults and in number of children, and are more often looking after older relatives, than the general population. More Caribbean households are of children living only with a mother than in the general population. Irish households are similar to those of the general population on these crude measures: despite stereotypes of high Catholic fertility, the mean number of dependant children in households of the Irish-born, who include a high proportion of Catholics, is currently identical to that of the general population.

Religion may be an important influence on many of these patterns. There are religious limits placed on smoking among Sikhs, on drinking alcohol among Muslims, and on both among evangelical Protestants. There was also a temperance movement among Catholics in Ireland in the last century which is still apparent in high levels of abstention there. The smoking levels of Pakistani and Bangladeshi men referred to above, which contrast with the low levels of smoking in South Asian groups otherwise, reflect the absence of a Muslim prohibition on smoking, although there is a general expectation of restraint for women.

In the same way, Sikh male levels of drinking reflect the absence of a specific Sikh prohibition on alcohol. Religion also influences diet, including the vegetarian patterns referred to earlier.

Language use has been considered an important influence on some health-related activities among South Asian groups.[45] However, the tendency to refer to this as a factor tends to mask more deep-seated difficulties of communication, some of which are related to racism.

There are special problems in using culture, behaviour or beliefs to explain health. The association of an ethnic group with a pattern of health does not indicate that the pattern of health is the result of a cultural difference. Crude assumptions of this sort, combined with the general tendency to focus on health problems more than health successes, have led to patterns of culture blaming which have received extensive criticism. A cultural explanation only becomes an initial possibility when particular beliefs or behaviours associated with the ethnic group concerned can be shown to account for the health pattern. For example, some observers consider the ethnic variation in drinking in the US to be accounted for through differing patterns of socialisation in the family.

Further exploration of these issues is needed. Many health-related behaviours have class or standard of living gradients, suggesting that they are also influenced by variations in income and wealth. Hence in relevant cases it may be necessary to test the possibility that any beliefs or behaviours concerned are influenced by class or standard of living. In a recent study, high levels of symptoms experienced by South Asian women were particularly elevated in Muslim groups and among those with poor English, suggesting cultural factors; however, when low standard of living, stress in work around the house and absence of kin and confidants were included in the analysis the cultural differences were explained.[52]

Where beliefs or behaviours and material factors are jointly involved, care has to be taken in interpreting the direction of causation, which may be complex. For example, bringing up children in deprived circumstances may lead to increased smoking as a way of reducing tension; however, the proportion of a group in deprived circumstances is increased by barriers to jobs and income, and access to jobs and income may be restricted by the racism. In this review racism is treated separately in a later section, but it provides an important illustration of ways in which cultural and material factors can interact.

Other requirements are also necessary for fully adequate cultural explanations. It is important that cultural factors are described in the terms used by cultural insiders, even if these descriptions are set beside other descriptions. Early research on reporting of symptoms assumed that South Asian languages lacked terms for identifying depressive states; but this assumption has been challenged by qualitative interviews with South Asian women.[53] Again, even when the behaviours or beliefs associated with an ethnic group can be shown to account for a particular health pattern, the fluidity of these factors and the way in which they are constantly refashioned within a culture need to be recognised, especially after migration when people have access to the resources of two different cultures. For example, western foods are more frequently eaten by the second generation of Muslim families in Britain, but there are considerable variations between Muslim groups, and the pattern is more common at lunch than at dinner.[54] Nor does the association of beliefs or behaviours with the health of an ethnic group in Britain guarantee that they are associated in the country of origin. Victorian explanations of Irish ill-health in Britain blamed Irish culture, yet levels of mortality in Ireland were much lower than in the receiving towns in Britain.[55] The situation in the new country, especially if hostile, may itself alter the beliefs and behaviour of incomers, or change their implications.

Racism

Racism and discrimination could possibly have an effect on health in three ways. First, there could be an indirect effect on health as a result of consequent socioeconomic disadvantage. Second, ethnic minority people will have a clear recognition of the relative disadvantage they face as a result of the obvious inequalities, discrimination and racism that they experience in virtually all spheres of their lives.[56] This sense of relative disadvantage, as Wilkinson has argued,[57] may have a significant impact on health.

Third, the experience of racial discrimination and harassment may have a direct detrimental effect on health. There has been recent evidence of both the nature and extent of the harassment members of ethnic minorities experience[56,58,59] and the multiple victimisation that some are subjected to could lead to mental distress and poor health. For example, it has been demonstrated that experiencing racial harassment is associated with reported acute illness (after controlling for other relevant variables) and that experiencing any form of discrimination at work is associated with both acute and longstanding illness.[60]

However, evidence is not consistent. For example, the Fourth National Survey showed that variations across ethnic minority groups in the reported experiences of racial harassment did not match those for health.[56] Bangladeshis, who had the poorest health, were less likely than both African Asians and Chinese, who had the best health, to report that they had been racially harassed. Part of the reason for this inconsistency in evidence is undoubtedly the difficulty of assessing the extent of racial harassment individuals experience. For example, studies in the US have shown that black Americans who report and challenge racial harassment and discrimination have *lower* blood pressure than those who say they would tolerate harassment and discrimination and do not report experiencing it.[61,62] The authors suggest that, in the case of hypertension at least, the negative health effect is a consequence of internalised anger, which would be more likely among those who experience, but do not report, racial harassment.

Biology

The use of studies of ethnic differences in health to point to presumed underlying biological – usually genetic – factors has been much discussed and criticised.[63] There is, however, generally more genetic variation within ethnic groups than between ethnic groups. This does not mean that differences in some health problems – for example haemoglobinopathies and melanoma – are not strongly influenced by genetic factors which alter propensity to disease. However, as contributors to overall health differentials between ethnic groups these play a relatively minor role. Several research groups are investigating whether differences in common chronic diseases, such as diabetes, coronary heart disease and hypertension, may be influenced by genetic factors which are differentially distributed between ethnic groups. Opinion on this differs with, for example, some researchers considering epidemiological evidence to demonstrate that the higher prevalence of hypertension among African Caribbean people and people of African origin in the UK or US is strongly influenced by genetic factors,[64] while focused studies of this issue find little support for this hypothesis, instead identifying environmental factors as of primary importance.[65] The 'racialisation' of research and health policy which focus on genetic differences is, and should be, resisted for many obvious reasons.

Similarly the failure of many approaches based on genetic factors to acknowledge the often necessary role of environmental factors in the expression of any genetic differences is particularly unhelpful.

The understandable reluctance – on both empirical and ideological grounds – to accept a major role for genetic differences in explaining health differentials between ethnic groups has sometimes led to a reluctance to consider biological factors as having any role in generating health differentials. However, many important determinants of health are physiological characteristics which are strongly influenced by socioeconomic and other environmental factors, and in turn have a long-lasting influence on health. Thus low birthweight, which is strongly influenced by adverse material circumstances acting over the lifetime of the mother, is associated with high rates of diabetes, coronary heart disease, respiratory disease and hypertension in adult life. Similarly short stature, influenced by nutrition in early life, is related to an increased risk of respiratory and cardiovascular mortality. Several aspects of bodily habitus, such as birthweight, growth in childhood, achieved height and lung function, are factors which are at the same time socially produced and biological. Similar considerations apply to the role of such factors in explaining socioeconomic differentials in health status within ethnic groups. An understandable tendency to reject any form of explanation presented in biological terms fails to recognise the extent to which socioeconomic and environmental forces become embodied and, through this embodiment, influence the health of people throughout their lives, and may even influence the health of subsequent generations.

Health service access and use

The role of health services in determining health status has often been underestimated in comparison to environmental and genetic factors. But surgery for heart disease or arthritis, medical treatment for diabetes, and immunisation can have a major impact. There are several reasons why people from minority ethnic groups have inequitable access to care. Studies from the US show large inequities in healthcare access, especially when comparing African American people to white people, largely due to the relationship between wealth and ability to obtain health care.

But equity in access to healthcare, particularly by ethnicity, has been poorly researched in the UK, as it is assumed that there should be no inequity in a service which is free at the point of delivery. Such a simplistic argument ignores the complexity of the route to obtaining appropriate care, so that barriers can occur at any stage of the care-seeking process. At the patient level, individuals differ in their perceptions of the severity of their symptoms, and the urgency with which they seek care. Once the decision has been made, physical barriers to the general practitioner (GP), such as lack of access to a car, and unavailability of an appointment at a convenient time, may also cause delay. The outcome of the consultation depends largely on the GP being able to arrive at a correct diagnosis, which is influenced by patient demographic characteristics, including social class, and the quality of the GP. These factors may also influence the receipt of hospital care, once a referral has been made.

Earlier studies have simply examined utilisation of primary or hospital services, and suffer from several methodological limitations which results in confused interpretations. GP consultations were found to be higher in Pakistani, Indian and Caribbean adults compared with the general population,[45,66] but no account was taken of differences in morbidity or need.

Consultations for specific conditions show that while Caribbean people attend more for diseases of the circulatory system, Asian attendance rates are similar to that of the general population.[67,68] The latter finding is not reassuring given the substantially higher rate of heart disease observed in South Asians.

Use of screening services, such as breast and cervical cancer screening, has often been reported to be low in people from minority ethnic groups, especially South Asian women.[45] The explanation provided for this is that there is a poor understanding of the value of preventative care, and a general lack of knowledge about such services. However, these explanations are contradicted by the finding that immunisation rates are generally higher in people from minority ethnic groups.[69]

These studies tell us very little about whether, or where, inequalities in access to care occur. More recent studies, generally focusing on a specific condition, have provided better information. In the management of chronic heart disease, South Asian people have to wait twice as long for specialist intervention than Europeans.[70] But again this study could not show where the barrier to care occurred. An examination of proposed action in the event of chest pain indicated that South Asian people were more likely to be concerned about such symptoms, and more likely to seek immediate care than the general population.[71] This finding is confirmed by a study of mothers, which showed that Bengali mothers were more likely to seek immediate care for an unwell child than their counterparts from other ethnic groups.[17] Thus it would appear that barriers are unlikely to occur before the healthcare service is approached. There is some evidence that physical access to the GP is more difficult, and obtaining an appointment is harder for South Asian people, particularly

Bangladeshi people, compared with the general population.[45] But at the consultation, South Asian people are more likely to report that they have satisfactorily communicated their needs.[72]

This is confounded by studies of the outcome of consultations. South Asian people are less likely to leave the surgery with a follow-up appointment,[67] and less likely to be offered services such as a district nurse, despite being keen to use these services once offered them.[72] Difficulties in communication between the doctor and patient have often been ascribed to language,[73] but this is less of a problem than it at first appears. Facility with English is now high in the younger South Asian groups,[72] and around 80% of South Asian people are registered with a South Asian GP.[45] But there are indications that cultural perceptions about symptoms may differ, and may make it hard for people from minority ethnic groups to articulate their needs within the framework used by the UK general population. In those who had a confirmed heart attack, South Asian people are less likely to present with classical symptoms, and the diagnosis is therefore often missed.[74] Others have shown that referral rates from general practice for a barium meal examination are higher in South Asian people than Europeans, but that abnormalities are reported much less often.[75] As a result of this, GPs may find it harder to arrive at an appropriate diagnosis.

It appears that people from minority ethnic groups may have poorer access to healthcare in the UK compared with the general population, but the reasons for this, its extent and the degree to which it influences health outcomes are unknown.

Conclusions

The empirical evidence on differentials in health status between ethnic groups in the UK remains somewhat patchy and limited. Data on some ethnic groups – for example Chinese and Irish people – are very limited and conclusions about even basic issues cannot be reached. Morbidity data for representative population samples are scarce, although the recent publication of results from the Fourth National Survey has provided important new information here. The collection of adequate data in which the association between ethnicity, health and health services utilisation can be investigated – and from which proposals for improvement can be generated – should be encouraged.

Influences considered under each of the explanatory categories we have discussed above will all make some contribution to the production of ethnic differentials in health. Different influences will act during different periods of people's lives and the accumulation of such factors over the entire lifecourse – and even the lifecourses of previous generations – must be considered if an adequate framework for understanding ethnic differentials in health is to be developed.

A key issue relates to the ways in which measurement and conceptual issues regarding socioeconomic position can influence studies of the contribution of socioeconomic differences to ethnic group differentials in health status, as has been discussed by several authors.[76-78] A failure to appreciate these problems when studying the contribution of socioeconomic position to health differences between ethnic groups produces a form of reasoning by elimination, which leads to explanations concentrating on assumed genetic or cultural differences.

For example, a recent study of ethnic group differences in stroke in London[79] compared stroke rates among two groups they defined as black (Afro-Caribbean, 'black African' and 'black other' according to the 1991 British Census categories) and white (a group they do not define). The stroke rates among black people were around twice as high as among white people, and statistical adjustment for occupational social class only partly accounted for this elevated stroke rate. On the basis of this the authors suggest that "Ethnic differences in genetic, physiological and behavioural risk factors for stroke require further elucidation". As discussed earlier, adjustment for occupational social class will capture only some of the aspects of socioeconomic environment that influence stroke risk and may not provide an index of social circumstances in the same way among the group Stewart et al refer to as blacks and whites. This then produces data which apparently – but spuriously – demonstrate that health differences are due to genetic or cultural/behavioural factors.

As some minority ethnic groups are among the most disadvantaged sections of British society, measures which misrepresent the standard of living of minority ethnic groups risk not only perpetrating but exacerbating disadvantage through inadequate investment of public resources. Equally, an improved understanding of the processes which underlie ethnic differences in socioeconomic position and health has the potential to lead to more appropriately targeted interventions. There is therefore a pressing need to develop more sensitive indicators of socioeconomic position, particularly for use in research into the causes of ethnic inequalities in health.

References

[1] Engels, F. (1987, first published 1845) *The condition of the working class in England*, Harmondsworth: Penguin.

[2] Trask, J.W. (1916) 'The significance of the mortality rates of the coloured population of the US', *American Journal of Public Health*, vol 6, pp 254-60.

[3] Bhopal, R. (1997) 'Is research into ethnicity and health racist, unsound, or important science?', *British Medical Journal*, vol 314, pp 1751-6.

[4] Harding, S. and Maxwell, R. (1997) 'Differences in mortality of migrants', in F. Drever and M. Whitehead (eds) *Health inequalities*, London: The Stationery Office.

[5] Harding, S. and Balarajan, R. (1996) 'Patterns of mortality in second generation Irish living in England and Wales: longitudinal study', *British Medical Journal*, vol 312, pp 1389-92.

[6] Harding, S. (1998) 'The incidence of cancers among second-generation Irish living in England and Wales', *British Journal of Cancer*, vol 78, pp 958-61.

[7] Abbotts, J., Williams, R., Ford, G., Hunt, K. and West, P. (1998) 'Morbidity and Irish Catholic descent in Britain: an ethnic and religious minority 150 years on', *Social Science and Medicine*, vol 45, pp 3-14.

[8] Balarajan, R., Soni Raleigh, V. and Botting, B. (1989) 'Sudden Infant Death Syndrome and postneonatal mortality in immigrants in England and Wales', *British Medical Journal*, vol 298, pp 716-20.

[9] Farooqi, S. (1994) 'Ethnic differences in infant care practices and in the incidence of Sudden Infant Death Syndrome in Birmingham', *Early Human Development*, vol 38, pp 209-13.

[10] Raleigh, V.S. and Balarajan, R. (1995) 'The health of infants and children among ethnic minorities', *The health of our children*, Decennial Supplement, pp 82-94.

[11] Pilgrim, S., Fenton, S., Hughes, T., Hine, C. and Tibbs, N. (1993) *The Bristol black and ethnic minorities health survey report*, Bristol: University of Bristol.

[12] McKeigue, P. (1992) 'Coronary heart disease in Indians, Pakistanis and Bangladeshis: aetiology and possibilities for prevention', *British Heart Journal*, vol 67, pp 341-2.

[13] McKeigue, P.M., Ferrie, J.E., Pierpoint, T. and Marmot, M.G. (1993) 'Association of early-onset coronary heart disease in South Asian men with glucose intolerance and hyperinsulinemia', *Circulation*, vol 87, pp 152-61.

[14] Chaturvedi, N., McKeigue, P.M. and Marmot, M.G. (1993) 'Resting and ambulatory blood pressure differences in Afro-Caribbeans and Europeans', *Hypertension*, vol 22, pp 90-6.

[15] Unwin, N., Harland, J., White, M., Bhopal, R., Winocour, P., Stephenson, P., Watson, W., Turner, C. and Alberti, K.G. (1997) 'Body mass index, waist circumference, waist-hip ratio, and glucose tolerance in Chinese and Europid adults in Newcastle', *Journal of Epidemiology and Community Health*, vol 51, pp 160-6.

[16] Duran-Tauleria, E., Rona, R.J., Chinn, S. and Burney, P. (1996) 'Influence of ethnic group on asthma treatment in children in 1990-1: national cross sectional study', *British Medical Journal*, vol 313, pp 148-52.

[17] Watson, E. (1994) 'Health of infants and use of health services by mothers of different ethnic groups in East London', *Community Medicine*, vol 6, pp 127-35.

[18] Jackson, S.H.D., Bannan, L.T. and Beevers, D.G. (1981) 'Ethnic differences in respiratory disease', *Postgraduate Medical Journal*, vol 57, pp 777-8.

[19] Williams, R., Bhopal, R. and Hunt, K. (1993) 'The health of a Punjabi ethnic minority in Glasgow: the comparison with the general population', *Journal of Epidemiology and Community Health*, vol 47, pp 96-102.

[20] McKeigue, P.M., Shah, B. and Marmot, M.G. (1991) 'Relation of central obesity and insulin resistance with high diabetes prevalence and cardiovascular risk in South Asians', *Lancet*, vol 337, pp 382-6.

[21] Harland, J.O., Unwin, N., Bhopal, R.S., White, M., Watson, B., Later, M. and Alberti, K.G.M.M. (1997) 'Low levels of cardiovascular risk factors and coronary heart disease in a UK Chinese population', *Journal of Epidemiology and Community Health*, vol 51, pp 636-42.

²² Williams, R., Bhopal, R. and Hunt, K. (1994) 'Coronary risk in a British Punjabi population: comparative profile of non-biochemical factors', *International Journal of Epidemiology*, vol 23, pp 28-37.

²³ Sorlie, P., Rogot, E., Anderson, R., Johnson, N.J. and Backlund, E. (1992) 'Black-white mortality differences by family income', *Lancet*, vol 340, pp 346-50.

²⁴ Menchik, P.L. (1993) 'Economic status as a determinant of mortality among black and white older men: does poverty kill?', *Population Studies*, vol 47, pp 427-36.

²⁵ **Davey Smith, G., Neaton, J.D., Wentworth, D., Stamler, R. and Stamler, J. (1998) 'Mortality differences between black and white men in the USA: contribution of income and other risk factors among men screened for the MRFIT', *Lancet*, vol 351, pp 934-9.**

²⁶ Marmot, M.G., Adelstein, A.M. and Bulusu, L. (1984) *Immigrant mortality in England and Wales 1970-78. OPCS studies of medical and population subjects no 47*, London: HMSO.

²⁷ Abbotts, J., Williams, R. and Davey Smith, G. (1998) 'Mortality in men of patrilineal Irish decent in Britain', *Public Health*, vol 112, pp 229-32.

²⁸ Davey Smith, G., Bartley, M. and Blane, D. (1994) 'Explanations for socioeconomic differentials in mortality: evidence from Britain and elsewhere', *European Journal of Public Health*, vol 4, pp 131-44.

²⁹ Andrews, A. and Jewson, N. (1993) 'Ethnicity and infant deaths: the implications of recent statistical evidence for materialist explanations', *Sociology of Health and Illness*, vol 15, pp 137-56.

³⁰ Chandola, T. and Jenkinson, C. (2000) 'Validating self-rated health in different ethnic groups', *Ethnicity and Health*, vol 5, pp 151-9.

³¹ Abraido-Lanza, A., Bruce, P., Dohrenwend, P., Daisy, S., Ng-Mak, M. and Blake Turner, J. (1999) 'The Latino mortality paradox: a test of the "Salmon Bias" and healthy migrant hypotheses', *American Journal of Public Health*, vol 89, no 10, pp 1543-8.

³² Williams, R. and Ecob Ecob, R. (1999) 'Regional mortality and the Irish in Britain', *Sociology of Health and Illness*, vol 21, pp 344-67.

[33] Hull, D. (1979) 'Migration, adaptation and illness', *Social Science and Medicine*, vol 13A, pp 25-36.

[34] Nazroo, J.Y. (1997) *The health of Britain's ethnic minorities: Findings from a national survey*, London: Policy Studies Institute.

[35] Townsend, P. and Davidson, N. (1982) *Inequalities in health: The Black Report*, Harmondsworth: Penguin.

[36] Smith, D. (1977) *Racial disadvantage in Britain*, Harmondsworth: Penguin.

[37] Heath, A. and Ridge, J. (1983) 'Social mobility of ethnic minorities', *Journal of Biosocial Science*, vol 8, suppl, pp 169-84.

[38] **Davey Smith, G., Shipley, M.J. and Rose, G. (1990) 'The magnitude and causes of socioeconomic differentials in mortality: further evidence from the Whitehall Study',** *Journal of Epidemiology and Community Health***, vol 44, pp 265–70.**

[39] Beishon, S., Virdee, S. and Hagell, A. (1995) *Nursing in a multi-ethnic NHS*, London: Policy Studies Institute.

[40] Lillie-Blanton, M. and Laveist, T. (1996) 'Race/ethnicity, the social environment, and health', *Social Science and Medicine*, vol 43, pp 83-91.

[41] Williams, D.R., Lavizzo-Mourey, R. and Warren, R.C. (1994) 'The concept of race and health status in America', *Public Health Reports*, vol 109, pp 26-41.

[42] Williams, R., Wright, W. and Hunt, K. (1998) 'Social class and health: the puzzling counter-example of British South Asians', *Social Science and Medicine*, vol 47, pp 1277-88.

[43] McKenzie, K. and Crowcroft, N.S. (1996) 'Describing race, ethnicity, and culture in medical research', *British Medical Journal*, vol 312, p 1054.

[44] Office for National Statistics (1996) *Social focus on ethnic minorities*, London: HMSO.

[45] Rudat, K. (1994) *Black and ethnic minority groups in England: Health and lifestyles*, London: Health Education Authority.

[46] Cochrane, R. and Bal, S. (1990) 'The drinking habits of Sikh, Hindu and white men in the West Midlands: a community survey', *British Journal of Addiction*, vol 85, pp 759-69.

[47] Balarajan, R. and Yuen, P. (1986) 'British smoking and drinking habits: variation by country of birth', *Community Medicine*, vol 8, pp 237-9.

[48] Pearson, M., Madden, M. and Greenslade, L. (1991) *Generations of an invisible minority*, Liverpool: Institute of Irish Studies, University of Liverpool.

[49] Mullen, K., Williams, R. and Hunt, K. (1996) 'Irish descent, religion and alcohol and tobacco use', *Addiction*, vol 91, pp 243-54.

[50] Bush, H., Williams, R., Sharma, S. and Cruickshank, K. (1997) *Opportunities for and barriers to good nutritional health among ethnic minorities*, London: DoH and Health Education Authority.

[51] Owen, D. (1994) *Black people in Great Britain*, Census Statistical Paper No 6, Warwick: Centre for Research in Ethnic Relations, University of Warwick.

[52] Williams, R. and Hunt, K. (1997) 'Psychological distress among British South Asians: the contribution of stressful situations and subcultural differences in the West of Scotland Twenty-07 Study', *Psychological Medicine*, vol 27, pp 1173-81.

[53] Fenton, S. and Sadiq-Sangster, A. (1996) 'Culture, relativism and the expression of mental distress: South Asian women in Britain', *Sociology of Health and Illness*, vol 18, pp 66-85.

[54] Kassam Khamis, T., Thomas, J. and Judd, P. (1996) 'Eating habits of second generation South Asians in the UK', *Scandinavian Journal of Nutrition*, vol 40, pp S84-6.

[55] Williams, R. (1994) 'Britain's regional mortality: a legacy from disaster in the Celtic periphery?', *Social Science and Medicine*, vol 39, pp 189-99.

[56] Modood, T., Berthoud, R., Lakey, J., Nazroo, J., Smith, P., Virdee, S. and Beishon, S. (1997) *Ethnic minorities in Britain: Diversity and disadvantage*, London: Policy Studies Institute.

[57] Wilkinson, R.G. (1996) *Unhealthy societies: The afflictions of inequality*, London: Routledge.

[58] Virdee, S. (1995) *Racial violence and harassment*, London: Policy Studies Institute.

[59] Hickman, M. and Walter, B. (eds) (1997) *Discrimination and the Irish community in Britain*, London: Commission for Racial Equality.

[60] Benzeval, M., Judge, K. and Solomon, M. (1992) *The health status of Londoners*, London: King's Fund Institute.

[61] Krieger, N. (1990) 'Racial and gender discrimination: risk factors for high blood pressure?', *Social Science and Medicine*, vol 30, pp 1273-81.

[62] Krieger, N. and Sidney, S. (1996) 'Racial discrimination and blood pressure: the CARDIA study of young black and white adults', *American Journal of Public Health*, vol 86, no 10, pp 1370-8.

[63] Herman, A.A. (1996) 'Toward conceptualisation of race in epidemiology research', *Ethnicity and Disease*, vol 6, pp 7-20.

[64] Wild, S. and McKeigue, P. (1997) 'Cross sectional analysis of mortality by country of birth in England and Wales, 1970-92', *British Medical Journal*, vol 314, pp 705-10.

[65] Cooper, R., Rotimi, C., Ataman, S., McGee, D., Osotimehin, B., Kadiri, S., Muna, W., Kingue, S., Fraser, H., Forrester, T., Bennett, F. and Wilks, R. (1997) 'The prevalence of hypertension in seven populations of West African origin', *American Journal of Public Health*, vol 87, pp 160-8.

[66] Balarajan, R., Yuen, P. and Raleigh, V.S. (1989) 'Ethnic differences in general practitioner consultations', *British Medical Journal*, vol 299, pp 958-60.

[67] Gillam, S.J., Jarman, B., White, P. and Law, R. (1989) 'Ethnic differences in consultation rates in urban general practice', *British Medical Journal*, vol 299, pp 953-7.

[68] McCormick, A., Fleming, D. and Charlton, J. (1995) *Morbidity statistics from general practice. Fourth national study 1991-1992*, London: HMSO.

[69] Baker, M.R., Bandaranayake, R. and Schweiger, M.S. (1984) 'Differences in rate of uptake of immunisation among ethnic groups', *British Medical Journal*, vol 288, pp 1075-9.

[70] Shaukat, N., de Bono, D.P. and Cruickshank, J.K. (1993) 'Clinical features, risk factors, and referral delay in British patients of Indian and European origin with angina matched for age and extent of coronary atheroma', *British Medical Journal*, vol 307, pp 717-18.

[71] Chaturvedi, N., Rai, H. and Ben-Shlomo, Y. (1997) 'Lay diagnosis and health care seeking behaviour for chest pain in South Asians and Europeans', *Lancet*, vol 350, pp 1578-83.

[72] Badger, F., Atkin, K. and Griffiths, R. (1989) 'Why don't general practitioners refer their disabled Asian patients to district nurses?', *Health Trends*, vol 21, pp 31-2.

[73] Ritch, A.E.S., Ehtisham, M., Guthrie, S., Talbot, J.M., Luck, M. and Tinsley, R.N. (1996) 'Ethnic influence on health and dependency of elderly inner city residents', *Journal of the Royal College of Physicians of London*, vol 30, pp 215-20.

[74] Lear, J.T., Lawrence, I.G., Pohl, J.E. and Burden, A.C. (1994) 'Myocardial infarction and thrombolysis: a comparison of the Indian and European populations on a coronary care unit', *Journal of the Royal College of Physicians of London*, vol 28, pp 143-7.

[75] Malcolm, P.N., Chan, T.Y.K., Li, P.-L., Richards, J. and Hately, W. (1995) 'Management of dyspepsia among Asians by general practitioners in East London', *British Medical Journal*, vol 10, pp 910-11.

[76] Kaufman, J.S., Cooper, R.S. and McGee, D.L. (1997) 'Socioeconomic status and health in blacks and whites: the problem of residual confounding and the resiliency of race', *Epidemiology*, vol 8, no 6, pp 621-8.

[77] **Davey Smith, G. (2000) 'Learning to live with complexity: ethnicity, socioeconomic position, and health in Britain and the US', *American Journal of Public Health*, vol 90, pp 1694-8.**

[78] Nazroo, J.Y. (1998) 'Genetic, cultural or socioeconomic vulnurability? Explaining ethnic inequalities in health', *Sociology of Health and Illness*, vol 20, pp 714-34.

[79] Stewart, J.A., Dundas, R., Howard, R.A., Rudd, A.G. and Woolfe, C.D.A. (1999) 'Ethnic differences in incidence of stroke: prospective study with stroke register', *British Medical Journal*, vol 318, pp 967-71.

25

Learning to live with complexity: ethnicity, socioeconomic position, and health in Britain and the US

George Davey Smith

Abstract

The relation between ethnicity, socioeconomic position, and health is complex, has changed over time and differs between countries. In the US there is a long tradition of treating ethnic group membership simply as a socioeconomic measure and differentials in health status between African Americans and groups of European origin have been considered purely socioeconomic. A contrary position sees the differences as either 'cultural' or due to inherent 'racial' differences.

Although conventional socioeconomic indicators statistically explain much of the health difference between African Americans and Americans of European origin, they do not tell the full story. Incommensurate measures of socioeconomic position across ethnic groups clearly contribute to this difference. Additional factors, such as the extent of racism, are also likely to be important.

The interaction of ethnicity, social position, and health in Britain is similarly complex. Studies that inadequately account for socioeconomic circumstances when examining ethnic group differences in health can reify ethnicity (and its supposed correlates), however, the reductionist attribution of all ethnic differences in health to socioeconomic factors is untenable. The only productive way forward is through studies that recognise the contingency of the relations between socioeconomic position, ethnicity, and particular health outcomes.

American Journal of Public Health, 2000, vol 90, pp 1694–8

Introduction

That health is related to what we now call ethnicity has been noted from the time when quantitative health data were first recorded in Britain. Thus, in 1845 Friederich Engels noted the poor health and mortality record of Irish people living in England.[1] Engels also drew attention to the miserable social and environmental circumstances in which the majority of the Irish population lived, and he clearly considered these circumstances to underlie their poor health. Similarly, in a 1916 US report, John W. Trask concluded that the lower death rates among white people than among black people reflected more favourable socioeconomic circumstances, rather than any inherent ethnic differences.[2] The associations between ethnicity, social position, and health were clearly apparent to these authors, but the complexity of these interrelationships has not been fully recognised in much of the research conducted over the past century.

In the US, ethnicity is often used as a proxy for socioeconomic position, owing, in part, to the relative absence of socioeconomic data in some routine data sources. Although there has been a long tradition of analysing socioeconomic position and health in the US,[3,4] this work went into abeyance, to a degree, after the Second World War. The availability of information on ethnicity in routine data sources has allowed the explicit use of ethnicity as a socioeconomic indicator. Thus, in a Department of Health and Human Services report titled *Health status of the disadvantaged*, a high proportion of tables present health indicators by what is referred to as 'race' and not by any explicitly socioeconomic measure.[5]

The use of ethnicity in this way is clearly problematic. First, it can lead to the ignoring of socioeconomic differences in health status within minority ethnic populations. Indeed, until relatively recently the association between socioeconomic position and mortality among minority ethnic groups was little examined in the US.[6-8] Second, the use of ethnicity as a proxy for socioeconomic position often makes the inappropriate assumption that all members of minority ethnic groups are economically disadvantaged or deprived, an implied identity that, understandably, many people would want to reject. Third, it assumes that common interests are shared within but not between ethnic groups, whereas the real interests of the working class, for example, may be shared across ethnic groups more than real interests are shared by the capitalist and working-class members within ethnic groups.[9,10]

Finally, this approach has difficulty accounting for cases in which minority ethnic groups who are economically disadvantaged compared with the majority population have better health outcomes – for example, the low mortality of Hispanic adults in the US,[11,12] of African Caribbean men in Britain,[13] and the low post-neonatal mortality among offspring of women of Bangladeshi or Indian origin in Britain.[14]

Recognition of the need to analyse ethnicity and socioeconomic position as separate variables in health studies raises several important issues. First, do conventional socioeconomic measures have the same association with health status within different ethnic groups? Second, to what degree does standardisation for conventional socioeconomic indicators account for health differences between ethnic groups? Third, what are the problems with this approach?

Socioeconomic position and health status within minority ethnic groups

Findings relating socioeconomic position to health status within minority ethnic groups are varied. Within the US, socioeconomic gradients in all-cause adult mortality appear similar among non-Hispanic white, non-Hispanic black, and Hispanic people.[6-8,11] In one study, a formal test of interaction found the socioeconomic gradient in mortality to be greater among black than among white men, particularly after adjustment for risk factors.[7] Socioeconomic gradients in infant mortality, uptake of vaccinations, activity limitation in children, teenage childbearing, blood lead levels in childhood and adulthood, homicide, and poor self-ratings of health are similar for males and females within the different groups for whom data are available, generally non-Hispanic white, non-Hispanic black, Asian or Pacific Islander, and American Indian or Alaska Native.[8]

For some health outcomes, socioeconomic gradients vary between ethnic groups. Thus the socioeconomic gradient in lung cancer mortality is greater in white than in black men, while the gradient in non-cardiovascular, non-cancer mortality is greater in black than in white men.[7] In San Francisco, there is a positive socioeconomic gradient (higher risk among the better-off) for breast cancer among Hispanics and Asians or Pacific Islanders, but no marked gradient among white or black people; for lung cancer incidence there is a positive gradient among Hispanic people and an inverse gradient among white and black people; and for cervical cancer, there are marked inverse gradients among white and Hispanic women and much weaker gradients among Asians or Pacific Islanders and black women.[15] There are several other health measures for which socioeconomic gradients are different in different ethnic groups, including low birthweight (little gradient among Hispanic and Asian or Pacific Island people but inverse gradients among white and black people), adolescent obesity (inverse gradient in white people and positive gradients among black and Mexican people), and suicide (inverse gradients among white and black people but a positive gradient among Hispanic people).[8]

In British health studies, ethnicity has often been indexed by country of birth because of the availability of this information in the Census.[16,17] This is clearly problematic for, say people born in Britain but of Caribbean family background, or people of British family background born on the Indian subcontinent. In many studies, the intention to categorise family or origin is evident in the separation of those born in West Africa (most of whom will be of African family origin) from those born in East Africa, who, within Britain, generally have Indian subcontinent family origins.

The 1991 British Census contained a question on ethnic group that proved controversial because of the external imposition of categories, leading many people to opt for the 'Any other ethnic group' or 'Black-other' categories (as opposed to 'Black-Caribbean' or 'Black-African').[18] The 2001 Census is likely to contain more categories than have been used previously – in particular, 'mixed' ethnicity categories[19] – and will lead to a marked change in the official description of the ethnic composition of Britain simply by providing more precoded choices.

This demonstrates the way in which methods of data collection construct ethnicity, and this relationship is equally true of the treatment of ethnicity in studies of health status.

In writing reviews such as this one, it becomes problematic to stick to the terminology used in the original sources cited, and reclassification of, say, 'Black' (as an original response category in a study) to 'African American' (or vice versa), as a way of allowing information to be summarised, occurs. This moves away from the principle that the exact details of how classification is carried out should always be reported (and, preferably, justified) in studies of ethnicity and health, to keep the constructed nature of the categories fully apparent.

British studies, like those in other places, have been constrained by data availability. There has until recently been little investigation of socioeconomic differences in health within minority groups in Britain, perhaps because of an influential study based on the 1971 Census that found no marked or consistent associations between occupational social class and mortality among migrants to England and Wales.[16] This study concluded that differences in social class did not contribute to mortality differences between migrant groups and the indigenous population.

More recently, social class differences in adult mortality at the time of the 1991 Census have been examined, and mortality differences in the conventional direction between manual social class and non-manual social class have been demonstrated among men living in England and Wales but born in the Caribbean, West or South Africa,

East Africa, India, Pakistan, Bangladesh, Scotland, or Ireland.[13] Similar social class gradients are seen for perinatal, neonatal, post-neonatal, and overall infant mortality among different country-of-birth groups.

For particular causes of death, however, exceptions to the pattern seen in the overall population are evident: there is no gradient in ischaemic heart disease mortality for men born in the Caribbean or West or South Africa, no gradient in respiratory disease mortality among men born in the Caribbean, and a reverse gradient for suicide among men born on the Indian subcontinent.[13]

A recent national study examined socioeconomic differences in self-reported overall health status, diagnosed heart disease, hypertension, respiratory symptom, and diabetes. With a few exceptions, similar gradients were found among the African Caribbean, Indian or African Asian, Pakistani or Bangladeshi, and white groups.[20] Similarly data have been reported in other British studies.[21]

Socioeconomic circumstances and ethnic group health differentials

In studies using the same socioeconomic measures within different ethnic groups, health differentials are generally – but not always – in a similar direction and of similar magnitude in the US and Britain. Several studies have reported on the influence of socioeconomic circumstances in health differentials between ethnic groups. For example, in some US studies, black–white mortality differentials have been reported to be almost entirely due to income or class inequalities,[22,23] while other studies suggest that this explanation is at best partial.[6,24] In one study, adjustment for an area-based income measure reduced a 47% higher all-cause mortality rate among black men to a rate that was 19% higher,[25] and very similar findings have been reported from other studies (eg, Sorlie et al,[26] and Menchik[27]). For particular causes of death, however, the situation is more complex, with socioeconomic adjustment reversing the black excess in coronary heart disease and essentially abolishing the black excess in lung cancer, but leaving considerable black excess in heart failure, myeloma, and prostate cancer mortality in men.[25]

In Britain, adjustment for social class fails to attenuate the adult mortality differentials according to place of birth; in fact, such adjustment generally increases the differentials, making an already lower rate lower still among Caribbean-born men and an elevated rate higher still among men born in East Africa.[13]

A common response to residual ethnic group differences in health status seen after adjustment for socioeconomic circumstances is illustrated in a recent study from London. Stewart et al[28] compared stroke rates among a group they defined as black (Afro-Caribbean,

Black African, and Black-other, according to the 1991 British Census categories) and white (a group the authors did not define). The stroke rates were about twice as high among black people as among white people, and statistical adjustment for occupational social class only partly accounted for the elevation: the relative risk of 1.71 among those of working age was reduced to 1.53 after adjustment. The authors concluded that 'ethnic' differences in genetic, physiological and behavioural risk factors for stroke require further elucidation. This conclusion – that if socioeconomic adjustment leaves a residual 'racial' effect, then genes, culture, or behaviours are to blame – is a common one in this field.

This approach has several important limitations. First, it assumes that the available socioeconomic indicators are adequate markers of current social circumstances. Several studies (eg Davey Smith et al[29] and Goldblatt[30]) have demonstrated that the introduction of additional socioeconomic indicators into studies relating occupational socioeconomic measures to health outcomes produces additional differentiation of health status. Studies adjusting for a single socioeconomic measure will therefore leave considerable scope for residual confounding by socioeconomic circumstances.[31] Models demonstrate the degree to which misclassification of confounders (as socioeconomic position is often treated in studies of ethnicity and health) can leave spurious, apparently 'independent' effects of variables on health status. The results found in this field are often entirely within the bounds of what may be expected as a result of such residual confounding.[32]

Second, socioeconomic indicators may have different meanings for members of different ethnic groups. Thus, at the same level of income, black households in the US have considerably lower wealth than white households;[33] within the same jobs, black people have greater levels of exposure than white people to work-related hazards;[34] education brings lower returns in terms of income, occupational status, and avoidance of unemployment among black people than among white people;[35] and the purchasing power of black people is less than that of white people at any given income level, with respect to food, housing, and other necessary expenditures.[36] At a given level of income, occupational position, or educational achievement, blacks people are disadvantaged in other domains with respect to white people, and adjustment for income, occupational position or educational achievement will not fully adjust for differences in socioeconomic circumstances between the groups.

A similar situation pertains in Britain.[37] For example, housing tenure – a commonly used socioeconomic indicator in British studies[30] – is not an adequate marker of housing quality, since South Asian owner-occupiers are at increased likelihood of living in houses that are older, unmodernised and overcrowded[38] or lacking in basic amenities.[20] Car ownership has been widely used as an indicator of available income, because income data are not routinely collected in UK data sources such as the Census. While car ownership has proved to be a powerful predictor of health status in many UK studies (eg, those of Davey Smith et al[29] and Goldblatt[30]), it cannot be used in any simple way to study differences in socioeconomic position between ethnic communities, because driver's license possession varies dramatically between ethnic groups and because different groups place different priorities on car ownership.

As another example, one study found that a considerably higher proportion of Indian origin men than of European origin men were in non-manual occupations, yet income was higher in the latter group.[39] Some preliminary evidence shows that the fact that social position measures have different meanings in different ethnic groups has important implications for studies of ethnicity and health.

In a British study, poorer general health status and an elevated prevalence of coronary heart disease were seen among those of Pakistani or Bangladeshi origin. These differences remained after adjustment for occupational social class, education, and housing tenure (indicators that will indeed have different implications for social circumstances in different ethnic groups), but were essentially abolished by adjustment for a comprehensive index of material conditions and living standards.[20,40]

Third, area-based measures of social circumstances, which are widely used in health studies, may not be directly comparable across ethnic groups. A British study concluded that tuberculosis was not associated with poverty among South Asians, because area-based deprivation indices that predicted tuberculosis rates among the majority white population did not do so among South Asians.[41] The indicators used in the area-based measures, such as overcrowded housing, housing tenure, and car ownership, are known to have different ethnic group level associations with income, occupation, and education.[39]

In the US, the mortality excesses seen in relation to poverty levels within areas show differences between black and white people, differences which themselves vary by geographical location within the country.[42,43] Furthermore, the ethnic group composition within an area may have health consequences. The proportion of the population that is African American is positively related to mortality rates for African American and other groups, whereas the proportion of the population that is Hispanic shows a U-shaped association with mortality.[44] These effects are independent of other area characteristics (including median income and educational level) and of individual-level socioeconomic characteristics, and could reflect the fact that some exposures – such as to solid waste sites, air-polluting plants, and alcohol retailers – are more prevalent for people living in predominantly black areas.[45] Conversely, in some circumstances the identification of areas with their ethnic minority residents can allow the development of strong community ties, enhance political influence, and provide resistance to racist attacks, all of which could act to improve health outcomes.[46,47]

Fourth, there is growing evidence that socioeconomic circumstances in early life (and even during the lives of previous generations) can influence health in adulthood.[48,49] Intergenerational influences – from the health and development of mothers – may exist, mediated through foetal development and birthweight, which are related to the adult health of the offspring.[50] Evidence of lower birthweights among minority groups within Britain and the US suggests that these influences may be important.[14] Deprivation in childhood is associated with increased risk for several important causes of death – including stroke, coronary heart disease, respiratory disease, and stomach cancer – in later life.[49] In many cases, members of minority ethnic groups will, independent of their social circumstances in adulthood, be more likely to bear the long-term effects of their mothers having been deprived during pregnancy, and also to have themselves been deprived in childhood.

Finally, there are forms of social influence – racism and its effects – that are experienced almost exclusively by members of minority ethnic groups. Racism may influence health through several potential mechanisms,[51] for example, by leading to less favourable socioeconomic circumstances (through educational, occupational, and residential discrimination), through constraints placed on life-style choices, or through more direct psychosocial stress effects. Racism cannot be taken to be a given feature of society; its historical roots and current social origins need to be explored.

As Raymond Franklin observed, the adoption of African slavery in the US – a supposedly democratic society – required the development of an extraordinary rationale; to "declare that all people are entitled to certain inalienable rights and then deny such rights to large numbers of persons needed an ideology that debases Blacks. Racism became such an ideology."[52] Perceptions of the general economic marginality of many black people from post-slavery times on – with overrepresentation of black people in low-status (or no) occupations and poor neighbourhoods – in turn feed into continuing segregation discrimination, and racism. Socioeconomic disadvantages and exclusionary social practices are, in this view, mutually constitutive; the 'shadows of race and class' cannot be easily separated.[52]

Learning to live with complexity

The social processes that influence health differences within and between ethnic groups are clearly complex and context-specific. One approach to this complexity has been to call for the abandonment of an issue that is impossible to examine, and that should perhaps remain unexamined.[53] Such an abandonment would leave the field peopled only by those keen to demonstrate genetic determinism or to identify cultural practices that require changing. At the same time, it would constitute a failure to take advantage of ways of learning how to improve the health of populations and to better understand the determinants of illness.[54]

In conceptualising the social determination of ethnic group differences in health we should ultimately aim to bridge the gap between the macrosocial and the molecular-biological. This is not an impossible task, as is shown by a consideration of how much nearer we are today to understanding the up, down, up, down patterns of adult mortality in Britain from 1850 to 1950 and to answering Jerry Morris' question, "What are the *social* changes that underline the *biological* changes…?"[55] than was possible when it was posed. It requires, however, a willingness to consider the particular aspects of these social and biological processes,[56] and not to rely on the illusory comfort of (perhaps metaphorical) metatheories that appear to explain everything (while accounting for nothing).[57]

With respect to the contribution of socioeconomic circumstances to ethnic group health differentials, this focus on the particular involves understanding the historical antecedents to any synchronic nexus of social and ethnic group membership. For example, in the face of a labour shortage in the postwar years, British capitalism was led, after attempts at alternative strategies and against considerable resistance, to motivated recruitment – through encouraged immigration – of labour from the Caribbean and the Indian subcontinent. For these labourers, access was limited to unpopular and often simply unpleasant jobs, and opportunities for training and promotion were severely restricted. The current form of socioeconomic disadvantage faced by British ethnic minorities, in an age when the 'reserve army of labour' is waiting to meet labour requirements that currently do not exist, can be understood only in the light of this history.[58]

In New York City, the application of microeconomic planning theory led to a reduction of services and the deterioration of ethnic minority neighbourhoods, which in turn exacerbated the tuberculosis, AIDS, and drug use epidemics.[59] In this way, a strategy to deal with the tendency for the rate of profit to fall has resulted in falling CD4 cell counts in people who are conspicuously failing to benefit from the economic growth enjoyed by the already privileged.

It is not surprising that the outcome of such macrosocial forces cannot be summed up by simple measures of individual socioeconomic position in adulthood. For minority ethnic groups, the social world will produce both social and biological effects with long-term impacts. Low birthweight, infections acquired in childhood, and suboptimal childhood development will all influence health in adulthood, as will socially determined less favourable educational outcomes (and the later social circumstances they provide access to) and the effects of discrimination in schooling and residential location. The disadvantages already existing when a member of an ethnic minority enters adulthood will be amplified by the less favourable social trajectory these very disadvantages lead to. This social trajectory includes a world in which there is a high level of inequality in economic resources, and increasing competition for social goods (such as good quality housing in favourable residential locations) to a level at which the less well-off cannot compete. Poorer members of highly unequal societies may thus live in less favourable environments than similarly poor members of more equal societies.[60] As W. E. B. Du Bois said long ago, "To be a poor man is hard, but to be a poor race in a land of dollars is the very bottom of hardship."[61]

Acknowledgements

Many thanks to Nancy Krieger, Margaret Kelaher, Helen Lambert, James Nazroo and Jane Ferrie for comments on an earlier draft of this article.

References

[1] Engels, F. (1987, originally published 1845) *The condition of the working class in England*, Harmondsworth: Penguin.

[2] Trask, J.W. (1916) 'The significance of the mortality rates of the coloured population of the US', *American Journal of Public Health*, vol 6, pp 254-60.

[3] Chaplin, C.V. (1924) 'Deaths among taxpayers and non-taxpayers: income tax, Providence 1865', *American Journal of Public Health*, vol 14, pp 647-51.

[4] Britten, R.H. (1934) 'Mortality rates by occupational class in the US', *Public Health Reports*, vol 49, pp 1101-11.

[5] Chartbook (1990) *Health status of the disadvantaged*, Washington, DC: US DHHS.

[6] Sorlie, P., Rogot, E., Anderson, R., Johnson, N.J. and Backlund, E. (1992) 'Black-white mortality differences by family income', *Lancet*, vol 340, pp 346-50.

[7] **Davey Smith, G., Wentworth, D., Neaton, J.D., Stamler, R. and Stamler, J. (1996) 'Socioeconomic differentials in mortality risk among men screened for the Multiple Risk Factor Intervention Trial, 2: black men',** *American Journal of Public Health*, **vol 86, pp 497-504.**

[8] Pamuk, E., Makuc, D., Heck, K., Reuben, C. and Lockner, K. (1998) *Socioeconomic status and health chartbook, Health, US*, Hyansville, MD: National Centre for Health Statistics.

[9] Buhle, P. (ed) (1998) *C.L.R. James: His life and work*, London: Verso Books.

[10] Callinicos, A. (1993) *Race and class*, London: Bookmarks.

[11] Sorlie, P.D., Backlund, E., Johnson, N.J. and Rogot, E. (1993) 'Mortality by Hispanic status in the US', *Journal of the American Medical Association*, vol 270, pp 2464-8.

[12] Abraido-Lanza, A.F., Dohrenwend, B.P., Ng-Mak, D.S. and Turner, J.B. (1999) 'The Latino mortality paradox: a test of the "Salmon Bias" and health migrant hypotheses', *American Journal of Public Health*, no 89, pp 1543-8.

[13] Harding, M.R. (1997) 'Differences in mortality of migrants', in F. Drever and M. Whitehead (eds) *Health inequalities: Decennial supplement*, Series DS No 15, London: The Stationery Office.

[14] Raleigh, V.S. and Balarajan, R. (1995) 'The health of infants and children among ethnic minorities', in B. Botting (ed) *The health of our children*, OPCS Series DS, vol 11, London: HMSO, pp 82-94.

[15] Krieger, N., Quesenberry, C., Peng, T. et al (1999) 'Social class, race/ethnicity, and incidence of breast, cervix, colon, lung and prostate cancer among Asian, black, Hispanic and white residents of the San Francisco Bay area, 1988-92 (US)', *Cancer Causes Control*, vol 10, pp 525-37.

[16] Marmot, M.G., Adelstein, A.M. and Bulusu, L. (1984) *Immigrant mortality in England and Wales 1970-78*, OPCS Studies of Medical and Population Subjects, vol 47, London: HMSO.

[17] Balarajan, R. (1991) 'Ethnic differences in mortality from ischaemic heart disease and cerebrovascular disease in England and Wales', *British Medical Journal*, vol 302, pp 560-4.

[18] Dorling, D. and Dixie, J. (2002) 'New questions for the 2001 Census', in P. Rees, D. Martin and P. Williamson (eds) *The census data system*, Chichester: John Wiley and Sons.

[19] Department of Health (2000) *Ethnicity* (available at: http://www.doh.gov.uk/ethdevlist3.htm, accessed 19 August 2000).

[20] Nazroo, J. (1997) *The health of Britain's ethnic minorities: Findings from a national survey*, London: Policy Studies Institute.

[21] **Davey Smith, G., Chaturvedi, N., Harding, S., Nazroo, J. and Williams, R. (2000) 'Ethnic inequalities in health: a review of UK epidemiological evidence', *Critical Public Health*, vol 10, pp 375-408.**

[22] Navarro, V. (1990) 'Race or class versus race and class: mortality differentials in the US', *Lancet*, vol 336, pp 1238-40.

[23] Sterling, T., Rosenbaum, W. and Weinkam, J. (1993) 'Income, race and mortality', *Journal of the National Medical Association*, vol 85, pp 906-11.

[24] Cooper, R.S. (1993) 'Health and the social status of blacks in the US', *Annals of Epidemiology*, no 3, pp 137-44.

[25] **Davey Smith, G., Neaton, J.D., Wentworth, D., Stamler, R. and Stamler, J. (1998) 'Mortality differences between black and white men in the USA: contribution of income and other risk factors among men screened for the MRFIT', *Lancet*, vol 351, pp 934-9.**

[26] Sorlie, P.D., Backlund, E. and Keller, J.B. (1995) 'US mortality by economic, demographic, and social characteristics: the National Longitudinal Mortality Study', *American Journal of Public Health*, vol 85, pp 949-56.

[27] Menchik, P.L. (1993) 'Economic status as a determinant of mortality among black and white older men: does poverty kill?', *Population Studies*, vol 47, pp 427-36.

[28] Stewart, J.A., Dundas, R., Howard, R.A., Rudd, A.G. and Woolfe, C.D.A. (1999) 'Ethnic differences in incidence of stroke: prospective study with stroke register', *British Medical Journal*, vol 318, pp 967-71.

[29] **Davey Smith, G., Shipley, M.J. and Rose, G. (1990) 'Magnitude and causes of socioeconomic differentials in mortality: further evidence from the Whitehall Study',** *Journal of Epidemiology and Community Health*, **vol 44, pp 260-5.**

[30] Goldblatt, P. (1990) *Mortality and social organisation: Longitudinal study 1971-1981*, London: HMSO.

[31] Davey Smith, G. and Phillips, A.N. (1992) 'Confounding in epidemiological studies: why "independent" effects may not be all they seem', *British Medical Journal*, vol 305, pp 757-9.

[32] Phillips, A.N. and Davey Smith, G. (1992) 'Bias in relative odds estimation due to imprecise measurement of correlated exposures', *Statistics in Medicine*, vol 11, pp 953-61.

[33] Blau, F.D. and Graham, J.W. (1990) 'Black–white differences in wealth and asset composition', *Quarterly Journal of Economics*, vol 105, pp 321-9.

[34] Robinson, J.C. (1984) 'Racial inequality and the probability of occupational-related injury or illness', *Milbank Memorial Fund Quarterly*, vol 62, pp 567-90.

[35] Hacker, A. (1995) *Two nations: Black and white, separate, hostile, unequal*, New York, NY: Ballantine Books.

[36] Williams, D.R. and Collins, C. (1995) 'US socioeconomic and racial differences in health: patterns and explanations', *Annual Review of Sociology*, vol 21, pp 349-86.

[37] Davey Smith, G., Charsley, K., Lambert, H., Paul, S., Fenton, S. and Ahmad, W. (2000) 'Ethnicity, health and the meaning of socioeconomic position', in H. Graham (ed) *Understanding health inequalities*, London: Open University Press, pp 23-37.

[38] Jones, T. (1993) *Britain's ethnic minorities*, London: Policy Studies Institute.

[39] Bhopal, R., Unwin, N., White, M. et al (1999) 'Heterogeneity of coronary heart disease risk factors in Indian, Pakistani, Bangladeshi, and European origin populations: cross sectional study', *British Medical Journal*, vol 319, pp 215-20.

[40] Nazroo, J.Y. (1998) 'Genetic, cultural or socioeconomic vulnerability? Explaining ethnic inequalities in health', in M. Bartley, D. Blane and G. Davey Smith (eds) *The sociology of health inequalities*, Oxford: Blackwell Publishers.

[41] Hawker, J.I., Bakhshi, S.S., Ali, S. and Farrington, C.P. (1999) 'Ecological analysis of ethnic differences in relation between tuberculosis and poverty', *British Medical Journal*, vol 319, pp 1031-4.

[42] Geronimus, A.T., Bound, J., Waidmann, T.A., Hillemeier, M.M. and Burns, P.B. (1996) 'Excess mortality among blacks and whites in the US', *New England Journal of Medicine*, vol 335, pp 1552-8.

[43] Geronimus, A.T., Bound, J. and Waidmann, T.A. (1999) 'Poverty, time and place: variation in excess mortality across selected US populations, 1980-1990', *Journal of Epidemiology and Community Health*, vol 53, pp 325-34.

[44] LeClere, F.B., Rogers, R.G. and Peter, K.D. (1997) 'Ethnicity and mortality in the US: individual and community correlates', *Social Forces*, vol 76, pp 169-98.

[45] Bryant, B. and Mohai, P. (1992) *Race and the incidence of environmental hazards*, Boulder, CO: Westview Press.

[46] Smaje, C. (1996) 'The ethnic patterning of health: new directions for theory and research', *Sociology of Health and Illness*, vol 18, pp 139-71.

[47] Halpern, D. and Nazroo, J. (2000) 'The ethnic density effect: results from a national community survey of England and Wales', *International Journal of Social Psychiatry*, vol 46, pp 34-46.

[48] Kuh, D. and Ben-Shlomo, Y. (1997) *A life course approach to chronic disease epidemiology*, Oxford: Oxford University Press.

[49] **Davey Smith, G., Hart, C., Blane, D. and Hole, D. (1998) 'Adverse socioeconomic conditions in childhood and cause-specific adult mortality: prospective observational study', *British Medical Journal*, vol 316, pp 1631-5.**

[50] Barker, D.J.P. (1998) *Mothers, babies and health in later life*, Edinburgh: Churchill Livingstone.

[51] Krieger, N. (1999) 'Embodying inequality: a review of concepts, measures and methods for studying health consequences of discrimination', *International Journal of Health Services*, vol 29, pp 295-352.

[52] Franklin, R.S. (1991) *Shadows of race and class*, Minneapolis, MN: University of Minnesota Press, p 38.

[53] Kaufman, J.S. and Cooper, R.S. (1999) 'Seeking causal explanations in social epidemiology', *American Journal of Epidemiology*, vol 150, pp 113-20.

[54] Krieger, N. and Davey Smith, G. (2000) 'Re: seeking causal explanations in social epidemiology', *American Journal of Epidemiology*, vol 151, pp 831-2.

[55] Morris, J.N. (1957) *Uses of epidemiology*, Edinburgh: Livingstone.

[56] Kunitz, S.J. (1994) *Disease and social diversity*, Oxford: Oxford University Press.

[57] **Davey Smith, G. and Egger, M. (1996) 'Understanding it all – health, meta-theories, and mortality trends', *British Medical Journal*, vol 313, pp 1584-5.**

[58] Harris, C. (1996) 'Post-war migration and the industrial reserve army', in W. James and C. Harris (eds) *Inside Babylon: The Caribbean diaspora in Britain*, London: Verso Books.

[59] Wallace, D. and Wallace, R. (1999) *A plague on your houses: How New York was burned down and national public health crumbled*, London: Verso Books.

[60] Lynch, J., Davey Smith, G., Kaplan, G. and House, J. (2000) 'Income inequality and mortality: importance to health of individual income, psychosocial environment, or material conditions', *British Medical Journal*, vol 320, pp 1200-4.

[61] Du Bois, W.E.B. (1995) quoted in M.L. Oliver and T.M. Shapiro, *Black wealth/white wealth*, London: Routledge.

26

Mortality differentials between black and white men in the US: contribution of income and other risk factors among men screened for the Multiple Risk Factor Intervention Trial (MRFIT)

George Davey Smith, James D. Neaton,
Deborah Wentworth, Rose Stamler and
Jeremiah Stamler for
the MRFIT Research Group*

Abstract

Objective: To determine the extent to which differences in socioeconomic status between black and white men contribute to differentials in all-cause and cause-specific mortality.

Methods: Of the 361,662 men screened for the MRFIT between 1973 and 1975, median family income of households in their zipcode of residence was available for 20,224 black and 300,685 white men. This socioeconomic measure has been added to the available data – age, cigarette smoking, blood pressure, serum cholesterol, previous heart attack and receipt of drug treatment for diabetes. Deaths over the 16-year follow-up period have been grouped into specific causes and differences in mortality between black and white men are compared with and without consideration of differences in income.

*This is a longer version of an article originally published in
The Lancet, 1998, vol 351, pp 934-9

Results: Over an average of 16 years of follow-up 31,737 white and 2,937 black men died. Age-adjusted relative risk (black/white) was 1.47 (95% CI: 1.42-1.53). Adjustment for risk factors (diastolic blood pressure, serum cholesterol, cigarette smoking, use of medication for diabetes and prior hospitalisation for heart attack) reduced this to 1.40 (95% CI: 1.35-1.46). Adjustment for income but not the other risk factors attenuated the relative risk to 1.19 (95% CI: 1.14-1.24); additional adjustment for risk factors did not alter this estimate. Adjustment for income reduced relative risk estimates for all major causes of death groups. For cardiovascular death, relative risk was reduced from 1.36 to 1.09; for cancer, from 1.47 to 1.25; for non-CVD, non-cancer deaths from 1.71 to 1.26. For some specific causes – prostate cancer, myeloma, and hypertensive heart disease – the higher mortality rates in black men did not seem to be simple reflections of income differentials. Rates from some causes of death (suicide, melanoma) were lower in black men than white men, as was coronary heart disease once income had been taken into account.

Conclusions: Socioeconomic position as measured by household median family income of area of residence is an important contributor to mortality differentials between black and white men. Black–white differences in mortality from some specific causes are not simple reflections of income differentials, however, and more detailed investigations are needed of how they are produced, by environmental exposures, lifetime socioeconomic conditions, life-style, effects of racism and other sociocultural and biological factors.

Introduction

The mortality gap between black and white men in the US is large and has increased over recent years.[1,2] The persistence of this stark inequality is of major public health concern and there is a long history of investigations within the social medicine framework of this issue.[3-7] Various approaches have been taken to the examination of black–white health differentials. First, 'race' has implicitly been used as a proxy for socioeconomic position in much official health data. Thus, in the Department of Health and Human Services report, *Health status of the disadvantaged*, many of the tabulations present health indicators by 'race' and not by any direct socioeconomic measures.[8] This tendency receives encouragement from the relative lack of socioeconomic data in many US government health statistics.[9] Second, black–white differentials in some specific diseases – such as coronary heart disease and hypertension – have been investigated in detail, in an attempt to better understand aetiology,[10] but again the axis of classification is generally 'race', without consideration of socioeconomic position. Third, some attempts have been made to quantify the contribution of socioeconomic position and other indicators of mortality risk to the black–white differential. Thus one large study demonstrated that family income makes an important contribution to black–white mortality differentials,[11] while several smaller studies have investigated the contribution of other risk factors, such as smoking and blood pressure.[12]

To date, studies of factors underlying black–white adult mortality differentials have been limited either by lack of data beyond basic demographic characteristics, or by small study size, which allows for investigation of only a few major cause of death groups.[12,13] In this paper we report data from the cohort of men screened for the Multiple Risk Factor Intervention Trial (MRFIT). The large size of this cohort facilitates examination of the contribution of socioeconomic position and other risk factors to black–white differentials in mortality from a wide variety of causes.

Methods

Methods used to recruit participants to the screening examination for the MRFIT have been reported.[14,15] In brief, from November 1973 to November 1975, 361,662 men aged 35-57 years were screened at 20 MRFIT clinical centres in 18 cities. For recruitment, centres used a variety of methods, including house-to-house canvassing; screening of government, industrial, or other employee populations; and through civic groups, unions, and churches.

Name, address, date of birth, social security number, and number of cigarettes smoked per day were recorded. Participants reported whether they were white, black, Hispanic, American Indian, oriental or 'Other'. Serum cholesterol level was determined at one of 14 local laboratories with an Auto Analyser II and with standardisation by the Lipid Standardisation Program, Centers for Disease Control in Atlanta.[16] Three blood pressure measurements were taken with a standard mercury sphygmomanometer. The average of the second and third readings is used in this report. Participants also reported whether they had been hospitalised for heart attack, or were taking medication for diabetes.

Although socioeconomic position of each participant was not recorded at the time of screening, this has been indexed by matching participants' postal zipcode with data from the 1980 US Census. Median family income specific for families headed by black and white householders within zipcode areas is used as an ecologic marker of socioeconomic position, as previously reported.[17,18] Thus for black men median income of families headed by black householders within their zipcode of residence is the income measure, while for white men the median income of families headed by white householders within their zipcode of residence is used. For the 325,384 white men and 23,490 black men who were screened, median family income of zipcode area of residence was available for 300,685 and 20,224 respectively; 4,644 zipcode areas were represented by the white men and 1,376 by the black men. The relatively small differences in characteristics recorded at screening between the men for whom income data are available and those for whom income data are not available are similar for the black and white men.[18] Systolic blood pressure readings were missing for one black and 38 white men for whom income data were available.

Of the 320,909 men for whom zipcode data are available, 228,893 – 209,089 white men and 19,804 black men – resided in zipcodes from which at least one white and one black man were included in the study. This group, residing in a total of 1,302 zipcodes, is referred to as the 'common zipcode' group. The analyses presented in this paper are primarily of the total cohort of 320,909 men with available zipcode data. However, since accurate matching of socioeconomic position – including when indexed by residential area[19,20] – is of major concern when examining black–white health differentials, analyses have also been performed for the common zipcode group.

The vital status of each man was determined through December 1990, an average of 16 years of follow-up (range 15 to 17 years).[21] For each decedent, the death certificate was obtained and underlying cause of death was coded by a trained nosologist using the Ninth Revision of the International Classifications of Diseases (ICD-9).[22]

Comparisons of black and white men for all-cause and cause-specific mortality are based on time-to-event methods, including Kaplan-Meier estimation, log-rank tests, and proportional hazards regression. Relative risks (black versus white) of mortality, with covariate adjustment for age, black/white specific median family income of zipcode of residence, diastolic blood pressure, serum cholesterol level, number of cigarettes smoked per day, prior history of hospitalisation for heart attack and medication for diabetes as covariates, were estimated with the proportional hazards regression model. Most analyses are stratified by 22 clinical centres (one centre had three clinical sites) to ensure that across clinical centre effects do not distort the black–white mortality differentials. In the common zipcode cohort, the proportional hazards analyses have been stratified by the 1,302 zipcodes, instead of clinical centre, so that exact matching by zipcodes occurs. Stratifying by individual zipcode matches closely on characteristics of the area of residence, and additional adjustment for income in such analyses takes into account differences in income between households headed by black and white people. Mortality rates cited in tables have been age-standardised by the direct method, using the total MRFIT study population as the standard, and are presented as rates per 10,000 person years of follow-up.

Results

Median family income of black householder families for the black men screened is compared with the median family income of white householder families for the white men screened in Table 1. Median income of black and white householder headed families in the zipcode area in which participants resided (henceforth referred to as income) differed markedly. For example, 58% of black men fell into the income strata below $15,000. In contrast, only 2% of white men fell into these strata.

Black men were slightly younger, had higher systolic and diastolic blood pressures and prevalence of hypertension, and had lower serum cholesterol, than white men (Table 2). More black men smoked, but among the smokers the white men reported using more cigarettes per day. A higher proportion of black men were taking medication for diabetes. Zipcode areas of residence were markedly different in several population characteristics: median family income of both black and white householder families, proportion of residents in professional and managerial occupations, average years of schooling, proportion unemployed, and proportion below the poverty line.

Table 1: Distribution of median family income for zipcode of residence[a] for black and white men screened for the MRFIT

Income ($)	Black men		White men	
	Number	%	Number	%
<10,000	2,628	13.0	397	0.1
10,000-12,499	4,278	21.2	892	0.3
12,500-14,999	4,799	23.7	4,480	1.5
15,000-17,499	2,529	12.5	11,729	3.9
17,500-19,999	2,285	11.3	32,200	10.7
20,000-22,499	1,963	9.7	60,502	20.1
22,500-24,999	762	3.8	56,458	18.8
25,000-27,499	376	1.9	45,311	15.1
27,500-29,999	221	1.1	36,580	12.2
30,000-32,499	146	0.7	25,265	8.4
32,500+	237	1.2	26,871	8.9
Total	20,224	100.0	300,685	100.0

[a] Based on data from the 1980 US Census; median income of black households for black men and median income of white households for white men.

Table 2: Characteristics of black and white men screened for the MRFIT, and of zipcode areas in which they reside

	Black men (*n*=20,224)		White men (*n*=300,685)	
	Mean or %	SD	Mean or %	SD
Characteristics of the men				
Age (years)	45.3	6.3	46.0	6.4
Serum cholesterol (mg/dl)	210.0	42.4	214.5	39.1
Systolic BP (mm Hg)	133.6	18.0	129.8	15.7
Diastoloic BP (mm Hg)	86.8	12.3	83.5	10.4
Stage 1 Hypertension[a] (%)				
(SBP 140-59 or DBP 90-9)	9.4	–	8.2	–
Stage 2-4 Hypertension[a] (%)				
(SBP ≥160 or DBP ≥100)	16.6	–	8.6	–
Cigarette smoker (%)	48.8	–	35.2	–
Cigarettes/day for smokers (no)	18.5	10.5	26.7	13.2
Prior hospitalisation for heart attack (%)	1.4	–	1.5	–
Medication for diabetes (%)	3.2	–	1.4	–
Characteristics of zipcode areas of residence[b]				
Median family income of white households ($)	19,635	5,874	25,028	5,918
Median family income of black households ($)	15,338	5,482	20,600	8,820
Professional/managerial occupation (%)	8.5	5.1	13.3	6.0
Years of schooling	13.5	0.8	14.2	0.8
Unemployed (%)	4.8	1.4	3.1	1.2
Below poverty line (%)	13.9	9.0	4.6	4.2

[a] Stages based on the report of the Fifth Joint National Committee on Detection, Evaluation and treatment of high blood pressure, although data on antihypertensive drug use, utilized in the JNC definitions, are not available. The definition of Stage 1 hypertension includes not being eligible for classification as stages 2-4 hypertension.

[b] Based on data from the 1980 US Census.

All-cause mortality

Over the 16 years of follow-up, 31,737 of the 300,685 white men and 2,937 of the 20,224 black men died. The crude black/white relative risk estimated from the stratified (by centre) proportional hazards model is 1.37. With age-adjustment this relative risk is 1.47 (95% confidence interval [CI]: 1.42-1.53). The relative risk of all-cause mortality adjusted for diastolic blood pressure, serum cholesterol, cigarette smoking, use of medication for diabetes and prior hospitalisation for a heart attack was 1.40 (95% CI: 1.35-1.46). Adjustment just for age and income yielded a much reduced relative risk of all-cause mortality of 1.19 (95% CI: 1.14-1.24). Further adjustment for the other risk factors did not change this estimate (relative risk 1.19; 95% CI: 1.14-1.25).

Analyses restricted to the 228,893 men from zipcodes represented by at least one black and one white cohort member yielded similar results. The age-adjusted relative risk of mortality for black compared to white men is 1.46 (95% CI: 1.41–1.52); this relative risk is reduced to 1.19 (95% CI: 1.13–1.24) on adjustment for income as well as age. Stratifying by the 1,302 zipcode areas, instead of clinical centre, yields an age-adjusted relative risk of 1.30 (95% CI: 1.23–1.37) which is reduced to 1.21 (95% CI: 1.12–1.31) after adjustment for both age and income.

With income adjustment, zipcode area and clinical centre stratification produce similar results. Thus all subsequent analyses are based on the full cohort of 320,909 men, with stratification by clinical centre.

Table 3 compares mortality of black and white men in each income stratum to white men in the upper income stratum. Mortality rates are higher for both black and white men living in lower income zipcodes; within each income stratum mortality rates are higher for black men. Black–white differences in mortality are greater at lower income levels than at the higher levels, although a formal test of this interaction is not significant at conventional levels ($p=0.12$). With adjustment for smoking, medication for diabetes, hospitalisation for previous heart attack, diastolic blood pressure, and serum cholesterol, together with age, this interaction is nominally significant ($p=0.03$). This suggests that after taking into account the distribution according to income group of these other risk factors among black and white men, the elevated risk of mortality for black compared to white men is greater for the men in the lower income strata. For the small percentage of black men in the two highest income strata, relative

Table 3: Mortality rates and relative risk estimates for black and white men screened for the MRFIT according to black or white household median family income for zipcode of residence

Income	Black men					White men				
	No of men	No of deaths	Rate[a]	Relative risk[b]	Relative risk[c]	No of men	No of deaths	Rate[a]	Relative risk[b]	Relative risk[c]
<10,000	2,628	469	123.2	2.14	1.89	397	72	112.8	1.98	1.72
10,000–14,999	9,077	1,467	112.3	1.92	1.71	5,372	802	94.8	1.64	1.47
15,000–19,999	4,814	602	90.0	1.55	1.42	43,929	5,749	83.5	1.42	1.29
20,000–24,999	2,725	319	86.7	1.52	1.38	116,960	12,985	72.7	1.25	1.17
25,000–27,499	376	32	64.4	1.15[d]	1.11[d]	45,311	4,486	65.8	1.13	1.08
27,500+	604	48	57.2	1.05[d]	1.03[d]	88,716	7,643	57.8	1.00	1.00

[a] Age-adjusted rate per 10,000 person years.

[b] Adjusted for age, diastolic blood pressure, serum cholesterol, cigarettes per day, use of medication for diabetes, and prior hospitalisation for heart attack; white men living in zipcodes with a median family income of $27,500 or more is the reference category.

[c] Adjusted for age; white men living in zipcodes with a median family income of $27,500 or more as the reference category.

Note: All relative risk estimates except those with [d] ($p>0.05$) are significantly greater than 1.0 ($p<0.0001$).

risks are only slightly increased, for example, multivariate adjusted relative risk of 1.03 for black men in the highest income stratum.

Age-adjusted and age and income-adjusted relative risk estimates for all-cause mortality were calculated for each of the 22 MRFIT clinical centres. In 21 of 22 centres, the age-adjusted death rate for black men exceeded that for white men ($p=0.12$ for 21 df test for heterogeneity among centres). With adjustment for income as well as age, relative differences between black and white men were reduced in each centre and differences among centres remained small ($p=0.12$ for 21 df test for heterogeneity among centres after adjustment for age and income).

Black–white differences in mortality were more marked for those in the younger age groups at time of screening (Table 4) ($p<0.001$ for interaction). For men under 50 years of age at baseline, black men had a 20 to 40% higher death rate after adjustment for income and other risk factors. For those aged 50-54 and 55-57, increased risks were small.

Cause-specific mortality

Rates and adjusted relative risks of mortality from 23 cause of death categories are presented in Table 5. Black men had higher death rates from stroke, hypertensive heart disease, prostate cancer, and myeloma.

Table 4: All-cause mortality rates and relative risk estimates according to age at screening of black and white men screened for the MRFIT

Age (years)	Black men			White men			Relative risk adjusted for:		
	No of men	No of deaths	Rate[a]	No of men	No of deaths	Rate[a]	Age[b]	Age, income[c]	Age, income, risk factors[d]
35-39	4,534	283	40.2	60,976	2,267	23.6	1.62	1.21[e]	1.30
40-44	4,940	517	68.3	65,054	4,082	40.3	1.65	1.36	1.40
45-49	4,794	739	102.5	71,055	7,245	66.5	1.51	1.20	1.22
50-54	4,237	902	145.9	71,285	11,203	104.8	1.37	1.09[e]	1.08[f]
55-57	1,719	496	203.6	32,315	6,940	147.2	1.38	1.15	1.13[e]

[a] Age-adjusted rate per 10,000 person years.

[b] Relative risks adjusted for age.

[c] Relative risks adjusted for age and black and white household median family income of zipcode of residence.

[d] Relative risks adjusted for age, black/white household median family income of zipcode of residence, diastolic blood pressure, serum cholesterol, cigarettes per day, use of medication for diabetes and prior hospitalisation for heart attack.

Note: All relative risks estimates are significantly greater than 1.0 ($p< 0.01$) except those marked [e] ($p<0.05$) and [f] ($p=0.06$).

Table 5: Mortality rates and relative risk estimates for specific causes of death for black and white men screened for the MRFIT

Cause of death (ICD Code)	Black men (n=20,224)		White men (n=300,685)		Adjusted relative-risk estimates (95% CI)		
	Number of deaths	Age-adjusted rate[a]	Number of deaths	Age-adjusted rate[a]	Age	Age and income	Age, income and other risk factors[b]
All deaths[c]	2,937	103.0	31,737	69.4	1.47 (1.42-1.53)	1.19 (1.14-1.24)	1.19 (1.14-1.25)
All CVD (390-459)	1,188	41.9	14,102	30.8	1.36 (1.28-1.44)	1.09 (1.02-1.17)	1.05 (0.98-1.12)
CHD (410-14, 429.2)	724	25.6	10,579	23.1	1.12 (1.04-1.21)	0.91 (0.83-0.99)	0.88 (0.81-0.95)
Myocardial infarction (410)	358	12.8	6,054	13.2	0.94 (0.84-1.05)	0.76 (0.68-0.86)	0.73 (0.65-0.83)
Other CHD (411-14, 429.2)	366	12.8	4,525	9.9	1.37 (1.23-1.53)	1.11 (0.99-1.25)	1.08 (0.96-1.22)
Heart failure (428)	21	0.6	173	4.8	1.89 (1.18-2.99)	1.14 (0.66-1.97)	1.03 (0.60-1.78)
Stroke (430-8)	143	5.1	986	2.2	2.23 (1.86-2.67)	1.78 (1.44-2.20)	1.57 (1.27-1.94)
Intracranial haemorrhage (431-2)	50	1.7	265	0.6	2.88 (2.10-3.94)	2.39 (1.65-3.48)	2.10 (1.44-3.06)
Non-haemorrhagic stroke (433-8)	82	3.0	560	1.2	2.28 (1.79-2.89)	1.65 (1.25-2.19)	1.41 (1.06-1.88)
Hypertensive heart disease (402)	79	2.8	296	0.6	4.21 (3.25-5.45)	3.37 (2.45-4.62)	2.80 (2.03-3.86)
All malignant diseases (140-209)	1,017	36.0	11,111	24.3	1.47 (1.38-1.58)	1.25 (1.16-1.34)	1.35 (1.25-1.45)

contd.../

Table 5: contd.../

Cause of death (ICD Code)	Black men (n=20,224)		White men (n=300,685)		Adjusted relative-risk estimates (95% CI)		
	Number of deaths	Age-adjusted rate[a]	Number of deaths	Age-adjusted rate[a]	Age	Age and income	Age, income and other risk factors[b]
Lung cancer (162)	372	13.1	3,729	8.2	1.53 (1.37-1.70)	1.14 (1.01-1.29)	1.48 (1.30-1.67)
Melanoma (172)	4	0.2	293	0.6	0.21 (0.08-0.57)	0.24 (0.09-0.67)	0.24 (0.09-0.66)
Prostate cancer (185)	102	3.9	658	1.4	3.04 (2.45-3.77)	2.73 (2.12-3.50)	2.73 (2.13-3.52)
Myeloma (203)	35	1.3	174	0.4	3.61 (2.48-5.27)	3.21 (2.05-5.02)	3.14 (2.00-4.93)
All non-CVD, noncancer	698	24.0	6,168	13.5	1.71 (1.58-1.86)	1.26 (1.15-1.38)	1.24 (1.13-1.36)
Infection (1-139)	62	2.1	351	0.8	2.45 (1.86-3.23)	1.76 (1.28-2.44)	1.77 (1.28-2.45)
Diabetes (250)	64	2.2	402	0.9	2.63 (2.00-3.46)	1.43 (1.03-1.98)	0.99 (0.71-1.37)
Respiratory (460-519)	131	4.7	1,270	2.8	1.74 (1.45-2.10)	1.14 (0.93-1.98)	1.27 (1.03-1.58)
Chronic obstructive pulmonary disease (490-6)	63	2.2	677	1.5	1.60 (1.22-2.08)	0.99 (0.73-1.33)	1.20 (0.89-1.63)
Pneumonia and influenza (480-7)	47	1.7	345	0.8	2.31 (1.69-3.17)	1.42 (0.99-2.06)	1.43 (0.99-2.07)
Symptoms and ill-defined causes (780-99)	23	0.8	227	0.5	1.51 (0.98-2.35)	1.07 (0.65-1.76)	1.12 (0.68-1.84)
Accidents and violence (800-999)	220	7.3	1,933	4.2	1.59 (1.38-1.84)	1.24 (1.05-1.46)	1.25 (1.06-1.48)
Accidents (800-949)	105	3.5	1,073	2.3	1.41 (1.15-1.73)	1.10 (0.87-1.38)	1.09 (0.87-1.38)
Suicide (950-9, 980-9)	35	1.2	705	1.5	0.70 (0.50-0.99)	0.62 (0.43-0.89)	0.64 (0.45-0.93)
Homicide (960-9)	80	2.6	153	0.3	6.13 (4.63-8.11)	2.99 (2.04-4.38)	3.02 (2.06-4.44)

[a] Per 10,000 person years.

[b] Diastolic BP, serum cholesterol level, cigarettes per day, prior hospitalisation for heart attack, and medication for diabetes.

[c] Cause of death was unknown for 356 deaths among white men and 34 deaths among black men.

Table 6: Relative risks of mortality associated with baseline characteristics for narrow and broad definitions of coronary heart disease (CHD)

Risk factor	Definite CHD[a] (11,303[b])	Possible CHD[c] (1,357[b])	Definite and possible CHD (12,660[b])
Black	0.88 (0.81-0.95)	1.81 (1.47-2.22)	0.97 (0.89-1.04)
Cigarettes (10 per day)	1.25 (1.24-1.27)	1.24 (1.20-1.28)	1.25 (1.24-1.26)
Cholesterol (1 mmol)	1.28 (1.26-1.29)	1.17 (1.11-1.23)	1.27 (1.25-1.28)
DBP (10 mm Hg)	1.34 (1.32-1.36)	1.44 (1.38-1.52)	1.35 (1.33-1.37)
Income ($10,000 lower)	1.17 (1.13-1.21)	1.18 (1.05-1.33)	1.17 (1.13-1.21)
Previous heart attack	5.14 (4.83-5.48)	2.40 (1.80-3.19)	4.89 (4.60-5.20)
Diabetes	3.18 (2.94-3.43)	2.58 (1.97-2.37)	3.12 (2.90-3.36)

[a] ICD-9 codes 410-14 and 429.2.

[b] Number of deaths.

[c] ICD-9 codes 402 (375 deaths), 427 (604 deaths), 429 codes other than 429.2 (67 deaths), 440 (75 deaths), and 797-9 (236 deaths).

Note: All variables in table, plus age, included in the models; DBP = diastolic blood pressure.

The elevated relative risks of mortality from these conditions were only moderately attenuated by adjustment for measured risk factors and income. For total stroke and its subcategories, and hypertensive heart disease, adjustment for systolic blood pressure, instead of diastolic blood pressure, did not alter the relative risk estimates.

Increased risks of death from heart failure and ill-defined conditions for black men were essentially abolished by adjustment for income, and those from respiratory disease, diabetes, and homicide were much attenuated. Deaths from melanoma and suicide were less common among black than white men. Risk of dying from coronary heart disease (CHD) was lower among black than white men after adjustment for income. This represented a reversal from an increased risk of CHD among black men when income was not taken into account.

Since it is possible that coding of CHD as a cause of death differs between black and white men, a category of possible CHD was created, which added hypertensive heart disease (ICD-9 code 402), cardiac dysrhythmia (ICD-9 427), ill-defined descriptions and complications of heart disease (remaining ICD-9 429 codes), atherosclerosis (ICD 440), and ill-defined or unknown causes of death (ICD-9 797-9), to the CHD-defining ICD codes (410-14 and 429.2). For this expanded category of possible CHD, there were 11,752 deaths among white men and 908 among black men. The age-adjusted relative risk was 1.25 (95% CI: 1.16-1.33); this was reduced to 1.01 (95% CI:0.93-1.09) after adjustment for income; and to 0.97 (95% CI: 0.90 to 1.05) after adjustment for other risk factors (Table 6). Excluding ill-defined or unknown causes of death (ICD codes 797-799) from the possible CHD category left these findings essentially unchanged. Major risk factors were significantly related to risk of CHD death with use of each of the three definitions (definite CHD, possible CHD, definite and possible CHD).

Discussion

Crude and age-adjusted death rates were significantly higher among black compared to white men. The consistency of the relative difference in mortality between black and white men across the 22 MRFIT clinical centres in 18 US cities indicates that these findings are robust and generalisable. With adjustment for income the black versus white differentials in all-cause mortality were substantially reduced, both in the overall data and within the individual clinical centres.

Several findings indicate that the mortality experience of the black and white men screened for the MRFIT provides a useful model for exploring factors underlying black–white mortality differentials in the general population. First, distinctive features of the samples of black and white men screened for the MRFIT are similar to those seen in representative population samples. The difference in median family income of white households in the zipcodes of residence of the white men, and black households in the zipcodes of residence of the black men, was $9,690 by 1980 figures. At this time the black–white difference in family income in the general population was around $10,000.[8] There was a higher prevalence of cigarette smoking among the black compared to the white men screened for the MRFIT, but the white smokers used more cigarettes per day than the black smokers. These differences are the same as those seen in representative population studies carried out around the same time.[23,24] Degree of elevation in prevalences of hypertension and diabetes seen among the black men screened for the MRFIT are also similar to those reported from representative population samples.[25,26]

Second, the black–white differentials in mortality seen among the men screened for the MRFIT closely mirror those seen in both the total US population[27] and in the representative National Longitudinal Mortality Study (NLMS).[28] Age at death of decedents in the present study ranged from 35 to 74 years, with most deaths occurring at the older end of this range. Overall, the black men experienced a 47% higher age-adjusted all-cause mortality rate. In 1980, mid-point of the follow-up period of this study, risk of death of black men in the general population was 66% above that of white men in the age range 55-64, and 27% higher in the age range 65-74.[27] Similar findings were reported from the NLMS.[28] Higher relative risks of black mortality at younger ages among the men screened for the MRFIT reflect similar findings for the US total population[27] and the NLMS.[28] When specific causes are examined, the striking findings of age-adjusted black–white relative risks of above 6 for death from homicide, of around 4 for hypertensive heart disease, around 3 for prostate cancer and multiple myeloma, and around 2 for stroke, pneumonia or influenza, and diabetes, are also seen in national data.[28,29]

Contribution of socioeconomic factors to black–white mortality differentials

It has long been contended that adverse socioeconomic conditions underlie black–white health differentials. Thus in 1859 Smith demonstrated that the prevalence of rickets, which was high among black people, was similarly elevated among poor white people.[30] In 1916, Trask concluded that the higher death rate of black people reflected their less favourable economic circumstances, rather than any inherent differences between black and white people.[3] The contribution of socioeconomic factors to black–white differences in mortality has been formally investigated in several databases. In the National Mortality Followback Survey black–white differentials in all-cause mortality were essentially abolished by adjustment for household income.[13] In the NLMS black men aged 45-64 had a 68% higher mortality rate than white men in this age group; this was reduced to 28% after adjustment for employment status, income, education, marital status, and household size.[31] A similar reduction in the increased risk of mortality among black men on adjustment for wealth, having lived in poverty, and area of residence was seen in the National Longitudinal Study of Older Men.[32] The effect of adjustment for socioeconomic factors on differentials in all-cause mortality in these studies is similar to that seen among the MRFIT screenees.

The residual elevation of mortality among black men seen after adjustment for socioeconomic factors may indicate that within a given socioeconomic stratum life circumstances for US black men compare unfavourably to those of white men. Thus at the same level of income, black households have considerably lower wealth than white households;[33] within the same job, black men have greater levels of exposure to work-related hazards;[34] education brings lower returns in terms of income, occupational status, and avoidance of unemployment in blacks than whites;[35,36] purchasing power of black men is less than white men at a given income level with respect to food, housing, and other necessary expenditures.[36] Furthermore, within any particular social category, lifecourse socioeconomic experiences of black men will be less favourable than those of white men. Recent research has demonstrated that adverse childhood socioeconomic conditions may have long-lasting influences on mortality risk,[37] ones not captured by measures of adulthood socioeconomic position alone. Childhood social circumstances appear to influence mortality risk among black people in the US,[38] particularly with respect to cardiovascular mortality.[39] The concept that lifetime social environment contributes to health status has been developed with respect to black–white differences in pregnancy outcome in the 'weathering hypothesis'.[40]

Use of an area-based indicator of socioeconomic position has implications for ability to adjust for socioeconomic factors in the present study. Two biases, generally countervailing, can be introduced by use of area-based measures.[17,41] If the area-based measure is taken simply as a proxy for individual socioeconomic characteristics, then misclassification of individual socioeconomic position occurs and attenuated associations result. If contextual influences of areas themselves affect health – as research on black–white health differentials in the US[20,21,42] and health inequalities in other contexts[43,44] suggest – then area-based measures may pick up effects over and above those of individual measures[41] (technically, residuals from analyses with individual-level data will be correlated with the area-based indicator).[41,45] In this case use of an area-based indicator can lead to larger differentials than use of individual-level measures. The degree to which these biases operate is an empirical question, and it appears to differ between population groups studied and health outcomes examined.[41,46-49] However, a tendency for area-based measures to be less adequate than individual-level measures to control for socioeconomic confounding has been noted in analyses of black–white differences in health.[41] Therefore in the present study it could be argued that residual differences in mortality risk between black men and white men reflect inadequate adjustment for current socioeconomic circumstances.

Two points have a bearing on this. First, we performed exact zipcode matched analyses for study participants who lived in zipcodes in which at least one black and one white study participant resided, and further adjusted for median income of black and white households within these zipcodes. These analyses yielded essentially identical results to those produced by the simple adjustment for income. Second, when causes of death are examined it is clear that some contributors to the overall black–white mortality differential (eg prostate cancer, myeloma) are not conditions which are strongly linked to socioeconomic position and further adjustment would leave the residual effects little changed.

Black–white mortality differentials for particular causes of death

Coronary heart disease was the most frequent single cause of death among both black and white men in this study, in line with national data. Coronary heart disease mortality in national statistics has been lower for black than white men since it was first recorded, but since 1989 a cross-over has occurred and rates have been higher among black men.[50] Given the combination of adverse risk factor profiles and the socioeconomic disadvantage among black men, higher rates of CHD mortality for black than white men would be expected. In line with this, statistical adjustments for income and CHD risk factors led to a 12% lower risk of CHD among black than white men as compared to a 12% greater risk before adjustment. Risk factor adjustment had less influence on relative risk than income because black men had higher blood pressure levels than white men and slightly lower serum cholesterol levels, and black smokers did not use as many cigarettes per day as white smokers. Similar findings of lower CHD mortality among black and white men after adjustment for risk factor profiles have been reported from the Evans County and Charleston studies.[51]

This lower risk of CHD mortality for black than white men after adjustment may be due, in part, to misclassification of cause of death.[50] We created a very broad definition of CHD by including a wide category of causes as 'possible CHD'. For this broad category of CHD, adjusted relative risk was closer to one. However, this category of deaths may be overly inclusive. Compared with definite CHD, the relationship between serum cholesterol and possible CHD was weaker, and the association between blood pressure and possible CHD was stronger (Table 6). This suggests that the possible CHD group contains many deaths which are not directly due to CHD but are associated with hypertension and are more frequent causes of death in black than white men. With this over-inclusive category of total possible CHD, the adjusted risk remained slightly lower for black men than white men. The lower CHD mortality among black men in the US general population before 1989 remains intriguing and a wholly adequate explanation has still not been found. Recent data, however, demonstrate higher CHD mortality rates among young black than young white men,[52,53] which, together with trends in CHD mortality and in CHD risk factors[50] indicate that an increasing excess in CHD mortality among black men will be seen in the future.

Stroke mortality for 35- to 74-year-old black men in the general population is around 2.5 times as high as that of white men;[54] this is similar to the age-adjusted findings in the present study. In line with national data, elevations in both intracranial haemorrhage and non-haemorrhagic stroke are seen. Adjustment for income produces some attenuation, but substantial elevation remains. These findings are in line with adjustment effects for income or occupational social class in other US studies.[55,56] A small study with risk factor data demonstrated residual elevated stroke risk among black women after systolic blood pressure and prevalent diabetes had been taken into account.[57] In this study, however, there was little elevation in the unadjusted stroke rate among men. In our analyses, risk factor adjustment led to relatively small additional decreases in risk once income had been taken into account. The higher stroke mortality among black men is accompanied by higher stroke incidence in various studies[54] and this increased risk has not been adequately accounted for. Long-term influences from childhood could be important, since place of birth appears to contribute to stroke risk among black men in the US,[39] in line with other data suggesting that adverse socioeconomic circumstances in early life can increase stroke risk.[58]

Although high prevalence of hypertension among black men does not seem to account entirely for the stroke excess, it still represents a serious health burden, reflected also in the present data in elevated rates of hypertensive heart disease mortality among black men. The increased risk of hypertensive heart disease mortality is reduced, but not abolished, by adjustment for income and blood pressure. In this cohort black men also have a considerably higher rate of end-stage renal disease than white men, which is attenuated, but remains substantial, after adjustment for blood pressure and income.[59] Blood pressure is related in a similar way to cardiovascular mortality and to end stage renal disease in black and white men in the present study,[14,59] as in other data.[60]

The higher prevalence of hypertension and higher average blood pressure among black than white men does not appear to be simply a reflection of socioeconomic position.[61] Preliminary evidence suggests that the experience of racism, especially when this is perceived as an inevitable 'fact of life', is associated with higher blood pressure among young black men.[62] Other studies have indicated that black men who strive hard against adversity, but with limited resources to succeed, have high blood pressure.[63] Differences in levels of obesity, consumption of salt, protein, magnesium, calcium, and potassium; heavy alcohol use; and insulin resistance may also contribute to the black–white differences in blood pressure.[64-67] Recently attention has focused on the possibility that poor intrauterine growth, as indexed by low birthweight – which is more prevalent among black than white people in the US – has long-term influences on blood pressure in adulthood, possible through both increasing prevalence of insulin resistance and through impaired maturation of the kidneys.[68]

There was a 50% higher rate of lung cancer mortality among black than white men. Adjustment for income greatly attenuated this elevated risk, while risk-factor adjustment (the primary effect being through smoking in this instance) increased the degree of elevation of risk among black men. This reflects the lower number of cigarettes smoked per day by black smokers and the steep graded association between numbers of cigarettes smoked per day and lung cancer mortality in this cohort.[69] Differences in smoking style – such as smoking more of each cigarette – could contribute to the higher lung cancer risk at a given level of smoking among black men.[70] Occupational, environmental, and dietary exposures which are related to income could also contribute to the elevated lung cancer mortality among black men. Place of birth is also of importance with respect to lung cancer mortality among black men in the US. Those born in the South, with on average more adverse socioeconomic conditions in childhood, have higher rates of lung cancer mortality, independent of their place of residence at death.[71] This is in line with other evidence relating to a possible influence of early life factors on lung cancer risk,[72] although evidence for this is equivocal.[37]

Prostate cancer mortality is over three times as high in black than white men in the present study, as in US national data.[29] It is not strongly associated with socioeconomic position in either the present cohort[17] or other studies[73] and adjustment for income has little effect. Like lung cancer, prostate cancer mortality shows strong place of birth relationships, with black men born in the South at increased risk wherever they reside in adulthood.[71] Circulating testosterone is a risk factor for prostate cancer and black men are reported to have higher serum testosterone levels than white men,[74,75] but determinants of this putatively higher testosterone level among black men are not known, although dietary factors and intrauterine environment have been implicated.[76,77]

As in other studies, myeloma mortality was substantially higher among black than white men. Income shows little association with myeloma in our data and, as in other studies,[78] adjustment for it had only a small effect. Despite considerable investigation, reasons for the high myeloma risk among black men remain unclear. Some authorities have strongly hypothesised that genetic factors are involved, although attempts to find these have been negative;[79] attention should also be paid to potential environmental, including occupational, causes, and early life factors.

Prevalence and mortality from diabetes, considerably higher among black than white men as in other US data,[80] mainly reflect non-insulin-dependent diabetus mellitus. Adjustment for income greatly attenuated the elevated risk of diabetes mortality, while additional adjustment for risk factors abolished the elevated risk. This included adjustment for prevalent diabetes at baseline. Diabetes mortality was also higher in black than white men after exclusion of those with diabetes at baseline. Adjustment for income greatly reduced this elevated risk (data not shown). Higher prevalence of obesity among black than white men makes a major, but not exclusive, contribution to the higher diabetes risk found in other studies[80]. Low birthweight has been implicated as an additional factor responsible for higher diabetes risk among black than white Americans.[68]

Chronic obstructive pulmonary disease (COPD) mortality is higher in US black than white men under age 60.[81] COPD mortality behaves similarly to lung cancer mortality in this cohort: adjustment for income essentially abolished the elevated risk, but adjustment for risk factors (in particular, smoking) yielded higher risks in black than white men. Similar factors – related to smoking style, occupational, environmental, and dietary exposures – could be involved in COPD and lung cancer. Measured lung function is lower among black than white men, and this difference can already be seen in early childhood.[82] Differences could be established at this age through a differential rate of respiratory infection in infancy,[83] as well as poor intrauterine growth.[84]

Death from homicide is considerably more common among black than white men, while suicide is a more frequent cause of death for white men.[85] Adjustment for income leads to a substantial attenuation of the elevated homicide risk among black men. Poverty is clearly central here[86] and in this instance the use of median income for zipcode area of residence may be an inadequate indicator. Homicide, like other crime, shows marked geographical segregation and studies which closely match for area of residence further attenuate, or abolish, black–white differences in homicide risk.[87]

Black–white mortality differentials: remaining issues

Several factors which could contribute to black–white differences in mortality could not be investigated in the present dataset. These include data on dietary and alcohol consumption patterns, on exercise, on occupational exposures, on body mass index and on the lifetime – rather than cross-sectional – patterns of blood pressure, circulating cholesterol and cigarette smoking. In other studies, differences in healthcare provision and utilisation have been extensively explored. In general, worse access, longer waiting times, lower satisfaction with consultations, poorer continuity of care, and lesser degrees of investigation have been seen for black than white people.[88] Thus utilisation of a wide range of clinical tests and facilities has been found to be lower for black people, in a way which could not be accounted for by differential prevalence of associated medical conditions.[89] Black MEDICARE beneficiaries make less physician visits, have lower rates of other forms of health service use, and receive less cardiovascular procedures than white MEDICARE beneficiaries.[90] Even after adjustment for disease severity, black people with coronary disease were less likely than white people to receive bypass surgery in the Duke University database and this appeared to contribute to the poorer survival of black people with CHD than white people in this study.[91] Lack of health insurance, or public rather than employer-provided insurance, is associated with higher mortality,[92,93] and non-insurance or public insurance is more frequently seen among black than white men.[93] Cancer survival after diagnosis has been found to be less favourable for black than white people for some sites.[94] The differences discussed above do not appear to be entirely explained by socioeconomic factors.[90,95] Taken together, these data suggest that there could be some role of differing experiences with healthcare in the black–white mortality differentials. However, given the magnitude of such effects in studies where these were ascertained, they are likely to produce only a relatively small component of the mortality differences reported here.

Several socioenvironmental factors which influence mortality risk may not be captured by use of median income of zipcode area of residence. First, lifetime exposures are not adequately captured by a single measure of adulthood socioeconomic position.[37] Thus intergenerational influences – from the health of the mothers of the men in our cohort – may exist, mediated through intrauterine development and birthweight.[68] Recent investigations of differences in birth outcomes between black and white people suggest that this process is continuing and that the foundations of black adulthood health disadvantage in the future are currently being laid down.[40] Poorer socioeconomic circumstances in childhood will also have been experienced by the black compared with the white men in the present cohort. These contribute to the overall adversity of lifetime socioeconomic experience and to mortality risk.[37] Future studies should aim to obtain data regarding socioeconomic factors acting across the lifecourse when attempting to account for black–white health differentials.

Second, some exposures appear to be more prevalent and severe for people living in predominantly black areas. Thus environmental hazards – such as solid waste sites and air polluting plants – are more likely to be located in areas where black people make up a high percentage of the population, even when other socioeconomic characteristics are taken into account.[96] Segregation also leads to concentration of unfavourable neighbourhood characteristics – poor schooling, high crime, poor facilities, high social disorganisation, poor housing stock, lack of local employment opportunities, and poor medical services.[97] Such segregation has been shown to relate to mortality: both the black–white mortality ratio and the overall level of black mortality are higher in areas which are more segregated.[42] Segregation means that socioeconomic indicators can have a different relationship to environmental exposures for black than white people: at a given level on any indicator the material conditions of existence may be less favourable for black people. We have attempted to address this issue in the present study by performing analyses matched for exact zipcode area. However this may be inadequate because of segregation effects within zipcode areas. This may apply particularly to homicide,[87] although the close correlation at the small area level between homicide mortality and several other health indicators suggests that it may be a more general phenomenon.[98]

Racism can be considered the 'missing variable' in research on black–white differences in health.[62,99] This may have direct psychologically mediated effects, but also could underpin differences in socioeconomic position, experience of medical care, and opportunities to take action to maintain and improve health. Racism needs to be investigated and combated at the individual, institutional, and societal level.

The major determinants of black–white differentials in mortality are apparently socioenvironmental, in the broadest sense. Action is therefore required at this level.

Endnote

* The principal investigators and senior staff of the clinical, coordinating and support centres, the National Heart, Lung, and Blood Institute project office, and members of the MRFIT Policy Advisory Board and Mortality Review Committee are listed in a previous report (*Journal of the American Medical Association*, 1982, vol 248, pp 1465-77). The mortality follow-up of the men screened for the MRFIT and data analysis for this report were supported by a National Institute for Health research grant, R01 HL28715. We are pleased to thank Anne Rennie and Claire Hjarne for help in preparation of the typescript.

References

[1] Rogers, R.G. (1992) 'Living and dying in the USA: socio-demographic determinants of death among blacks and whites', *Demography*, vol 29, pp 287-303.

[2] Kochanek, K.D., Maurer, J.D. and Rosenburg, H.M. (1994) 'Why did black life expectancy decline from 1984-1989 in the USA?', *American Journal of Public Health*, vol 84, pp 938-44.

[3] Trask, J.W. (1916) 'The significance of the mortality rates of the coloured population of the US', *American Journal of Public Health*, vol 6, pp 254-60.

[4] Moriyama, I., Woolsey, T. and Stamler, J. (1958) 'Observations on possible causative factors responsible for the sex and race trends in cardiovascular-renal diseases mortality in the US', *Journal of Chronic Diseases*, vol 7, pp 401-12.

5 Stamler, J., Kjelsberg, M. and Hall, Y. (1960) 'Epidemiologic studies on cardiovascular-renal diseases: I. Analysis of mortality by age-race-sex-occupation', *Journal of Chronic Diseases*, vol 12, pp 440-55.

6 Kjelsberg, M. and Stamler, J. (1960) 'Epidemiologic studies on cardiovascular-renal diseases: II. Analysis of mortality by age-race-sex-place of residence, including urban-rural comparisons', *Journal of Chronic Diseases*, vol 12, pp 456-63.

7 Krieger, N., Rosley, D.L., Herman, A.A., Avery, B. and Phillips, M.T. (1993) 'Racism, sexism, and social class: implications for studies of health, disease, and well-being', *American Journal of Preventative Medicine*, vol 9, suppl, pp 82-122.

8 DHHS (Department of Health and Human Services) (1990) *Health status of the disadvantaged: Chart book 1990*, Washington, DC: DHHS.

9 Krieger, N. (1992) 'The making of public health data: paradigms, policies and policy', *Journal of Public Health Policy*, vol 13, pp 412-27.

10 Editorial (1992) 'Hypertension in black and white', *Lancet*, vol 339, pp 28-9.

11 Sorlie, P.D., Rogot, R., Anderson, R., Johnson, N.J. and Buckland, E. (1992) 'Black–white mortality differences by family income', *Lancet*, vol 340, pp 346-50.

12 Otten, M.W., Teutsch, S.M., Williamson, D.F. and Marks, J.S. (1990) 'The effect of known risk factors on the excess mortality of black adults in the US', *Journal of the American Medical Association*, vol 263, pp 345-50.

13 Sterling, T., Rosenbaum, W. and Weinkam, J. (1993) 'Income, race, and mortality?', *Journal of the National Medical Association*, vol 85, pp 906-11.

14 Neaton, J.D., Kuller, L.H., Wentworth, D. and Borhani, N.O. (1984) 'Total and cardiovascular mortality in relation to cigarette smoking, serum cholesterol concentration, and diastolic blood pressure among black and white males followed for up to five years', *American Heart Journal*, vol 108, pp 759-69.

15 Neaton, J.D., Grimm, R.H. and Cutler, J.A. (1987) 'Recruitment of participants for the Multiple Risk Factor Intervention Trial (MRFIT)', *Controlled Clinical Trials*, vol 8, pp 415-535.

[16] Lipid Research Clinics Program (1974) *Manual of operations, Volume 1: Lipid and lipoprotein analysis*, Washington, DC: US Department of Health Education and Welfare.

[17] Davey Smith, G., Neaton, J.D., Wentworth, D., Stamler, R. and Stamler, J. (1996) 'Socioeconomic differentials in mortality risk among men screened for the Multiple Risk Factor Intervention Trial: Part I – results for 300,685 white men', *American Journal of Public Health*, vol 86, pp 486-96.

[18] Davey Smith, G., Wentworth, D., Neaton, J.D., Stamler, R. and Stamler, J. (1996) 'Socioeconomic differentials in mortality risk among men screened for the Multiple Risk Factor Intervention Trial: Part II – results for 20,224 black men', *American Journal of Public Health*, vol 86, pp 497-504.

[19] Lillie-Blanton, M., Anthony, J.C. and Schuster, C.R. (1993) 'Probing the meaning of racial/ethnic group comparisons in crack cocaine smoking', *Journal of the American Medical Association*, vol 269, pp 993-7.

[20] Geronimus, A.T., Bound, J., Waidmann, T.A., Hillemeier, M.M. and Burns, P.B. (1996) 'Excess mortality among blacks and whites in the US', *New England Journal of Medicine*, vol 335, pp 1553-9.

[21] Wentworth, D.N., Neaton, J.D. and Rasmussen, W.L. (1983) 'Evaluation of SSA master beneficiary files and the National Death Index in ascertainment of vital status', *American Journal of Public Health*, vol 73, pp 1270-4.

[22] *International Classification of Diseases Ninth Revision: Clinical modification* (1981), Ann Arbor, MI: Edwards Bros.

[23] Office on Smoking and Health (1989) *Reducing the health consequences of smoking: 25 years of progress*, A report of the Surgeon General, Washington, DC: US DHHS.

[24] Sterling, T.D. and Weinkam, J.J. (1989) 'Comparison of smoking-related risk factors among black and white males', *American Journal of Industrial Medicine*, vol 15, pp 319-33.

[25] Manton, K., Clifford, P. and Johnson, K. (1987) 'Health differentials between blacks and whites: recent trends in mortality and morbidity', *Millbank Quarterly*, vol 65, suppl 1, pp 129-99.

[26] Harris, M.I., Hadden, W.C., Knowler, W.C. and Bennett, P.H. (1987) 'Prevalence of diabetes and impaired glucose tolerance and plasma glucose levels in US population aged 20-74 yr', *Diabetes*, vol 36, pp 523-34.

[27] DHHS (Department of Health and Human Services) (1993) *Health: US 1992*, Washington, DC: DHHS.

[28] Rogot, E., Sorlie, P.D., Johnson, N.J. and Schmitt, C. (1993) *A mortality study of 1.3 million persons by demographic, social and economic factors: 1979-1985. Follow-up, US National Longitudinal Mortality Study*, Washington, DC: NIH.

[29] Clayton, L.A. and Buird, W.M. (1993) 'The African-American cancer crisis, Part I: the problem', *Journal of Health Care for the Poor and Underserved*, vol 4, pp 83-101.

[30] Krieger, N. (1987) 'Shades of difference: theoretical underpinnings of the medical controversy on black/white differences in the US, 1830-1870', *International Journal of Health Services*, vol 17, pp 259-78.

[31] Sorlie, P.D., Backlund, E. and Keller, J.B. (1995) 'US mortality by economic, demographic, and social characteristics: the National Longitudinal Mortality Study', *American Journal of Public Health*, vol 85, pp 949-56.

[32] Menchik, P.L. (1993) 'Economic status as a determinant of mortality among black and white older men: does poverty kill?', *Population Studies*, vol 47, pp 427-36.

[33] Blau, F.D. and Graham, J.W. (1990) 'Black-white differences in wealth and asset composition', *Quarterly Journal of Economics*, vol 105, pp 321-39.

[34] Robinson, J.C. (1984) 'Racial inequality and the probability of occupational-related injury or illness', *Milbank Memorial Fund Quarterly*, vol 62, pp 567-90.

[35] Hacker, A. (1992) *Two nations: Black and white, separate, hostile and unequal*, New York, NY: Ballantine Books.

[36] Williams, D.R. and Collins, C. (1995) 'US socioeconomic and racial differences in health: patterns and explanations', *Annual Review of Sociology*, vol 21, pp 349-86.

[37] **Davey Smith, G., Hart, C., Blane, D. and Hole, D. (1997) 'Adverse socioeconomic conditions in childhood and cause-specific adult mortality: prospective observational study', *British Medical Journal*, vol 316, pp 1631-5.**

[38] Greenberg, M. and Schneider, D. (1992) 'Region of birth and mortality of blacks in the US', *International Journal of Epidemiology*, vol 21, pp 324-8.

[39] Fang, J., Madhavan, S. and Alderman, M. (1996) 'The association between birthplace and mortality from cardiovascular causes among black and white residents of New York City', *New England Journal of Medicine*, vol 335, pp 1545-51.

[40] Geronimus, A.T. (1996) 'Black/white differences in the relationship of maternal age to birthweight: a population-based test of the weathering hypothesis', *Social Science and Medicine*, vol 42, pp 589-97.

[41] Geronimus, A.T., Bound, J. and Neidert, L.J. (1996) 'On the validity of using Census geocode characteristics to proxy individual socioeconomic characteristics', *Journal of the American Statistical Association*, vol 91, pp 529-37.

[42] Polednak, A.P. (1996) 'Segregation, discrimination and mortality in US blacks', *Ethnicity and Disease*, vol 6, pp 99-108.

[43] Sooman, A., Macintyre, S. and Anderson, A. (1993) 'Scotland's health – a more difficult challenge for some? The price and availability of healthy foods in socially contrasting localities in the West of Scotland', *Health Bulletin*, vol 51, pp 276-84.

[44] Kaplan, G.A. (1996) 'People and places: contrasting perspectives on the association between social class and health', *International Journal of Health Services*, vol 26, pp 507-19.

[45] Firebaugh, G. (1978) 'A rule for inferring individual-level relationships from aggregate data', *American Sociological Review*, vol 43, pp 557-72.

[46] Krieger, N. (1992) 'Overcoming the absence of socioeconomic data in medical records: validation and application of a Census-based methodology', *American Journal of Public Health*, vol 82, pp 703-10.

47 Carr-Hill, R. and Rice, N. (1995) 'Is enumeration district level an improvement on ward level analysis in studies of deprivation and health?', *Journal of Epidemiology and Community Health*, vol 49, suppl 2, pp 28-9.

48 Hyndman, J.C.G., Holman, C.D.J., Hockey, R.L., Donovan, R.J., Corti, B. and Rivera, J. (1995) 'Risk classification of social disadvantage based on geographical areas: comparison of postcode and collector's district analyses', *International Journal of Epidemiology*, vol 24, pp 165-76.

49 Anderson, R.T., Sorlie, P., Johnson, N. and Kaplan, G. (1997) 'Individual and area-based indicators associating economic status and mortality: the National Longitudinal Mortality Study', *Epidemiology*, vol 8, pp 42-7.

50 Liao, Y. and Cooper, R.S. (1995) 'Continued adverse trends in coronary heart disease mortality among blacks, 1980-91', *Public Health Reports*, vol 110, pp 572-9.

51 Keil, J.E., Sutherland, S.E., Hames, C.G., Lackland, D.T., Gazes, P.C., Knapp, R.G. and Tyroler, H.A. (1995) 'Coronary disease mortality and risk factors in black and white men', *Archive of International Medicine*, vol 155, pp 1521-7.

52 Traven, N.D., Kuller, L.H., Ives, D.G., Rutan, G.H. and Perper, J.A. (1996) 'Coronary heart disease mortality and sudden death among the 35-44 year age group in Allegheny County, Pennsylvania', *Annals of Epidemiology*, vol 6, pp 130-6.

53 Escobedo, L.G., Giles, W.H. and Anda, R.F. (1997) 'Socioeconomic status, race, and death from coronary heart disease', *American Journal of Preventative Medicine*, vol 13, pp 123-30.

54 Gillum, R.F. (1988) 'Stroke in blacks', *Stroke*, vol 19, pp 1-9.

55 Howard, G., Russell, G.B., Anderson, R., Evans, G.W., Morgan, T., Howard, V.J. and Burke, G.L. (1995) 'Role of social class in excess black stroke mortality', *Stroke*, vol 26, pp 1759-63.

56 Casper, M.L., Barnett, E.B., Armstrong, D.L., Giles, W.H. and Blanton, C.J. (1997) 'Social class and race disparities in premature stroke mortality among men in North Carolina', *Annals of Epidemiology*, vol 7, pp 146-53.

[57] Kittner, S.J., White, L.R., Losonczy, K.G., Wolf, P.A. and Hebel, J.R. (1990) 'Black–white differences in stroke incidence in a national sample', *Journal of the American Medical Association*, vol 264, pp 1267-70.

[58] Davey Smith, G. and Ben-Shlomo, Y. (1997) 'Geographical and social class differentials in stroke mortality: the influence of early-life factors', *Journal of Epidemiology and Community Health*, vol 51, pp 134-7.

[59] Klag, M.J., Whelton, P.K., Randall, B.L., Neaton, J.D., Brancati, F.L. and Stamler, J. (1997) 'End stage renal disease in African-American and white men: 16-year MRFIT findings', *Journal of the American Medical Association*, vol 277, pp 1293-8.

[60] Cooper, R.S., Liao, Y. and Rotimi, C. (1996) 'Is hypertension more severe among US blacks, or is severe hypertension more common?', *Annals of Epidemiology*, vol 6, pp 173-80.

[61] Dressler, W.W. (1993) 'Health in the African-American community: accounting for health inequalities', *Medical Anthropology Quarterly*, vol 7, pp 325-45.

[62] Krieger, N. and Sidney, S. (1996) 'Racial discrimination and blood pressure: the CARDIA study of young black and white women and men', *American Journal of Public Health*, vol 86, pp 1370-8.

[63] James, S.A. (1994) 'John Henryism and the health of African-Americans', *Cultural Medical Psychiatry*, vol 18, pp 163-82.

[64] Williams, D.R. (1992) 'Black–white differences in blood pressure: the role of social factors', *Ethnicity and Disease*, vol 2, pp 126-41.

[65] Rutledge, D.R. (1994) 'Race and hypertension – what is clinically relevant?', *Drugs*, vol 47, pp 914-32.

[66] Stamler, J., Caggiula, A., Grandits, G.A., Kjelsberg, M. and Cutler, J.A. for the MRFIT Research Group (1996) 'Relationship to blood pressure of combinations of dietary macronutrients: findings of the Multiple Risk Factor Intervention Trial (MRFIT)', *Circulation*, vol 94, pp 2417-23.

[67] Stamler, J. (1997) 'The INTERSALT Study: background, methods, findings, and implications', *American Journal of Clinical Nutrition*, vol 65, suppl 2, pp 626-42.

68 Lopes, A.A.S. and Port, F.K. (1995) 'The low birth weight hypothesis as a plausible explanation for the black/white differences in hypertension, non-insulin-diabetes, and end-stage renal disease', *American Journal of Kidney Diseases*, vol 25, pp 350-6.

69 Davey Smith, G. and Phillips, A.N. (1996) 'Passive smoking and health: should we believe Philip Morris's "experts"?', *British Medical Journal*, vol 313, pp 929-33.

70 Clark, P.I., Gautam, S.P., Hlaing, W.M. and Gerson, L.W. (1996) 'Response error in self-reported current smoking frequency by black and white established smokers', *Annals of Epidemiology*, vol 6, pp 483-9.

71 Greenberg, M. and Schneider, D. (1995) 'The cancer burden of southern-born African Americans: analysis of a social-geographic legacy', *Milbank Quarterly*, vol 73, pp 599-620.

72 Hole, D.J., Gillis, C.R. and Watt, G. (1995) 'Does early respiratory environment influence lung cancer risk? Evidence from studies in the west of Scotland', *Journal of Epidemiology and Community Health*, vol 49, pp 548-9.

73 **Davey Smith, G., Leon, D., Shipley, M.J. and Rose, G. (1991) 'Socioeconomic differentials in cancer in men',** *International Journal of Epidemiology***, vol 20, pp 339-45.**

74 Ross, R., Bernstein, L., Judd, H., Hanisch, R., Pike, M. and Henderson, B. (1986) 'Serum testosterone levels in healthy young black and white men', *Journal of the National Cancer Institute*, vol 76, pp 45-8.

75 Ellis, L. and Nyborg, H. (1992) 'Racial/ethnic variations in male testosterone levels: a probable contributor to group differences in health', *Steroids*, vol 57, pp 72-5.

76 Henderson, B.E., Bernstein, L., Ross, R.K., Depue, R.H. and Judd, H.L. (1988) 'The early in utero oestrogen and testosterone environment of blacks and whites: potential effects on male offspring', *British Journal of Cancer*, vol 57, pp 216-18.

77 McIntosh, H. (1997) 'Why do African-American men suffer more prostate cancer?', *Journal of the National Camcer Institute*, vol 89, pp 188-9.

[78] Koessel, S.L., Theis, M.K., Vaughan, T.L., Koepsell, T.D., Weiss, N.S., Greenberg, R.S. and Swanson, G.M. (1996) 'Socioeconomic status and the incidence of multiple myeloma', *Epidemiology*, vol 7, pp 4-8.

[79] Pottern, L.M., Gart, J.J., Nam, J., Dunston, G., Wilson, J. et al (1992) 'HLA and multiple myeloma among black and white men: evidence of a genetic association', *Cancer Epidemiology Biomarkers and Prevention*, vol 1, pp 177-82.

[80] Carter, J.S., Pugh, J.A. and Monterrosa, A. (1996) 'Non-insulin-dependent diabetes mellitus in minorities in the US', *Annals of Internal Medicine*, vol 125, pp 221-32.

[81] Gillum, R.F. and Maryland, H. (1990) 'Chronic obstructive pulmonary disease in blacks and whites: mortality and morbidity', *Journal of the National Medical Association*, vol 82, pp 417-28.

[82] Gillum, R.F. and Maryland, R. (1991) 'Chronic obstructive pulmonary disease in blacks and whites: pulmonary function norms and risk factors', *Journal of the National Medical Association*, vol 83, pp 393-401.

[83] Mann, S.L., Wadsworth, M.E.J. and Colley, J.R.T. (1992) 'Accumulation of factors influencing respiratory illness in members of a national birth cohort and their offspring', *Journal of Epidemiology and Community Health*, vol 46, pp 286-92.

[84] Barker, D.J.P., Godfrey, K.M., Fall, C. et al (1991) 'Relation of birthweight and childhood respiratory infections adult lung function and death from chronic obstructive airways disease', *British Medical Journal*, vol 303, pp 671-5.

[85] Griffith, E.E.H. and Bell, C.C. (1989) 'Recent trends in suicide and homicide among blacks', *Journal of the American Medical Association*, vol 262, pp 2265-9.

[86] Williams, K.R. (1984) 'Economic sources of homicide: reestimating the effects of poverty and inequality', *Annual Sociological Review*, vol 49, pp 283-9.

[87] Centrewall, B.S. (1984) 'Race, socioeconomic status and domestic homicide: Atlanta, 1971-72', *American Journal of Public Health*, vol 74, pp 813-15.

[88] King, G. (1996) 'Institutional racism and the medical/health complex: a conceptual analysis', *Ethnicity and Disease*, vol 6, pp 30-46.

[89] Escarce, J.J., Epstein, K.R., Colby, D.C. and Schwartz, J.S. (1993) 'Racial differences in the elderly's use of medical procedures and diagnostic tests', *American Journal of Public Health*, vol 83, pp 948-54.

[90] Gornick, M.E., Eggers, P.W., Reilly, T.W., Mentnech, R.M., Fitterman, L.K., Kucken, L.E. and Vladeck, B.C. (1996) 'Effects of race and income on mortality and use of services among MEDICARE beneficiaries', *New England Journal of Medicine*, vol 335, pp 791-9.

[91] Peterson, E.D., Shaw, L.K., Delong, E.R., Pryor, D.B., Califf, R.M. and Mark, D.B. (1997) 'Racial variation in the use of coronary-revascularization procedures: are the differences real? Do they matter?', *New England Journal of Medicine*, vol 336, pp 480-6.

[92] Franks, P., Clancy, C.M. and Gold, M.R. (1993) 'Health insurance and mortality', *Journal of the American Medical Association*, vol 270, pp 737-41.

[93] Sorlie, P.D., Johnson, N.J., Backlund, E. and Bradham, D.D. (1994) 'Mortality in the uninsured compared with that in persons with public and private health insurance', *Archive of Internal Medicine*, vol 154, pp 2409-16.

[94] Hardy, R.E. and Hargreaves, M.K. (1991) 'Cancer prognosis in black Americans: a mini-review', *Journal of the National Medical Association*, vol 83, pp 574-9.

[95] Fichtenbaum, R. and Gyimah-Brempong, K. (1997) 'The effects of race on the use of physicians' services', *International Journal of Health Services*, vol 27, pp 139-56.

[96] Bryant, B. and Mohai, P. (1992) *Race and the incidence of environmental hazards*, Boulder, CO: Westview Press.

[97] Massey, D.S. (1990) 'American apartheid: segregation and the making of the underclass', *American Journal of Sociology*, vol 96, pp 329-57.

[98] Wilson, M. and Daly, M. (1997) 'Life expectancy, economic inequality, homicide and reproductive timing in Chicago neighbourhoods', *British Medical Journal*, vol 314, pp 1271-4.

[99] Davey Smith, G. and Egger, M. (1992) 'Socioeconomic differences in mortality in Britain and the US', Editorial, *American Journal of Public Health*, vol 82, pp 1079-81.

Section VII
Diversions

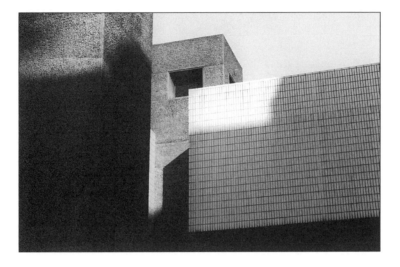

Photograph by Mary Shaw.

27

Socioeconomic differentials in the mortality of pets: probably reflect the same differences in material circumstances as in their owners

George Davey Smith and Brenda Bonnett

Factors associated with mortality among dogs have not been extensively studied, although recent work has examined age, breed, and sex distributions of mortality.[1] There has, however, been little investigation of socioeconomic differentials in pet mortality. The study by Moloo et al[2] is therefore welcome, although the results should be interpreted with caution. They show that the probability of reporting the death of a pet in the past year is greater for young people from less favourable socioeconomic backgrounds than for those from more favourable backgrounds.

Pet ownership may have some influence on psychological health,[3] but it does not itself seem to influence mortality[4] and therefore the dynamics of mortality among pet owners are likely to reflect those of the total population. In this regard the socioeconomic inequalities in mortality – shown in a wide range of populations – will be a key feature. There has been considerable research into explanations of socioeconomic differentials in mortality among humans,[5] and similar categories of explanation may account for such differentials in pet mortality.

The 'artefact' explanation suggests that socioeconomic differentials in mortality are more apparent than real, resulting from the way data are collected and analysed. In Moloo et al's study a potential artefact is created by the fact that the experience of a pet's death is analysed without information on whether the study household actually possessed a pet. Thus the results may simply reflect socioeconomic

British Medical Journal, 1998, vol 317, pp 1671-3

differences in pet ownership. In the US[6] and in Sweden (A Egenvall, personal communication) ownership of a pet is positively associated with household income, although this plateaus at high incomes.[7] This pattern might, therefore, create higher probabilities of pet death in the past 12 months for affluent than for poor households and this will lead to the data of Moloo et al under-estimating the true socioeconomic gradient in pet mortality. A second artefact could relate to the type of pet. If poorer households were more likely to have pets with shorter lifespans – gerbils, mice, or birds – than richer ones, then a higher probability of experiencing a death of a pet in the past 12 months would be expected. Evidence from the US suggests that ownership of most types of pets is higher among better-off families. Finally, pets often die as the result of euthanasia, and poorer families might be more likely to put down their pets because of an inability to support the animal. Thus several reasons exist why the socioeconomic gradient in pet mortality might be artefactual.

Health-related selection has been extensively investigated as an underlying cause of socioeconomic differentials in health among humans.[8] The basic proposition is that poor health leads to unfavourable social circumstances rather than vice versa. With respect to pet mortality, possible health-related selection would occur if poorer people took on pets who were less healthy or older at the time of acquisition. If this were so then higher mortality among the pets of less affluent families would be expected. This suggestion has some plausibility since one determinant of the cost of pets may be their health potential (although aesthetics seems more important). In humans evidence suggests that health-related selection makes only a small contribution to overall health inequalities,[8] but the situation in pets is unclear.

A third category of explanation suggests that health-related behaviour is responsible for socioeconomic differentials in health. Clearly the usual suspects – smoking and drinking – are unlikely to apply to pets. Differences in diet and exercise levels may exist between pets belonging to more or less affluent families. In humans it is important to recognise that health-related behaviours do not simply reflect individual choice but relate to structural constraints on the lives of people in straitened circumstances.[9] This is even clearer with respect to the health-related behaviours of pets. Socioeconomic differentials in medical care may contribute to human health inequalities, but are not considered key determinants.[10] There is some evidence of socioeconomic inequalities in veterinary care, although the degree to which this contributes to differentials in pet mortality is not known. Psychological and psychosocial factors have been advanced to explain inequalities in health among humans. These include social support[11] and work stress.[12] More affluent families may have more pets than less affluent households, providing their pets with more elaborate social networks, but greater social support is not necessarily health inducing;[13] indeed, cats in multicat households may be more stressed. Work stress is clearly not a candidate factor. Indeed, pets serve as an additional largely non-working group (along with unemployed and retired people, and, earlier this century, many women) among whom socioeconomic differentials in health are seen which are at least as great as those in working populations.[14]

A final category of explanation relates to material and structural factors, the importance of which has probably been underestimated with respect to socioeconomic differentials in human health.[5] Advantage clusters cross sectionally and longitudinally across the course of people's lives, with those born in adverse circumstances having a higher risk of embodied inequality (in the form of low birth weight and short stature) and a lower probability of succeeding educationally. This leads to entry into less privileged sections of the labour market, exposure to low pay and hazardous work, and reliance on limited welfare payments in old age. Within this framework the way in which apparent 'life-style' factors are outcomes of social processes which generate disadvantage in a wide variety of spheres becomes clear. For pets, the material circumstances they encounter will largely depend on the socioeconomic wellbeing of their owners.

The study by Moloo et al has many limitations and does not firmly establish the existence of socioeconomic differentials in pet mortality. However, if extrinsic – particularly violent – causes of death are put aside, then humans and other animals show some similarities in mortality dynamics.[15] A parsimonious explanation of health inequalities should perhaps account for differentials seen in different species, as well as for the fact that inequalities in mortality among humans are seen in different epochs and in different countries. In this light explanations solely in terms of artefact, selection, health-related behaviours, or particular stresses seem parochial. The structuring of advantage and disadvantage in the material and social environment across the course of a life could reflect a more stable process of social differentiation. Further research into socioeconomic differentials in the mortality of animals other than humans may play a role in advancing our understanding of this basic process.

References

[1] Bonnett, B.N., Egenvall, A., Olson, P. and Hedhammar, A. (1997) 'Mortality in insured Swedish dogs: rates and causes of death in various breeds', *Veterinary Record*, vol 141, pp 40-4.

[2] Moloo, J., Jackson, K.L., Waller, J.L., McKeown, R.E., Addy, C.L., Cuffe, S.P. et al (1998) 'Xenotransmission of the socioeconomic gradient in health? A population based study', *British Medical Journal*, vol 317, p 1686.

[3] Raina, P., Waltner-Toews, D., Bonnett, B., Woodward, C. and Abernathy, T. (2002) 'Influence of companion animals on the physical and psychological health of older people: an analysis of a one-year longitudinal study', *Journal of the American Geriatrics Society*, vol 47, pp 323-9.

[4] Tucker, J.S., Friedman, H.S., Thsi, C.M. and Martin, L.R. (1995) 'Playing with pets and longevity among older people', *Sociology and Ageing*, vol 10, pp 370-5.

[5] Blane, D.B., Bartley, M. and Davey Smith, G. (1997) 'Disease aetiology and materialist explanations of socio-economic mortality differentials', *European Journal of Public Health*, vol 7, pp 385-91.

[6] Veterinary Service Market for Companion Animals (1992) 'Part I: companion animal ownership and demographics', *Journal of the American Veterinary Medical Association*, vol 201, pp 990-2.

[7] *US pet ownership and demographics sourcebook* (1997) Schaumberg, IL: Centre for Information Management, American Veterinary Medical Association.

[8] Blane, D., Davey Smith, G. and Bartley, M. (1993) 'Social selection: what does it contribute to social class differences in health?', *Sociology of Health Illness*, vol 15, pp 1-15.

[9] Davey Smith, G. and Morris, J.N. (1994) 'Increasing inequalities in the health of the nation', *British Medical Journal*, vol 309, pp 1453-4.

[10] **Davey Smith, G. and Ben-Shlomo, Y. (1997) 'Inequalities in health: what is happening and what can be done?', in G. Scally (ed) *Progress in public health*, London: FT Healthcare.**

[11] House, J.S., Landis, K.R. and Umberson, D. (1988) 'Social relationships and health', *Science*, vol 241, pp 540-5.

[12] Marmot, M.G. and Theorell, T. (1988) 'Social class and cardiovascular disease: the contribution of work', *International Journal of Health Services*, vol 18, pp 659-74.

[13] Kunitz, S.J. and Levy, J.E. (1988) 'A prospective study of isolation and mortality in a cohort of elderly Navajo Indians', *Journal of Cross-Cultural Gerontology*, vol 3, pp 71-85.

[14] **Davey Smith, G. and Harding, S. (1997) 'Is control at work the key to socio-economic gradients in mortality?', *Lancet*, vol 350, pp 1369-70.**

[15] Olshansky, S.J. and Carnes, B.A. (1997) 'Ever since Gompertz', *Demography*, vol 34, pp 1-15.

28

Death in Hollywood: life-style excess, social comparisons or publication bias?

George Davey Smith

Death in Hollywood brings to mind the page-turning pleasures of Kenneth Anger's classic tales of a contemporary Babylon.[1,2] The mixture of drugs, drink, sex, violence, monstrous egos, gangsterism, speed and madness is often most starkly revealed in the premature deaths of (sometimes has-been) stars. The suicides can be particularly indicative of the roller coaster nature of fame. Albert Dekker, who wrote sections of the poor reviews from his last film in crimson lipstick on his body before hanging himself; Lou Tellegen, stabbing himself with gold scissors engraved with his name, surrounded by film posters, photographs and newspaper cuttings from his days of triumph; or Peg Enwistle who jumped to her death from one of the giant letters of the Hollywood sign (setting off a spate of copycat leaps into oblivion). Among the better known are (probably) Marilyn Monroe, or her Oscar-winning co-star in *All About Eve*, George Sanders, whose note read "Dear World: I am leaving you because I am bored. I am leaving you with your worries in this sweet cesspool". To these can be added the long list of those for whom the road to excess lead to premature demise, from the stars of the silent screen such as Wally Reid (morphine), John Gilbert (drink), Alma Rubens (heroin), Olive Thomas (barbiturates), Marie Prevost (drink), Barbara La Marr (everything), through to more recent times, with Oscar-winner and heroin enthusiast Bobby Driscoll, found dead in a New York tenement, or River Phoenix collapsing after his last speedball outside Johnny Depp's *Viper Room* club in Los Angeles.

The overdose at 50 of Don Simpson – actor and producer (of *Flashdance*, *Beverly Hills Cop* and *Top Gun*, among others) – encapsulates the Hollywood version of it being better to burn out than to fade away.[3] With his $60,000 a month drug habit, orgies, fights, and busts, we hear that "Don was never afraid of getting old. He was afraid of

British Medical Journal, 2001, vol 323, pp 1441-2

getting fat", and that his death "bore a completely organic connection to the circumstances of his life.... He died at a remarkably old age, given the way he was living".[4] Despite their sometimes squalid nature, these Hollywood deaths retain their glitter – surely this is a better way to go than to stagger on through to the boring three score years and ten? As a reader of a Don Simpson biography writes, "Why is it I love people who live their lives like sick maniacs and then burn out in a blaze of glory?"[5]

In a recent *British Medical Journal* article, however, the impossible is achieved, and Hollywood deaths are robbed of their glamour and excitement, by the simple expedient of turning such deaths into epidemiological end-points. In an ingenious analysis, Redelmeier and Singh examined the mortality records of screenwriters who were nominated at least once for an Oscar to see if those who win live longer than the also-rans.[6] Their motivation for this analysis is to test the hypothesis that socioeconomic differentials in health are largely determined by the psychological consequences of perceived social standing and the psychoneuroendocrinological consequences of these perceptions.[7] Some authorities consider that feelings of shame, humiliation, disrespect and social anxiety are major determinants of population health and of health differentials in rich countries[7] and that psychotherapy may be the solution to health inequalities.[8] Winning an Oscar, it is reasoned, should have a positive effect on feelings of perceived social standing. Indeed, as almost as many Americans watch the Oscar ceremony as vote in presidential elections[9] it is difficult to think of many greater public validations of self-worth in the US.

The findings, however, ran in the opposite direction to the expected: the Oscar-winning screenwriters have shorter life expectancies than the losing nominees. Why could this be? The obvious way to look at this is to see if it is a general finding or is specific to screenwriters. Clearly the Oscar ceremonies are largely about acting awards rather than writing credits – this is what the audience is tuning in for. So why was mortality among writers rather than actors and actresses examined? The answer, unsurprisingly, is that the influence on life expectancy of winning an acting Oscar was examined by the same authors,[9] but appropriately, since the acting Oscars are more prestigious than the writing Oscars, the findings with respect to the former were published in the *Annals of Internal Medicine* (Impact factor 9.8)[10] rather than the *British Medical Journal* (Impact factor 5.3).[10] In the acting domain, Oscar winners had longer life expectancy than nominees who did not win. There was no influence of being nominated but not winning an Oscar on life expectancy; a matched control group of actors or actresses who were in the same film as each Oscar nominee had equal life expectancy.

Thus there seems to be no general connection between the status-enhancing effect of Oscar winning and either increased or reduced life expectancy. Is this because there is something special about writers? Eminent creative writers have shorter life expectancies than artists in other fields,[11,12] one suggestion being that writers receive less immediate reward or sensory stimulation than other artists, which leads to greater stimulation-seeking and risk taking.[11] However, tortured creative souls are probably more likely to write slim volumes of poetry or gnostic novels than screenplays, and screenwriting is anyway often a collaborative activity.[6] The possible connection between creativity and psychopathology has long been discussed,[11] and the role of alcohol and suicide in the deaths of writers highlighted.[13] However, the overall life expectancies of the screenwriters were closely similar to those of the actors, suggesting that the former were not being crucified by their over-sensitivity. Redelmeier and Singh suggest that screenwriters can behave badly, unlike actors whose lives are under external scrutiny. Readers of the *National Enquirer* might doubt whether this is true, a view again backed up by the similar overall life expectancy of actors and screenwriters. Perhaps the difference lies in the meaning of an Oscar for the future life and career of a screenwriter and actor. For an actor an Oscar "can do wonders for ... negotiating a salary".[14] While more income may not do much for already wealthy actors – although for some an Oscar has meant escape from periods of hardship – this will also translate into more secure future employment, a longer acting career[9] and the ability to negotiate the terms and conditions of work. Screenwriters are, notoriously, a heavily exploited branch of the movie industry and for a screenwriter an Oscar may give a considerable immediate psychological boost, but will not guarantee future success or employment; this was particularly true during the Communist witch-hunt of the McCarthy era (which is covered by the present study), in which screenwriters (including many Oscar winners and nominees) were particularly persecuted. While all Oscars are 13.5 inches tall[14] and may bring increased feelings of self-worth, they may translate differently in actors and screenwriters into those factors that increase or decrease life expectancy.

References

[1] Anger, K. (1981) *Hollywood Babylon*, New York, NY: Dell Books.

[2] Anger, K. (1984) *Hollywood Babylon II*, London: Arrow Books.

[3] Fleming, C. (1998) *High concept: Don Simpson and the Hollywood culture of excess*, New York, NY: Doubleday.

[4] http://www.bbc.co.uk/works/s2/simpson/subjinfo.shtml

[5] http://www.amazon.com/exec/obidos/ASIN/0385486952/ref=ase_avsearch-bkasin-20/104-2290832-2956716

[6] Redelmeier, D.A. and Singh, S.M. (2001) 'Longevity of screenwriters who win an academy award: a longitudinal study', *British Medical Journal*, vol 323, pp 1491-6.

[7] Wilkinson, R. (2000) *Mind the gap: Hierarchies, health and human evolution*, London: Weidenfled and Nicolson.

[8] Stewart-Brown, S. (2000) 'What causes social inequalities: why is this question taboo?', *Critical Public Health*, vol 10, pp 233-42.

[9] Redelmeier, D.A. and Singh, S.M. (2001) 'Survival in academy-award winning actors and actresses', *Annals of Internal Medicine*, vol 134, pp 955-62.

[10] http://wos.mimas.ac.uk

[11] Kaun, D.E. (1991) 'Writers die young: the impact of work and leisure on longevity', *Journal of Economic Psychology*, vol 12, pp 381-99.

[12] Cassandro, V.J. (1998) 'Explaining premature mortality across fields of creative endeavor', *Journal of Personality*, vol 66, pp 805-33.

[13] Lester, D. (1991) 'Premature mortality associated with alcoholism and suicide in American writers', *Perceptual and Motor Skills*, vol 73, p 162.

[14] Katz, E., Klein, F. and Nolen, R.D. (2001) *The Macmillan international film encyclopaedia* (4th edn), London: Macmillan.

29

Sex and death: are they related? Findings from the Caerphilly Cohort Study

George Davey Smith, Stephen Frankel and John Yarnell

Abstract

Objective: To examine the relation between frequency of sexual intercourse and mortality.

Study design: Cohort study with a 10-year follow up.

Setting: The town of Caerphilly, South Wales, and five adjacent villages.

Participants: 918 men aged 45-59 at time of recruitment between 1979 and 1983.

Main outcome measures: All deaths and deaths from coronary heart disease.

Result: Mortality risk was 50% lower in the group with high frequency of sexual intercourse than in the group with low frequency, with evidence of a dose-response relation across the groups. Age-adjusted odds ratio for all-cause mortality was 2.0 for the group with low frequency of sexual intercourse (95% CI: 1.1-3.5, test for trend $p=0.02$). With adjustment for risk factors this became 1.9 (CI: 1.0-3.4, test for trend $p=0.04$). Death from coronary heart disease and from other causes showed similar associations with frequency of sexual intercourse, although the gradient was most marked for deaths from coronary heart disease. Analysed in terms of actual frequency of sexual intercourse, the odds ratio for total mortality associated with 100 more acts per year was 0.64 (0.44-0.95).

Conclusion: Sexual activity seems to have a protective effect on men's health.

British Medical Journal, 1997, vol 315, pp 1641-5

Introduction

Even for a group not especially known for humour, the epidemiologist's standard joke about 'being broken down by age and sex' is rather tired. It is also conceptually colourless, for the non-epidemiologist takes more interest in sex as an activity than as a stratification variable. Sexual behaviour as an exposure has been little investigated, outside its capacity for transmitting communicable disease. Few data exist on the association between patterns of sexual behaviour and later mortality, despite sex and death – the joint obsessions of adolescence[1,2] – being frequently linked in youthful interpretations of the human condition.[3-6] One barrier to the study of frequency of sexual intercourse as an exposure may be that observational epidemiology tends to be conducted on middle-aged and ageing populations by middle-aged or ageing researchers. The fading imaginations of researchers – assumed to be shared by their subjects – renders the whole area apparently uninteresting. This is an instance of a more general phenomenon of epidemiologists studying what interests other epidemiologists, and not always being drawn to areas of more general public concern. There may be more exciting issues for the public than determining exactly how many servings of fruit and vegetables a day may confer enhanced health, or discovering that smoking is even worse for people than was once thought.

A few exceptions to the general epidemiological silence on the association between sexual behaviour and later mortality exist. In the Duke first longitudinal study of ageing, frequency of sexual intercourse was inversely associated with mortality in men, and enjoyment of intercourse was inversely related to mortality among women.[7] This finding is compatible with a perception that the quantity of sexual activity is of more importance to men, while a greater concern with quality is seen among women.[8,9] In a Swedish study, early cessation of sexual intercourse was found to be associated with an increased mortality risk among men over a five-year follow-up.[10] Sexual dissatisfaction was found to be a risk factor for myocardial infarction in a case-control study of women, with premature ejaculation and impotence in husbands being the major underlying factor.[11] From a different perspective, the assumption that Catholic priests and nuns are celibate renders another epidemiological design relevant here. A retrospective cohort analysis involving 10,026 priests in the US revealed a marginally increased overall standardised mortality ratio (SMR) of 103 (95% CI: 100-106), although mortality for arteriosclerotic heart disease was more substantially raised (118, 113-22).[12] Interestingly, mortality for cirrhosis of the liver was greatly increased, with a SMR of 147 (CI: 122-173). A study of nuns found opposite findings, with lower overall mortality than in the general population.[13] Low rates of smoking among the nuns was considered to be key in this case.

Unfortunately all of these studies have contained only limited data on potential confounding factors and could thus say little about whether the observed associations were causal. In view of the dearth of evidence on this question we have examined the association between sexual behaviour and mortality in a cohort of men for whom data on health-related behaviours, existing coronary disease at baseline, social class, and physiological risk factors are available.

Participants and methods

The Caerphilly study is based on a 100% sample of men selected from the town of Caerphilly and five adjacent villages. The men were chosen by date of birth so that they were aged 45-59 years when examined between 1979 and 1983. A total of 2,512 men were seen – 89% of the 2,818 who were found to be eligible. At recruitment the men were invited to a clinic at which a standard medical history was obtained and a detailed questionnaire administered. At examination, height was measured with a Holtain stadiometer, blood pressure was measured, and a 12-lead electrocardiogram was recorded. Existing coronary heart disease at baseline was defined as either probable ischaemia detected by electrocardiogram or angina on the Rose questionnaire. The subjects were then asked to return, after an overnight fast, to an early morning clinic where a blood sample was taken with minimal venous stasis. Total cholesterol was assayed on these samples. Full details of the procedures used in the Caerphilly study have been reported previously.[14-16]

Following a brief explanation of the purpose of the question, men at each clinic were asked about frequency of sexual intercourse by a medical interviewer. The responses were classified into categories ranging from never through to daily. These were reduced to three categories: less than monthly; twice a week or more; and an intermediate category. Recalled number of orgasms has been shown previously to offer a reliable measure of male sexual activity.[17] The question was asked only in the first period of the survey; it was abandoned, after discussions with local GPs, because of a possible effect on the overall response rate. Responses were provided by 918 of the 1,222 men who were interviewed before the question was removed from the questionnaire.

The records of all men at the NHS Central Registry were flagged so that notification of death was automatic and a copy of the death certificate was received. Ten-year follow-up data for mortality are reported here. All death certificates were coded according to ICD-9 (International Classification of Diseases, Ninth Revision). Deaths due to coronary heart disease are those coded ICD 410-14.

Statistical methods

Age adjustment for risk factors was to the age structure of the population with usable data on frequency of sexual intercourse. Multiple logistic regression was used to explore the effects of other risk factors on the association between mortality and frequency of sexual intercourse. In these models age, systolic blood pressure, and cholesterol were entered as continuous variables, and social class (manual or non-manual), coronary heart disease at baseline, and smoking behaviour as categorical variables.

Results

Data regarding frequency of sexual intercourse were available on 918 men (response rate 75%). Differences between the men for whom responses were and were not obtained during the period the question was asked were considerable; those who gave responses that could be coded were younger, taller, had less evidence of coronary heart disease at screening, and were more likely to be in non-manual occupations than the men who refused to, or could not, answer the question. The odds ratio for all-cause mortality for the men from whom data on frequency of sexual intercourse were not obtained compared to those from whom they were was 2.05 (CI: 1.51-2.78). Adjusting for age, coronary heart disease at baseline, social class, and height reduced this to 1.73 (CI: 1.24-2.39).

Characteristics of the respondents according to reported frequency of sexual intercourse are presented in Table 1. The reported frequency decreased with age and was higher among men in non-manual occupations. No other risk factor was significantly related to frequency of sexual intercourse, although the tendency was for blood pressure and cholesterol concentrations to be more favourable among those reporting lower frequency, whereas smoking history and prevalent coronary heart disease at baseline showed an opposite pattern. Over 10 years of follow-up, 150 of the respondents died: 67 from coronary heart disease and 83 from other causes. Age-adjusted odds ratios for deaths from all causes, coronary heart disease, and other causes according to frequency of sexual intercourse group are given in Table 2. Mortality risk in the group with high frequency of sexual intercourse was less than half of that of the group with low frequency, with evidence of a dose-response relation across the groups. The patterns for deaths from all-causes, coronary heart disease, and other causes were similar, although the gradient was steepest for deaths from coronary heart disease. Adjusting for social class, smoking, blood pressure, and coronary heart disease at baseline (and for cholesterol in

Table 1: Characteristics of men (with standard error) in relation to frequency of sexual intercourse

	Frequency of sexual intercourse			
	Low (*n*=199)	Medium (*n*=490)	High (*n*=229)	*p* for trend
Age	54.1 (0.3)	51.8 (0.2)	49.8 (0.3)	<0.0001
Height (m)	1.71 (0.005)	1.72 (0.003)	1.71 (0.004)	0.69
Body mass index (kg/m²)	26.3 (0.2)	25.9 (0.2)	26.5 (0.2)	0.59
Systolic blood pressure (mm Hg)	140.7 (1.4)	142.1 (0.8)	143.9 (1.3)	0.22
Cholesterol (mmol/l)	5.55 (0.09)	5.68 (0.05)	5.66 (0.08)	0.54
Non-manual[a]	29.1 (3.6)	42.4 (2.2)	41.5 (3.3)	0.02
Existing coronary heart disease[a]	20.5 (2.7)	15.7 (1.7)	14 1 (2.5)	0.16
Never smoked[a]	13.2 (2.7)	17.5 (1.7)	18.2 (2.5)	0.15

[a] Prevalence per 100.

Notes: All age adjusted except the age variable. Standard error in parenthesis.

Table 2: Odds ratios (95% CI) for mortality adjusted for age and risk factors

Frequency of sexual intercourse	Age-adjusted	Fully adjusted[a]
All-cause mortality		
Low	2.0 (1.1-3.5)	1.9 (1.0-3.4)
Medium	1.6 (1.0-2.6)	1.6 (1.0-2.8)
High	1.0	1.0
p value for trend	0.02	0.04
Coronary heart disease		
Low	2.2 (1.0-5.2)	2.1 (0.9-5.1)
Medium	1.7 (0.8-3.6)	1.8 (0.8-4.0)
High	1.0	1.0
p value for trend	0.06	0.10
Other causes		
Low	1.7 (0.8-3.5)	1.6 (0.7-3.3)
Medium	1.5 (0.8-2.8)	1.5 (0.8-3.0)
High	1.0	1.0
p value for trend	0.19	0.27

[a] Age, social class, systolic blood pressure, smoking, coronary heart disease at baseline. Odds ratios for mortality from coronary heart disease also adjusted for cholesterol at baseline.

the case of death from coronary heart disease) attenuated the associations to a relatively small degree.

The association between frequency of sexual intercourse and all-cause mortality was also examined using the mid-point of each response category recoded as number of acts per year. The age-adjusted odds ratio for 100 more acts per year was 0.64 (CI: 0.44-0.95).

Discussion

Sex and death: is the association causal?

This study reveals an inverse relation between frequency of sexual intercourse and mortality and is consistent with most,[7,10-12] but not all,[13] previously published work. Before this finding can be considered as suggesting a causal relation, several aspects of the data must be considered. Relevant data were available on 75% of the original sample examined before the question about frequency of sexual intercourse was dropped from the study. The men with full data were younger, taller, had less coronary heart disease at baseline, were more likely to be in non-manual occupations, and had an overall lower mortality than those for whom frequency of sexual intercourse was not known. The possibility of bias must therefore be considered, though there is no reason to suspect that the subset of men without full data included a disproportionate number with either a high frequency of sexual intercourse and high mortality risk or a low frequency of sexual intercourse and a low mortality risk. The relation between frequency of sexual intercourse and mortality is clearly confounded by age and social class, and to a lesser extent by smoking habit and health status at baseline. The association between frequency of sexual intercourse and mortality was, as expected, attenuated somewhat when these variables were entered into the models. Nevertheless, a strong and statistically significant association remains in the adjusted models. Reverse causation must also be considered. Although this is likely to have strengthened the association found here, with early signs of later serious disease leading to a decreased frequency of sexual intercourse, existing coronary heart disease at baseline was adjusted for. We found an inverse association between death from coronary heart disease and frequency of sexual intercourse even though myocardial ischaemia and myocardial infarction can be triggered by sexual activity.[18,19]

Despite this, confounding may well account for our findings. Multivariable models are seriously limited in their ability to control for confounding, especially with covariates that are imprecisely measured.[20,21] Furthermore, unmeasured or unknown confounders can create strong, apparently 'independent', associations between risk factors and mortality.[22] However, the association between frequency of sexual intercourse and mortality in the present study is at least – if not more – convincing on epidemiological and biological grounds than many of the associations reported in other studies[23-25] and deserves further investigation to the same extent. Intervention programmes could also be considered, perhaps based on the exciting 'At least five a day' campaign aimed at increasing fruit and vegetable consumption[26] – although the numerical imperative may have to be adjusted. The disappointing results observed in health promotion programmes in other domains[27] may not be seen when potentially pleasurable activities are promoted.

Sex and death in other times and other places

This epidemiological indifference to the question of whether patterns of sexual behaviour influence general well-being contrasts with wider interest in this issue. Long-standing expressions of such concerns are codified in ritual practices and religious texts. Within the Christian tradition, Paul's assertion that "It is good for a man not to touch a woman"[28] is in continuity with one tradition of the Hellenistic world, where celibacy offered the opportunity to pursue philosophy and achieve virtue and well-being.[29] The view that the male pleasure of sexual intercourse is secured at the cost of vigour and wellbeing is common in a wide range of cultures. One of the extreme expressions of this idea is found among the Huli people of Papua New Guinea. Here young men were sent to secret bachelor houses hidden in the forest and taught by celibate specialists of the mortal dangers of succumbing to women's desires; if sexual contact had to occur at all, it should be restricted to the needs of procreation.[30] In North India any loss of semen is considered to be debilitating, leading to skin problems, lack of concentration, anxiety, painful joints, palpitations, headaches, pains in the chest, swollen gums, and halitosis.[31] The biological mechanism considered to be involved is that the production of one tablespoon of semen requires 40 kilograms of food.

The entropic idea that sexual restraint retains vigour also has a strong scientific tradition. This reached its most forceful expression in the work of Eugen Steinach, who became 'Professor Extraordinarius' in Prague in 1895, before returning to Vienna as professor of physiology.[32] The key outcome of his work in this context was the acceptance in surgical practice of the view that ligation of the vas deferens led to rejuvenating increases in the output of male sex hormones. Surgery thus produced a physiological form of celibacy that was compatible with, and was understood to stimulate, sexual performance. It is not surprising that such a powerful, and for surgeons lucrative,[33] placebo became very popular in the days before evidence-based surgery became the norm. Even some rather publicly unfavourable evidence did not dissuade hopeful and desperate old men in their search for 'rejuvenation'. A celebrated case was a certain Mr Wilson, one of Steinach's own patients, who died on the day before he was to have delivered a public lecture at the Albert Hall entitled 'How I was made twenty years younger'.[34] One of the most famous recipients of the Steinach operation was W.B. Yeats. Stephen Lock's account of this suggested that, at least in Yeats' case, the operation was highly successful.[35] Indeed, Yeats became known to Dubliners as 'the gland old man'.

Contradictory notions of how sexual activity should be related to health exist in the popular domain. Our finding that sexual activity may be protective of middle-aged men's health contrasts with some of the strictures dominant in a wide range of current and historical cultures. What may be regarded as good for societies may be bad for individuals. For example, it seems that the changes in living conditions that followed the first agricultural revolution disadvantaged the new farmers and resulted in deteriorating nutrition, however much it advantaged their rulers.[36] Sexual behaviour and social structures are closely intertwined. We do not know whether the public position promoting relative continence accords with people's actual views in this or other societies, and as far as we are aware this question has not been researched. In an earlier study that examined public ideas about the prevention of coronary heart disease we described a lay epidemiology that is in some ways closer to the true epidemiology of risk than to the strictures that are disseminated through health education.[37,38] It remains for other epidemiologists to offer supportive or contrasting findings on the issue considered here, although the likely absence of randomised controlled trial data will make the matter difficult to resolve. If these findings are replicated and confirm that sexual activity is indeed protective for middle-aged men, it is for anthropologists to judge whether the lay epidemiology supports the true epidemiology. It would be interesting to know whether people are privately convinced that the conventional case for relative abstinence is in their own interest, as well as that of an ordered society.

References

[1] Joyce, J. (1956) *A portrait of the artist as a young man*, London: Cape.

[2] Cohen, L. (1963) *The favourite game*, London: Secker and Warburg.

[3] SCUM Auxiliary. Con/text 119. (1983) On: *Obscure independent classics*, vol 6, Ipswich: Hamster Records.

[4] Easton Ellis, B. (1988) *American psycho*, New York, NY: Simon and Schuster.

[5] Acker, K. (1984) *Blood and guts in high school*, New York, NY: Random House.

[6]   Purdy, J. (1961) *Color of darkness*, New York, NY: Random House.

[7]   Palmore, E.B. (1982) 'Predictors of the longevity difference: a 25-year follow-up', *Gerontologist*, vol 6, pp 513-18.

[8]   Solanas, V. (1971) *SCUM manifesto*, Paris: Olympia Press.

[9]   Greer, G. (1968) *The female eunuch*, London: MacGibbon and Kee.

[10] Persson, G. (1981) 'Five-year mortality in a 70-year old urban population in relation to psychiatric diagnosis, personality, sexuality and early parental death', *Acta Psychiatr Scand*, vol 64, pp 244-53.

[11] Abramov, L.A. (1976) 'Sexual life and frigidity among women developing acute myocardial infarction', *Psychosomatic Medicine*, vol 38, pp 418-25.

[12] Kaplan, S.D. (1988) 'Retrospective cohort mortality study of Roman Catholic priests', *Preventive Medicine*, vol 17, pp 335-43.

[13] Butler, S.M. and Snowdon, D.A. (1996) 'Trends in mortality in older women: findings from the nun study', *Journal of Gerontology Series B*, vol 51, pp S201-8.

[14] Caerphilly and Speedwell Collaborative Group (1984) 'Caerphilly and Speedwell Collaborative heart disease studies', *Journal of Epidemiology and Community Health*, vol 38, pp 259-62.

[15] Yarnell, J.W.G., Sweetnam, P.M., Marks, V., Teale, J.D. and Bolton, C.H. (1994) 'Insulin in ischaemic heart disease: are associations explained by triglyceride concentrations? The Caerphilly prospective study', *British Heart Journal*, vol 71, pp 293-6.

[16] Yarnell, J.W.G., Beswick, A.D., Sweetnam, P.M. and Riad-Fahny, D. (1993) 'Endogenous sex hormones and ischaemic heart disease in men: the Caerphilly prospective study', *Arteriosclerosis Thrombrosis*, vol 13, pp 517-20.

[17] Davidson, J.M., Chen, J.J., Crapo, L., Gray, G.D., Greenleaf, W.J. and Catania, J.A. (1983) 'Hormonal changes and sexual function in aging men', *Journal of Clinical Endocrinology and Metabolism*, vol 57, pp 71-7.

[18] Drory, Y., Shapira, I., Isman, E.Z. and Pines, A. (1995) 'Myocardial ischaemia during sexual activity in patients with coronary artery disease', *American Journal of Cardiology*, vol 7, pp 835-7.

[19] Muller, J.E., Mittleman, M.A., Maclure, M., Sherwood, J.B. and Tofler, G.H. (1996) 'Triggering of myocardial infarction by sexual activity', *Journal of the Amercian Medical Association*, vol 275, pp 1405-9.

[20] Phillips, A.N. and Davey Smith, G. (1991) 'How independent are independent effects? Relative risk estimation when correlated exposures are measured imprecisely', *Journal of Clinical Epidemiology*, vol 44, pp 1223-31.

[21] Davey Smith, G. and Phillips, A.N. (1992) 'Confounding in epidemiological studies: why "independent" effects may not be all they seem', *British Medical Journal*, vol 305, pp 757-9.

[22] Davey Smith, G., Phillips, A.N. and Neaton, J.D. (1992) 'Smoking as "independent" risk factor for suicide: illustration of an artefact from observational epidemiology', *Lancet*, vol 340, pp 709-12.

[23] Knekt, P., Järvinen, R., Reunanen, A. and Maatela, J. (1996) 'Flavanoid intake and coronary mortality in Finland: a cohort study', *British Medical Journal*, vol 312, pp 478-81.

[24] Nyyssönen, K., Parviainen, T., Salonen, R., Tuomilehto, J. and Salonen, J.T. (1997) 'Vitamin C intake and risk of myocardial infarction: prospective population study of men from eastern Finland', *British Medical Journal*, vol 314, pp 634-8.

[25] Whiteman, M.C., Deary, I.J., Lee, A.J. and Fowkes, F.G. (1997) 'Submissiveness and protection from coronary heart disease in the general population: Edinburgh Artery Study', *Lancet*, vol 350, pp 541-5.

[26] Sharp, I. (ed) (1997) *At least five a day: Strategies to increase fruit and vegetable consumption*, London: The Stationery Office.

[27] Ebrahim, S. and Davey Smith, G. (1997) 'Systematic review of randomised controlled trials of multiple risk factor interventions for preventing coronary heart disease', *British Medical Journal*, vol 314, pp 1666-74.

[28] *Holy Bible*, 'I Corinthians', vii, 1 (King James Version).

[29] Deming, W. (1995) *Paul on marriage and celibacy*, Cambridge: Cambridge University Press.

[30] Frankel, S. (1986) *The Huli response to illness*, Cambridge: Cambridge University Press.

[31] Alter, J.S. (1997) 'Seminal truth: a modern science of male celibacy in north India', *Medical Anthropology Quarterly*, vol 11, pp 275-98.

[32] Schutte, H., Herman, J.R. and Eugen Steinach, 1861-1944 (1975) *Investigative urology*, vol 12, pp 330-1.

[33] Fraser, I. (1984) 'Steinach operation', *British Medical Journal*, vol 288, p 242.

[34] Haire, N. (1924) *Rejuvenation*, London: George Allen & Unwin.

[35] Lock, S. (1983) '"O that I were young again": Yeats and the Steinach operation', *British Medical Journal*, vol 287, pp 1964-8.

[36] Cohen, K.N. and Armelagos, G.J. (eds) (1984) *Paleopathology at the origins of agriculture*, New York, NY: Academic Press.

[37] Frankel, S.J., Davison, C. and Davey Smith, G. (1991) 'Lay epidemiology and the rationality of responses to health education', *British Journal of General Practice*, vol 41, pp 428-30.

[38] Davison, C., Davey Smith, G. and Frankel, S.J. (1991) 'Lay epidemiology and the prevention paradox – the implications of coronary candidacy for health education', *Sociology of Health and Illness*, vol 13, pp 1-19.

30

Health, health services and health politics in Britain: 1952-2002-2052

George Davey Smith

Then: 1952

Looking back over the previous 50 years from a mid-20th century vantage point the Chief Medical Statistician, Percy Stocks, saw a period of tremendous progress, with infant and child mortality rates having fallen to around one fifth of their 1900 level. Recent progress had been less encouraging with respect to death rates in middle age, especially among men, with the male excess in risk of dying between ages 55-64 having increased from less than a quarter to more than three quarters from 1900 to 1950. The rising problems were lung cancer, coronary heart disease (CHD) and peptic ulcer, which were threatening to counterbalance continuing falls in deaths from infectious diseases. Epidemiology was rapidly being transformed from a communicable disease discipline to one almost exclusively concerned with non-communicable diseases.

Socioeconomic inequalities in health were little discussed, and the 1951 *Decennial supplement* – which provided the first social class data since 1931 – suggested that inequalities in premature mortality rates were at an all-time low, and in any case, the recently introduced National Health Service (NHS) was thought to be the solution to any inequalities that remained.

The NHS, only a few years old, remained a contentious political issue. General practitioners had voted 2 to 1 against participation in the NHS in December 1946, had applauded when Nye Bevan – the architect of the NHS – was compared to Adolf Hitler, and fell behind a British Medical Association whose leadership had strong Conservative Party links. However, with pay guarantees, together with the promise that a salaried general practice service would not be

British Journal of General Practice, 2002, vol 51, pp 1032-3

introduced, the large majority of general practitioners finally agreed to work within the NHS.

The first successful attack on the principles of Bevan's NHS came from within the Labour Party, when the Chancellor, Hugh Gaitskell, announced he would introduce charges for dental and optical services; Bevan resigned as a cabinet minister in April 1951 in response. The Labour Prime Minister, Clement Attlee, claimed that there was no backing off from the principles of the NHS, that the charges would merely increase efficiency and reduce waste in the system, and that they may anyway only be a temporary expedient. By 1952 the newly elected Conservative government appeared to have policies little different from the Labour government that fell in October 1951.

A host of (now embarrassing) projections about health and healthcare in the year 2000 were published by those safe in the knowledge that they would not live to see the refutation of their predictions.

Now: 2002

At the beginning of the 21st century, life expectancy at birth is over 75 for men and over 80 for women – with increases of around 12 years for men and 10 years for women from the mid-20th century, that are continuing in a year-on-year fashion. These improvements are now being driven by falling mortality rates in middle-aged and older adults, rather than among infants and children as had been the case in the first 50 years of the 20th century. Treatments that substantially improve the prognosis for some of the major killers – breast cancer and coronary heart disease (CHD) – are now available, and a substantial reduction in smoking among older adults has occurred. The declines in death rates from the chronic diseases perceived to be the emerging problems in 1952 are spectacular, for example a 17% decline in male CHD and 18% decline in female CHD deaths in just six years from 1994 to 1999; equivalent figures for other causes being 15% for male lung cancer and an end to the rise in female lung cancer, at a level much below the peak reached among men; and an 11% fall in breast cancer mortality. Trends for less common causes – accidents and violence (and suicide in younger adults in particular) – are much less favourable, and morbidity measures – difficult to standardise over time – suggest that the increasing proportion of people who are staying alive do not feel healthier. Infectious diseases have also failed to disappear in the manner predicted, with HIV/AIDS, chlamydia, other sexually transmitted diseases and hepatitis C infection being direct causes of ill health, and diseases long thought to be of a classic non-communicable kind – such as peptic ulcer, cervical cancer and stomach cancer – now appearing to have an important infectious origin.

Inequalities in health became an important political football with the publication of the Black Report in 1980, and under the Thatcher and Major regimes official discussion of inequalities was strongly discouraged. The disparities between social groups increased substantially from the mid-century, and at the end of the 20th century were larger than they had been at any time since comparable records were collected. New Labour established several inquiries into inequalities in health, produced lists of literally hundreds of responses they were making to them, and the Health Minister Alan Milburn declared that their ambition "is to do something no government – Tory or Labour – has ever done. Not only to improve the health of the nation but to improve the health of the worst off at a faster rate". Early indications regarding this ambition are not good, however. The poorest constituencies in Britain are those in which Labour obtains its highest votes, and these were the ones that showed a relative worsening in mortality rates after the 1997 Election that returned Labour to office. Mr Milburn's own constituency of Darlington, for example, experienced a 6% relative increase in premature mortality rates after 1997.

The NHS also appears to be in perpetual crisis. Far from being a temporary expedient, the initial user charges introduced by the Labour government in 1951 expanded greatly. The continuing privatisation of healthcare now comes in the guise of the Private Finance Initiative (PFI), branded "perfidious financial idiocy" by the editor of the *British Medical Journal*. These schemes for mortgaging the future for temporary gain have become a shibboleth for New Labour, and no criticisms are tolerated. The Labour Prime Minister, Tony Blair, however, claims that there is no backing off from the principles of the NHS and that the charges would merely increase efficiency and reduce waste in the system – and are certainly not the backdoor to privatisation.

A host of projections about health and healthcare in the year 2050 are published by those reasonably safe in the knowledge that they would not live to see the refutation of their predictions.

Future: 2052

Scenario one

Life expectancies continued to grow, and in 2052 men can expect to live to 80 and women to 85. There is less and less focus on mortality rates, and the introduction of more reliable sources of morbidity data show that people are living longer with chronic conditions and limitations to activities of daily life; however, the increasing levels of obesity have already constrained the range of such activities. Morbidity levels from asthma, eczema and diabetes are such that the majority of people have maintenance treatment for one or other of these conditions at some stage of their lives. Aging-related problems – including dementia, macular degeneration and deafness – are commonplace. The major contributors to adult mortality are non-smoking related cancers (colorectal, prostate, breast, lymphomas, etc), diabetes, suicide and deaths at such advanced ages that the discredited term of 'senility' is making a comeback. Screening for genetic susceptibility is widely used for detecting those who could benefit from (mainly) pharmacological interventions.

Health inequalities continued to grow, as the inequality reduction targets set in 2001 fail to be realised. Increasingly, differential healthcare access feeds into inequalities in health outcomes. The health service is slowly privatised as meeting PFI lease-back charges and defaulting private sector concerns destabilise the possibility of coherent public sector funding of the NHS. In 2024 the last remaining university department of Public Health become a department of Health Care Financing. The *British Journal of General Practice* ceases publication in 2028, its function having been superseded by the web versions of *Medeconomics* and *Investors Chronicle*.

A host of projections about health and healthcare in the year 2100 are published by those already planning where would be the most fashionable place for a non agenarian to see in the next century.

Scenario two

The first case of smallpox occurred in early 2003, from suicide smallpox-carriers operating in crowded parts of London and other major British cities. The outbreak was worse than predicted, and the efforts to select virulent strains for dissemination were certainly successful. Simultaneous outbreaks in other parts of the world – combined with other precipitators – lead to the most serious global economic recession since the 1930s. The health trajectory of Britain resembles that of Eastern Europe during the restoration of free market capitalism, with considerable declines in male life expectancies (mainly due to increasing mortality in young and middle-aged men) and smaller falls in female life expectancy. Sexually transmitted diseases, HIV/AIDS and multi-drug resistant tuberculosis rates show rapid increases, and the Government of National Unity – a coalition of Labour, Conservative and British National Party – soon abandoned any attempts to maintain welfare medical care. The *British Journal of General Practice* ceases publication in 2014, its function having been superseded by the web versions of *Medeconomics* and *Soldier of Fortune*.

Nobody bothers to make any projections regarding health and healthcare in the year 2100.

Section VIII
Health inequalities – past and present

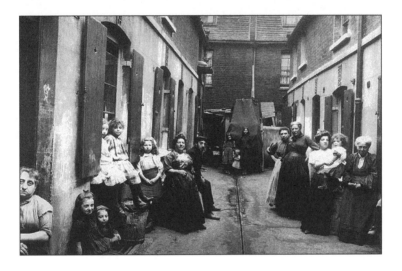

Providence Place, London, c.1900.

Socioeconomic differentials in mortality: evidence from Glasgow graveyards

George Davey Smith, Douglas Carroll, Sandra Rankin and David Rowan

Introduction

In 1842 the average age of death for "gentlemen and persons engaged in the professions and their families" was 45 years, for "tradesmen and their families" it was 26 years, whereas for "mechanics, servants and labourers and their families" it was only 16 years.[1] In 1904, the report of the Inter-Departmental Committee on Physical Deterioration noted the paucity of data available on social status and mortality, commenting in particular on the failure of the Registrar General's routine statistical returns in this regard.[2] Responding in part to this demand, T.H.C. Stevenson, one-time superintendent of statistics at the General Register Office, analysed mortality for the years 1910-12 according to eight occupationally-based social class groups.[3] He noted that this was unsatisfactory, since it was too dependent on classifications according to industry, with "all grades of worker, master and man, skilled and unskilled" grouped together in some cases. In 1921 "a determined attempt was made to purge the occupational classification of its industrial taint",[3] and it is from the reports of social class differentials in mortality around the 1921 Census that the continuing series of decennial supplements on occupational mortality are generally dated.

Since 1921 these reports have revealed a more or less consistent pattern of risk in all-cause mortality increasing from the professional groups in social class I to the unskilled labourers in social class V.[4,6-10] More recent studies focusing on non-occupational measures of material well-being, such as housing tenure and car ownership, have

British Medical Journal, 1992, vol 305, pp 1554-7

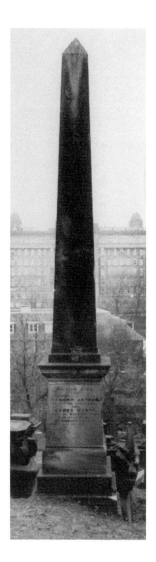

generally been able to differentiate mortality risk better than analysis by social class alone.[11] Indices such as these are not recorded on death certificates, so mortality rates cannot be computed by comparing death registrations (numerator) to census figures for the population at risk (denominator). Showing large differentials in mortality according to asset-based measures of available income has therefore depended on following up large cohorts[12,13] – but such data cannot be obtained for earlier periods.

One way the issue can be explored is through commemorative obelisks of a uniform design (found in burial grounds in Glasgow). The height of these obelisks varies greatly, yet their shape remains standard. As the height would influence the cost of the obelisk, it is reasonable to assume that more wealthy decedents would be commemorated by taller obelisks. We set out to determine whether a more favourable socioeconomic position, indexed by taller obelisks, was associated with greater longevity during the period 1801-1920.

Methods

A standard form of obelisk is a common marker of graves in the graveyards of Glasgow. All such obelisks were inspected in eight graveyards in Glasgow: the Cathedral, Eastern, Southern, and Western Necropolises, and Sighthill, Vennel, Rutherglen and Craigton graveyards. From the obelisk, details were taken of the year of death and age at death of the first generation of the family commemorated by the obelisk. In general, the obelisk would have been erected in memory of the first deceased of these; their year of death was taken to be the year of construction of the obelisk. Some obelisks commemorated only a male or female family elder; from these only one set of dates were recorded. Only people dying before 1921 were

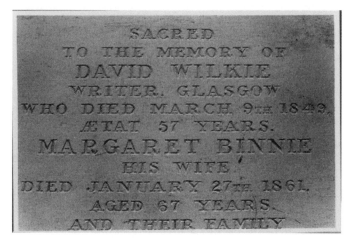

included in this study as the Registrar General started reporting death rates by five social class groups for the period around the 1921 Census. If one of a couple commemorated on an obelisk died before 1921 and one after, only data for the former were used.

If data were incomplete – on some obelisks the date of death, but not age at death, was recorded – a record of the burial was consulted.[14] Even so, complete data could not be obtained for 60 people. The inscriptions were illegible on 95 obelisks, usually because of weathering, although some could not be read because they had collapsed with the inscription facing downwards and could not be turned over.

The height of each obelisk was measured with a set of chimney sweep rods, each 90cm long, with gradations added. Height was measured from the base of the plinth to the crest of the pyramidal top piece, to the nearest 5cm. The principal material the obelisk was made of – granite, marble, or sandstone – was recorded. Four obelisks made of different materials (three iron, one concrete) were not included in the study. Granite was, and is, the most expensive of these materials and sandstone the least expensive (R. Taylor, personal communication).[15] The price differential between the materials depends on the exact source of the material and has varied over time, so no precise quantification of costs can be made. Therefore the three materials have been simply treated as giving an ordering of the cost for each obelisk at any given height.

The relations between continuous variables were examined by correlation and linear regression analyses. Differences in means were examined through analysis of variance and difference in medians by the Mann-Whitney U test.

Results

Data were obtained from 843 obelisks, 264 from the Cathedral Necropolis, 191 from Sighthill graveyard, and 388 from the six other graveyards combined. The earliest obelisk was constructed in 1805, and the median year of construction was 1883. Table 1 presents the number and proportion of obelisks built during 20-year periods from 1801-1920.

Height of the obelisks ranged from 1.75m to 11.40m, with a mean of 3.91m (standard deviation 1.11). Granite was the principal material for 514 (61%) of the obelisks, marble for 171 (20%), and sandstone for 158 (19%). The median year of construction of the sandstone obelisks was 1873, earlier than the median of 1884 for the granite ones, which in turn is earlier than 1890 for the marble ones (all differences $p<0.01$ by Mann-Whitney U test). The mean heights of

Table I: Period of construction of obelisk

	Number (%) built
1801-20	7 (1)
1821-40	20 (2)
1841-60	94 (11)
1861-80	267 (32)
1881-1900	282 (33)
1901-20	173 (21)

the three types of obelisk (3.89m for granite, 3.91m for marble, and 3.98m for sandstone) are similar (p=0.7 by analysis of variance).

The 843 obelisks yielded data for 725 men and 624 women dying before 1921. The median year of death of these 1,349 people was 1889. The mean ages at death are presented according to year of death and gender in Table 2 (range 20-98). Men had a higher mean age of death than women during all but the most recent time period. After 1860 there is a steady increase in mean age at death. If deaths occurring during the main childbearing years are excluded, a female advantage emerges earlier and is more pronounced (Table 3).

Correlations between height of obelisk, age at death, and year of death are presented in Table 4. As shown in Table 2, age at death increased over the time period. The average height of the obelisks decreased with year of death, but increased with age at death. Table 5 presents age at death according to tertile of the height of the obelisks,

Table 2: Age at death (years)

	Men		Women	
	Number	Mean age	Number	Mean age
1801-60	89	59.7	57	53.4
1861-80	194	57.5	147	52.6
1881-1900	252	65.4	234	63.6
1901-20	190	67.5	186	70.2

Table 3: Mean age at death of men and women aged over 45 years

	Men		Women	
	Number	Mean age	Number	Mean age
1801-60	71	65.1	37	62.5
1861-80	153	63.0	90	64.0
1881-1900	234	67.4	201	68.5
1901-20	184	68.5	171	73.2

together with the coefficient from simple linear regression of age at death against height of obelisk. The regression analyses show that every metre in height of obelisk translates into 1.42 years later age at death (95% CI: 0.53-2.31) for men and 2.19 (CI: 0.93-3.45) for women.

The average height of obelisks fell over time, whereas mean age at death increased. Correlations between height of obelisk and age at death are presented for different time periods in Table 6. These are generally higher than the overall correlations. Multiple regression was performed, with age at death as the dependent variable and height of obelisk and year of death as the independent variables. These analyses reveal that, adjusted for year of death, each metre in height of obelisk translates into 1.93 (CI: 1.06-2.80) years later age at death for men and an equivalent value of 2.92 (CI: 1.76-4.08) years for women.

Table 4: Correlations between height of obelisk, age at death, and year of death (men above diagonal, women below diagonal)

	Age at death	Year of death	Height of obelisk
Age at death		0.25**	0.12**
Year of death	0.40**		−0.15**
Height of obelisk	0.14**	−0.11*	

Note: *p<0.05; **p<0.005.

Table 5: Age of death according to height of obelisks

		Age at death	
	Mean height (m)	Men	Women
Lowest third	2.99	61.6	58.3
Middle third	3.77	62.8	63.1
Highest third	5.10	64.8	65.1
Regression coefficient per metre height		1.42*	2.19*

Note: *p<0.005.

Table 6: Mean age at death related to height of obelisks

	Men	Women
1801-60	0.34**	0.15
1861-80	0.15*	0.23**
1881-1900	0.16*	0.12
1901-20	0.07	0.28**

Note: *p<0.05; **p<0.005.

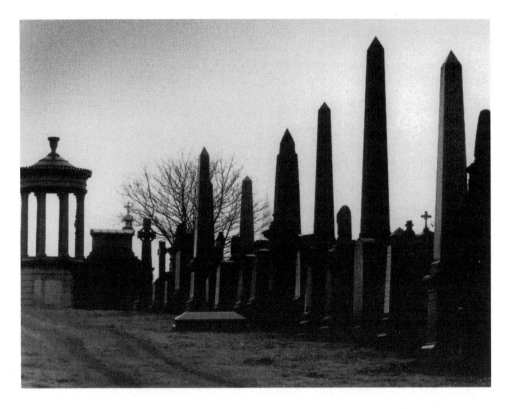

The mean ages at death according to the material of the obelisk are presented in Table 7. The trend is in the expected direction – that is, higher mean age at death is seen for the more expensive materials – but the effect is weak and not significant at conventional levels for either men (analysis of variance $p=0.1$; as trend in regression analysis $p=0.06$) or women (analysis of variance $p=0.7$; as trend in regression analysis $p=0.4$).

The main analyses were repeated separately for the two largest graveyards, which supplied 54% of obelisks in this study. As shown in Table 8, the pattern of results which emerged from these analyses was much the same as in the whole sample.

Table 7: Mean age at death according to material of obelisk

	Men	Women
Granite	63.7	62.6
Marble	63.5	61.3
Sandstone	60.9	61.3

Table 8: Analyses for the two major burial grounds

	Cathedral Necropolis		Sighthill graveyard	
	Men	Women	Men	Women
Age at death correlated with height	0.21**	0.14*	0.11	0.16*
Regression coefficient	1.93**	1.75*	1.41	3.12*
Regression coefficient (including year of death as a covariate)	2.45**	2.09*	1.87*	4.60**

Note: $*p<0.05$; $**p<0.005$.

Discussion

We used the average age at death as the indicator of mortality risk, as it was in the 1840s and is currently,[16] because denominator data are not available. This index is sensitive to the age structure of the population. Even with internal comparisons and with analyses in which year of death is controlled, as in the present study, different age distributions for adults in different socioeconomic groups could be due to factors other than differential survival. When mortality differences between regions of Scotland at this time are considered both in terms of average age at death and death rates in given age categories, similar differentials are seen despite large differences in age distribution. When numerator and denominator data are not available the average age at death can be a useful index, although it must be interpreted carefully.[16]

With this caveat in mind, we can consider reasons for height of obelisk being associated with age at death for people buried in the main graveyards of Glasgow. It is likely that one of two processes is involved – either higher socioeconomic position, as indexed by height of obelisk, is associated with greater longevity, or living longer leads to greater accumulation of assets, which are in part exchanged for a larger memorial after death. If the latter were the case, it would be expected that the height of obelisk would be more strongly related to men's than women's age at death, since for the middle-class groups who were commemorated in this manner, few women would have been independent wage earners.[18] If anything, however, the association between obelisk height and age at death was greater for women than men.

It is commonly understood that Victorian society was obsessed with class. A historian of the period describes the "multiple gradations or ranks in a pyramidal order" but sees a crucial distinction between the respectable and the non-respectable.[18] Burial arrangements could clearly reflect respectability and social aspirations as well as economic position. In this respect, height of obelisks is no different from the Registrar General's social class, which is based on the notion of the general standing of an occupation within the community rather than on economic rewards of particular jobs or a theoretical understanding of the class structure. The present data do not allow us confidently to separate social display from ability to pay.

The subjects of this study were in general from the privileged strata of society. On some of the obelisks, occupations were recorded for the men commemorated, who were predominantly merchants and various professionals – engineers, doctors, ministers. As might be expected, the average age at death from those buried in these grounds was old for the times. In the period 1881-1900 the mean ages at death for the study population were 65.4 for men and 63.3 for women. In 1890,[17] the mid-point of this range, for people dying at 20 years or over in Glasgow the mean ages at death were calculated to be 50.1 for men and 52.4 for women.

Although in 1815 Milne stated that "There can be no doubt but that the mortality is greater among the higher than the middle class of society",[19] the scattered evidence available suggests that in the 19th century there was apparently a graded relation, such that lower occupational standing was associated with higher mortality risk.[20,21] An exception is sometimes made for members of the peerage, who some observers thought had lower life expectancy than the general population.[19] If this were the case, then it seems to be a specific property of the aristocracy, rather than showing that the relation between socioeconomic position and mortality did not exist outside of the truly poor.

This study suggests that socioeconomic differentials in mortality existed among the relatively well-off during an earlier era. Absolute poverty, as discussed by Chadwick[1] and Booth,[22] presumably played no part in generating the differentials reported here. Although a continuous gradation of mortality risk accompanying the fine stratification of British society is seen currently,[23,24] for earlier periods more attention is generally paid to notions of absolute impoverishment.

In Glasgow, James Burn Russell, who served as the city's first full-time medical officer of health from 1872 to 1898, wrote numerous reports for the *Glasgow Medical Journal* and the *Sanitary Journal for Scotland*, with titles such as 'Local vices of buildings as affecting the death rate' and 'Public health and pauperism'.[25] Showing that mortality differentials persisted into privileged groups presents the same challenge for the interpretation of the factors underlying health inequalities then as it does now.[26]

A few other studies have examined the relation between non-occupational indicators of material well-being and mortality risk during an earlier age for which routine data are not available. Records of dowry investments made at birth for daughters of relatively affluent families in Florence from 1425 to 1442 have been related to ages at death for the girls concerned.[27] A gradient of decreasing mortality risk was seen from those accompanied by a dowry of less than 49 florins to those with dowries greater than 100 florins. In Providence, Rhode Island, mortality for taxpayers and non-taxpayers in 1865 could be calculated. Less than a quarter of the population were taxpayers, who constituted the affluent section of Providence society. In most age groups, death rates for non-taxpayers were two to three times higher than for taxpayers.[28]

Studies such as these help document the existence of socioeconomic differentials in mortality risk. The existence of such differentials among privileged groups suggest that notions of absolute poverty do not, on their own, provide an adequate explanatory framework. Further, the existence of the usual mortality gradient at a time when the familiar triad of sin – sloth, smoking and fatty food – may well have been a characteristic more of the rich than of the poor emphasises the parochial nature of explanations in terms of heath-related behaviours, as does the existence now of such differentials in societies with very different social structures to those of Britain today. When Chapin documented mortality differentials in Providence in 1924 he hoped that such a demonstration would be preparation for "what should be of great value, namely a study of the habits of life and environment which make for the longevity of the well-to-do".[28] This still pertains.

References

[1]   Chadwick, E. (1965) *Report on the sanitary condition of the labouring population of Great Britain, 1842*, Edinburgh: Edinburgh University Press.

[2]   Inter-Departmental Committee on Physical Deterioration (1904) *Report*, London: HMSO.

[3]   Stevenson, T.H.C. (1923) 'The social distribution of mortality from different causes in England and Wales, 1910-12', *Biometrika*, vol 15, pp 382-400.

[4]   Stevenson, T.H.C. (1928) 'The vital statistics of wealth and poverty', *Journal of the Royal Statistical Society*, vol 91, pp 207-20.

[5]   Pamuk, E.R. (1985) 'Social class inequality in mortality from 1921 to 1972 in England and Wales', *Population Studies*, vol 39, pp 17-31.

[6] Stocks, P. (1938) 'The effects of occupation and of its accompanying environment on mortality', *Journal of the Royal Statistical Society*, vol 101, pp 669-708.

[7] Logan, W.P.D. (1954) 'Social class variations in mortality', *British Journal of Preventive Social Medicine*, vol 8, pp 128-37.

[8] Hart, J.T. (1972) 'Data on occupational mortality, 1959-63: too little and too late', *Lancet*, vol I, pp 192-3.

[9] Morris, J.N. (1979) 'Social inequalities undiminished', *Lancet*, vol I, pp 87-90.

[10] Blane, D., Davey Smith, G. and Bartley, M. (1990) 'Social class differences in years of potential life lost: size, trends and principal causes', *British Medical Journal*, vol 301, pp 429-32.

[11] Davey Smith, G., Bartley, M. and Blane, D. (1990) 'The Black Report on socioeconomic inequalities in health: 10 years on', *British Medical Journal*, vol 301, pp 373-7.

[12] Fox, J. and Goldblatt, P.O. (1982) *Longitudinal study: Socio-demographic mortality differentials*, London: HMSO.

[13] **Davey Smith, G., Shipley, M.J. and Rose, G. (1990) 'The magnitude and causes of socioeconomic differentials in mortality: further evidence from the Whitehall Study',** *Journal of Epidemiology and Community Health***, vol 44, pp 265-70.**

[14] Willing, J.A. and Fairie, J.S. (1986) *Burial grounds of Glasgow: A brief guide for genealogists*, Glasgow: Glasgow and West of Scotland Family History Society.

[15] *Spon's architects' and builders' price book* (1990) London: Spon.

[16] Jannerfeldt, E. and Horte, L.-G. (1986) 'Median age at death as an indicator of premature mortality', *British Medical Journal*, vol 296, pp 678-81.

[17] *Thirty-sixth detailed annual report of the Registrar-General of births, deaths and marriages in Scotland* (1892), Edinburgh: HMSO.

[18] Best, G. (1979) *Mid-Victorian Britain 1851-1875*, London: Fontana.

[19] Titmuss, R. (1943) *Birth, poverty and wealth*, London: Hamish Hamilton Medical Books.

[20] Morris, J.N. (1957) *Uses of epidemiology*, London: Livingstone.

[21] Antonovsky, A. (1967) 'Social class, life expectancy and overall mortality', *Milbank Memorial Fund Quarterly*, vol 45, pp 31-73.

[22] Booth, C. (1969) *Charles Booth's London: A portrait of the poor at the turn of the century*, London: Hutchinson.

[23] Moser, K., Pugh, H. and Goldblatt, P. (1990) 'Mortality and the social classification of women', in P. Goldblatt (ed) *Longitudinal study: Mortality and social organisation*, London: HMSO, pp 145-62.

[24] Goldblatt, P. (1990) 'Mortality and alternative social classifications', in P. Goldblatt (ed) *Longitudinal study: Mortality and social organisation*, London: HMSO, pp 163-92.

[25] Checkland, O. and Lamb, M. (1982) 'Bibliography', in O. Checkland and M. Lamb (eds) *Health care as social history: The Glasgow case*, Aberdeen: Aberdeen University Press.

[26] Davey Smith, G. and Egger, M. (1992) 'Socioeconomic differences in mortality in Britain and the US', *American Journal of Public Health*, vol 82, pp 1079-81.

[27] Morrisson, A.S., Kirshner, J. and Molho, A. (1977) 'Life cycle events in 15th century Florence: records of the Monte Delle Doti', *American Journal of Epidemiology*, vol 106, pp 487-92.

[28] Chapin, C.V. (1924) 'Deaths among taxpayers and non-taxpayers of income tax: Providence, 1865', *American Journal of Public Health*, vol 14, pp 647-51.

32

The ghost of Christmas past: the health effects of poverty in London in 1896 and 1991

Daniel Dorling, Richard Mitchell,
Mary Shaw, Scott Orford
and George Davey Smith

Abstract

Objectives: To compare the extent to which late 20th century patterns of mortality in London are predicted by contemporary patterns of poverty and by late 19th century patterns of poverty. To test the hypothesis that the pattern of mortality from causes known to be related to deprivation in early life can be better predicted by the distribution of poverty in the late 19th century than by that in the late 20th century.

Design: Data from Charles Booth's survey of inner London in 1896 were digitised and matched to contemporary local government wards. Ward level indices of relative poverty were derived from Booth's survey and the 1991 UK Census. All deaths which took place within the surveyed area between 1991 and 1995 were identified and assigned to contemporary local government wards. Standardised mortality ratios (SMRs) for various causes of death were calculated for each ward for all ages, under age 65 and over age 65. Simple correlation and partial correlation analysis were used to estimate the contribution of the indices of poverty from 1896 and 1991 in predicting ward level SMRs in the early 1990s.

Setting: Inner London.

Results: For many causes of death in London, measures of deprivation made around 1896 and 1991 both contributed strongly to predicting their current spatial distribution. Contemporary mortality from diseases

British Medical Journal, 2000, vol 321, pp 1547-51

which are known to be related to deprivation in early life (stomach cancer and stroke) is predicted more strongly by the distribution of poverty in 1896 than that in 1991. In addition, all-cause mortality among people aged over 65 is slightly more strongly related to the geography of poverty in the late 19th century than to its contemporary distribution.

Conclusions: Contemporary patterns of some diseases have their roots in the past. The fundamental relationship between spatial patterns of social deprivation and spatial patterns of mortality is so robust that a century of change in inner London has failed to disrupt it.

Introduction

> They [left the busy scene, and] went into an obscure part of the town, where Scrooge had never penetrated before, although he recognised its situation, and its bad repute. The ways were foul and narrow; the shops and houses wretched; the people half-naked, drunken, slip-shod, ugly. Alleys and archways, like so many cesspools, disgorged their offences of smell, and dirt, and life, upon the straggling streets; and the whole quarter reeked with crime, with filth, and misery.[1]

With these words Charles Dickens describes Scrooge's journey with the Spirit of Christmas Yet to Come into the poorest streets of London to view the body of Tiny Tim, the child his miserliness will kill if it continues unchecked. Dickens' *A Christmas carol* also helped open the eyes of non-fictitious Londoners to the extent of poverty in their city at a time when social views were rapidly changing. Charles Booth was a contemporary chronicler of fact rather than fiction; together with his researchers, he surveyed these same streets so that we can see today where the Tiny Tims of the past lived. Using Booth's map of poverty at the end of the 19th century we test the hypothesis of the Spirit of Christmas Yet to Come: that miserliness in the past and present leads to future inequalities in health.

Today, poverty at all stages of life is implicated in determining the risk of mortality,[2] and relationships between the spatial distribution of poverty and mortality are well-known and robust.[3] It is also clear that there are specific relationships between adverse circumstances in childhood and the subsequent risk of particular causes of death in adulthood.[4] We seek to illustrate here one example of where the spirits of Christmases past – even those before childhood – have a strong influence on inequalities in health today.

Charles Booth's study of poverty in London was published between 1889 and 1903 in 17 volumes under the title of *Life and labour of the people of London.*[5-19] Booth's survey covered over 120,000 households, an area bounded by Pentonville prison to the north, Millwall docks to the east, Stockwell smallpox hospital to the south and Kensington Palace to the west. The information that Booth and his 20 researchers collected was projected as a series of detailed and exact maps, the most important of which was the 'Descriptive Map of London Poverty'[20] (see Figure 1). This map shows the streets of London, building by building, coloured to correspond to a classification of the resident population of the time. Booth's seven category classification scheme is described in Table 1.

This area of London was surveyed again in 1991, as part of the UK Census. The Registrar General's social classification scheme used in the Census is similar to Booth's scheme,[21] indeed the former was in part derived from Booth's work.[22-24] The similarity between the two schemes makes it possible to derive a hybrid which can be used as the basis for comparison between the two time periods. Table 1 shows how these two class schemes fit together.

Methods

To create an empirical measure of Dickens' fictitious description of 19th century London, Booth's map was digitised and its street-by-street data aggregated to contemporary ward boundaries using a geographical information system. Wards are administrative area units

Figure 1: Detail of Booth's descriptive map of London poverty

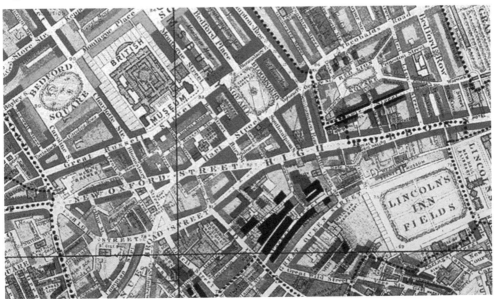

Table I: Booth's classes (1896) and Registrar General's social classes (1991)

Colour on 1896 map	Booth's description	% of households in 1896	Equivalent Registrar General's social class	% of households in 1991[a]	1896 SEP indicator[b]	1991 SEP indicator[b]
Black	Lowest class: vicious, semi-criminal	1.5[c]				
Blue	Very poor: casual labour, chronic want	3.7[c]	V[d]	6.9	0.937	0.965
Light blue	Poor: 18-21 shillings a week for a moderate family	7.4[c]				
Purple	Mixed: some comfortable, others poor	16.2	IV	12.8	0.794	0.867
Pink	Fairly comfortable: good ordinary earnings	35.2	III	33.8	0.537	0.634
Red	Well to do: middle class	27.7	II	37.3	0.223	0.278
Yellow	Wealthy: upper middle and upper classes	8.4	I	9.2	0.042	0.046

[a] Excludes households with no social class allocation in the 1991 Census (those described as in the army, inadequately described, and others without a social class allocation).

[b] Socioeconomic position (SEP) indicators are cumulative proportions: for class I, (I/2)/(I+II+III+IV+V); for class II, (I+II/2)/(I+II+III+IV+V); for class III, (I+II+III/2)/(I+II+III+IV+V); for class IV, (I+II+III+IV/2)/(I+I+II+III+IV+V); for class V, (I+II+III+IV+V/2)/(I+II+III+IV+V).

[c] Poor families made up 12.6% of households in 1896.

[d] Includes people of working age who have not worked in the last 10 years.

used by UK local government. Booth's survey area included 104 complete modern wards and the major part of 28 additional wards on its edge. The distribution of household social class within each ward was calculated for both 1896 and 1991.

A ward index of poverty was calculated by computing the proportion of households in each social class, weighting that proportion by the relative position of the class in the social hierarchy of the time, and summing the weighted proportions. The index of poverty thus assumes (as Booth showed) that social class is a proxy for poverty and that the extent of poverty in a class is related to its position within the class hierarchy. The extent of poverty within a class has thus been estimated using the number of people in higher social classes. The index for a particular ward is:

$$\text{Ward Poverty Index} = (I \star wI + II \star wII + III \star wIII + IV \star wIV + V \star wV)/(I + II + III + IV + V)$$

Where I is the number of households in class I in the ward at that time and wI is the socioeconomic position indicator associated with that class shown in Table 1. This indicator relates to the proportion of the population that is at a higher socioeconomic level than the midpoint of the group. For 1991 9.2% of households are in social class I so 4.6% of them are above the mid-point of this category and the indicator is 0.046. 37.3% of households are in social class II and it is assumed that all social class I households and half of social class II households are at a higher socioeconomic level than the mid-point of this group. Thus the indicator for social class II households is 0.092 + 0.186 = 0.278. Similar logic is applied to calculation of the indicators for social classes III to V. The formulae to calculate socioeconomic position indicators are given in the footnote to Table 1.

The index was low (approaching 0) in areas where large numbers of the resident households were in more affluent social classes, and high in areas where they were in less affluent social classes. Similar logic was applied to the calculation of the 1896 indicators. The use of such indicators takes into account the fact that the distribution of socioeconomic groups in 1896 and 1991 were different (such indicators have been widely used in inequalities in health research[25-27]). This index measures level of affluence for each ward in the study area and not inequality within them.

Figure 2 shows two images of Providence Place in Islington, North London, taken more than 100 years apart. Note how the number of people has fallen, as it has fallen in London as a whole over this period, and that the open drain has been covered. However, the social position of Providence Place in the geographical ranking of London streets remains much the same.

We compared the relative predictive power of the two poverty measures as they varied for specific causes of death and for different age groups. In particular, stroke and stomach cancer, as causes shown to be related to deprivation in early life, may be better predicted by an historical poverty measure.[5,28] Age-gender standardised mortality ratios (SMRs) for each ward were thus calculated for the causes of death shown in Table 2 and for all deaths which took place between 1991 and 1995. The analysis comprised of simple weighted and partial correlations in which ward mortality ratios were predicted by the two measures of poverty. The population of each ward provided the weights. Partial correlation analysis was also used to ascertain the

Figure 2: Providence Place (Islington) circa 1900 and 2000

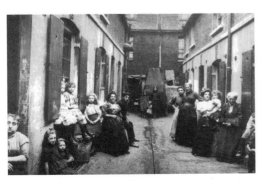
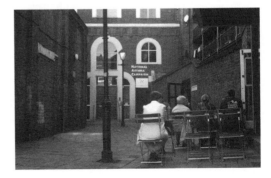

Table 2: Strength of relation between poverty in 1896 (Booth index) and 1991 (modern index) and SMRs for all ages for deaths in 1991-95

	Correlation of Booth index and mortality		Partial correlation of Booth index and mortality (controlling for modern index)		Correlation of modern index and mortality		Partial correlation of modern index and mortality (controlling for Booth index)	
	r value	p value	r value	p value	r value	p value	r value	p value
All causes	0.56	<0.001	0.22	0.012	0.60	<0.001	0.35	<0.001
Coronary heart disease	0.58	<0.001	0.21	0.015	0.65	<0.001	0.41	<0.001
Stroke	0.40	<0.001	0.22	0.013	0.36	<0.001	0.11	0.20
All cardiovascular disease	0.56	<0.001	0.20	0.023	0.61	<0.001	0.37	<0.001
Chronic obstructive pulmonary disease	0.58	<0.001	0.24	0.005	0.61	<0.001	0.35	<0.001
Pneumonia	0.26	0.002	0.07	0.45	0.30	<0.001	0.17	0.055
Lung cancer	0.61	<0.001	0.30	0.001	0.62	<0.001	0.33	<0.001
Stomach cancer	0.49	<0.001	0.24	0.007	0.47	<0.001	0.20	0.020
Accidents and suicide	0.05	0.56	−0.14	0.10	0.21	0.012	0.24	0.005

extent to which predictive power was duplicated between the indices. All analyses were carried out using the SPSS statistical package.

Results

Figure 3 shows three maps of the study area in Inner London allowing a comparison of the geography of poverty in the late 19th century (Map 1 in Figure 3), with that in the late 20th century (Map 2) and with mortality ratios for all causes for all ages (Map 3). The correlation coefficient between the two measures is 0.73 ($p<0.001$).

The blank area in the middle of the maps marks the City of London, which was not surveyed by Charles Booth. Figure 3 shows that there has been little change in the distribution of poverty in Inner London between the 19th and 20th centuries. Areas in which some groups of immigrants settled in the middle of the 20th century have moved down the social scale slightly, notably south of the River Thames, while others have gentrified. On the whole, however, affluent places have remained affluent and poor places have remained relatively poor – two images of the Albert Bridge 100 years apart (Figure 4) show part of the reason for this continuity – the perseverance of transport infrastructure. The map of all-age, all-cause SMRs demonstrates the close relation between poverty and mortality.

Table 2 shows the simple and partial correlations between poverty

Figure 3: London poverty (1896 and 1991) and mortality (1990s)

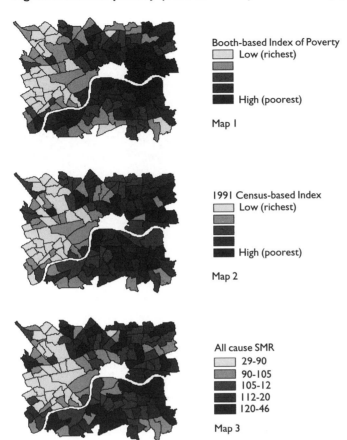

Booth-based Index of Poverty
Low (richest)

High (poorest)

Map 1

1991 Census-based Index
Low (richest)

High (poorest)

Map 2

All cause SMR
29-90
90-105
105-12
112-20
120-46

Map 3

and the SMRs for 1991-95. Both indices of poverty were related to all-cause SMRs. The partial correlation coefficients in the table also show that the index of poverty derived from Booth's 19th century observations (Booth index) contributed more to predicting deaths from stroke and stomach cancer in the late 20th century than that derived from the 1991 Census (modern index). For other causes of death, the modern index contributed more.

The results of further correlation analyses suggest that for deaths under the age of 65 the modern index makes a slightly greater contribution to predicting all-cause mortality in 1991-95 ($r=0.56$, $p<0.001$) than does the Booth index ($r=0.46$, $p<0.001$). This is substantiated by the results of the partial correlation analyses, where $r=0.39$ ($p=<0.001$) when mortality is correlated with the modern index, controlling for the Booth index, but $r=0.08$ ($p=0.36$) when mortality is correlated with the latter, controlling for the former.

When only deaths at ages greater than 65 are considered, however, both indices make a similar contribution to the model; the correlation

Figure 4: Albert Bridge (Chelsea) circa 1900 and 2000 (these two images show that the main change is that the trees have grown)

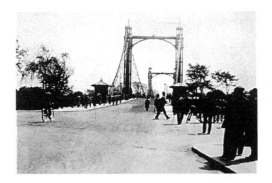 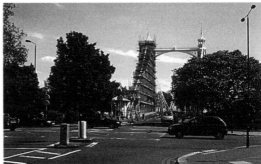

coefficients are $r=0.56$ ($p<0.001$) and $r=0.57$ ($p<0.001$) for the Booth and modern index respectively. Here the results of the partial correlations also suggest a similar contribution from each index ($r=0.26$, $p=0.002$ for the Booth index, controlling for the modern; $r=0.28$, $p=0.001$ when the indices are reversed).

Discussion

Almost everyone who was surveyed by Booth at the end of the 19th century will have died or left London before 1991. This means that the 19th century poverty index is truly ecological – it describes 'area-type' rather than the aggregate characteristics of the resident population. The fact that it performs so strongly as a predictor of mortality is perhaps partly because the median age of death of the people dying in the period 1991-95 is approximately 78. This means that, while very few would have been alive at the time Booth surveyed London, approximately half of these people would have been born before 1915. The Booth index is thus an indicator of the early life circumstances of those dying in the period 1991-95. Many of those people, however, will have migrated in the intervening period. Thus the predictive power of the Booth index is also an illustration of how the nature (and hierarchy) of different parts of London has remained relatively stable despite constant changeover of the resident individuals (illustrated by the similarities between Maps 1 and 2 in Figure 3). One might have expected to see considerable change in London's social and spatial structure given a century which included the Blitz in the Second World War and the development of London into an ever more dynamic major world city, but it is perhaps the continuity over this period which is most remarkable. Even the big wheel built to celebrate the millennium is not new – one just three quarters of its size was built a century ago in London (see Figure 5).

Figure 5: Big Wheel at Earl's Court (1896) and the London Eye (2000)

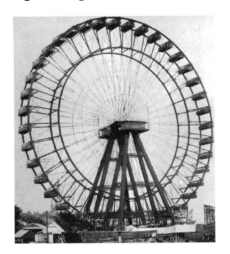 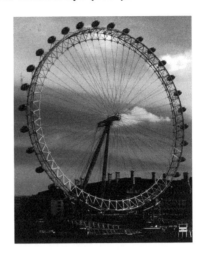

The social segregation of London is maintained through many processes. One that is particularly important is through the maintenance of differential housing values across the capital, which help steer patterns of migration within London. However, we have no way of knowing the migration histories of the individuals who died between 1991 and 1995.

Thus, these results will not reveal whether the high rates of mortality found in areas which have been continuously poor throughout are due to the continuous in-ward migration of a population at relatively higher risk of mortality (perhaps forced into cheaper accommodation, for example), or to some accumulative mortality risk raising the effects of day-to-day life in the area.

The fact that the index of poverty derived from Booth's survey is related more strongly to causes of death that have previously been shown to be sensitive to deprivation in early life – that is stroke and stomach cancer[5,28] – suggests that to some degree the ecological associations with past and present deprivation levels of areas do reflect individual level associations of deprivation at different stages of the lifecourse and health outcomes. In short, the longer people spend both in poverty and in poor places the earlier they tend to die. The maps and models also show that 100 years of policy initiatives have had almost no impact on the patterns of inequality in Inner London and on the relationship between people's socioeconomic position and their relative chances of dying.

We thus have a different ending to *A Christmas carol* than that given by Dickens below. The hypothesis of the Spirit of Christmas Yet to Come seems to be true – inequalities in health have not declined, partly because miserliness in the past does lead to future inequalities in health. Dickens advocated redistribution of wealth at the end of his tale. Wilkinson has suggested that greater income equality is beneficial for the health of the whole population – including the relatively affluent – not just for those who are badly off. In Dickens' story such redistribution not only aided the family of Tiny Tim, it also benefited Scrooge himself:

> "A merrier Christmas, Bob, my good fellow, than I have given you for many a year! I'll raise your salary, and endeavour to assist your struggling family."... Scrooge was better than his word. He did it all, and infinitely more; and to Tiny Tim, who did NOT die, he was a second father.... His own heart laughed: and that was quite enough for him.[1]

Acknowledgements

The authors would like to thank Kevin Holohan for digitising work, Nichola Tooke for historical research and Jonathan Tooby for photographic advice.

References

[1] Dickens, C. (1843) *A Christmas carol*, London: Chapman and Hall.

[2] **Davey Smith, G., Hart, C., Gillis, C. and Hawthorne, V. (1997) 'Lifetime socioeconomic position and mortality: prospective observational study', *British Medical Journal*, vol 314, p 547.**

[3] Shaw, M., Gordon, D., Dorling, D. and Davey Smith, G. (1999) *The widening gap: Health inequalities and policy in Britain*, Bristol: The Policy Press.

[4] **Davey Smith, G., Hart, C., Blane, D. and Hole, D. (1998) 'Adverse socioeconomic conditions in childhood and cause specific adult mortality: prospective observational study', *British Medical Journal*, vol 316, pp 1631–5.**

[5] Aves, E. (1916) 'Obituary: Charles Booth', *Economic Journal*, vol 26, December, pp 537-42.

[6] Bales, K. (1996) 'Lives and labours in the emergence of organised research, 1886-1907', *Journal of Historical Sociology*, vol 9, pp 113-38.

[7] Bales, K. (1999) 'Popular reactions to sociological research: the case of Charles Booth', *Sociology*, vol 33, pp 153-68.

[8] Booth, C. (1887) 'The inhabitants of Tower Hamlets (School Board Division), their condition and occupations', *Journal of the Royal Statistical Society Series*, vol 50, pp 326-401.

[9] Booth, C. (1969, first published 1889) *Life and labour of the people. First series, Poverty (I): East, Central and South London*, London: Macmillan.

[10] Booth, C. (1969, first published 1902) *Life and labour of the people. First series, Poverty (II): Streets and population classified*, London: Macmillan.

[11] Booth, C. (1902) *Life and labour of the people in London. Final volume. Notes on social influences and conclusions*, London: Macmillan.

[12] Cullen, M. (1979) 'Charles Booth's poverty survey: some new approaches', in T.C. Smout (ed) *The search for wealth and stability: Essays in economic and social history presented to MV Flinn*, London: Macmillan.

[13] Davies, W.J.D. (1978) 'Charles Booth and the measurement of urban social character', *Area*, vol 10, pp 290-6.

[14] Fried, A. and Elman, R.M. (1969) *Charles Booth's London: A portrait of the poor at the turn of the century, drawn from his 'Life and labour of the people in London'*, London: Hutchinson.

[15] O'Day, R. and Englander, D. (1993) *Mr Charles Booth's inquiry: 'Life and labour of the people in London' reconsidered*, London: The Hambledon Press.

[16] Pfautz, H.W. (1967) *On the city: Physical pattern and social structure: Selected writing of Charles Booth*, Chicago, IL: Chicago University Press.

[17] Spicker, P. (1990) 'Charles Booth: the examination of poverty', *Social Policy and Administration*, vol 24, pp 21-38.

[18] Simey, T.S. and Simey, M.B. (1960) *Charles Booth: Social scientist*, London: Oxford University Press.

[19] Townsend, P., Corrigan, P. and Kowarzik, U. (1987) *Poverty and labour in London: Interim report of a centenary survey*, Survey of Londoners' Living Standards No 1, London: Low Pay Unit.

[20] Reeder, D.A. (1984) *Charles Booth's descriptive map of London poverty 1889*, London: London Topographical Society, publication no 130.

[21] Gillie, A. (1996) 'The origin of the poverty line', *Economic History Review*, vol 49, pp 715-30.

[22] Stevenson, T.H.C. (1928) 'The vital statistics of wealth and poverty', *Journal of the Royal Statistical Society Series*, vol 91, pp 207-30.

[23] Szreter, S.R.S. (1984) 'The genesis of the Registrar-General's social classification of occupations', *The British Journal of Sociology*, vol 35, pp 522-46.

[24] Szreter, S.R.S. (1986) 'The first scientific social structure of modern Britain 1875-1883', in L. Bonfield, R.M. Smith and K. Wrightson (eds) *The world we have gained: Histories of population and social structure*, Oxford: Blackwell, pp 337-54.

[25] Pamuk, E.R. (1985) 'Social class inequality in mortality from 1921 to 1972 in England and Wales', *Population Studies*, vol 39, pp 17-31.

[26] Kunst, A.E. and Mackenbach, J.P. (1994) 'The size of mortality differences associated with educational level in 9 industrialised countries', *American Journal of Public Health*, vol 84, pp 932-7.

[27] **Davey Smith, G., Hart, C., Hole, D., MacKinnon, P., Gillis, C. et al (1998) 'Education and occupational social class: which is the more important indicator of mortality risk?', *Journal of Epidemiology and Community Health*, vol 52, pp 153-60.**

[28] Leon, D. and Davey Smith, G. (2000) 'Infant mortality, stomach cancer, stroke, and coronary heart disease: ecological analysis', *British Medical Journal*, vol 320, pp 1705-6.

33

Does early nutrition affect later health? Views from the 1930s and 1980s

George Davey Smith and Diana Kuh

Introduction

Recently there has been a shift in the focus of investigations of the causes of chronic disease from health-related behaviours and risk factors acting during adulthood to experiences occurring during early life: in childhood, infancy and during intra-uterine development. The work of the Medical Research Council (MRC) Environmental Epidemiology Unit in Southampton, under the direction of Professor David Barker, has been largely instrumental in this. The unit's work has occasioned an editorial in the *British Medical Journal* claiming that the 'early life experience' paradigm is a strong candidate for the replacement of the 'lifestyle paradigm' of chronic disease aetiology.[1]

The speed with which the findings of this research programme have entered policy discussions is noteworthy. The first publication[2] of the now extensive series[3] from Barker's team appeared only in 1986, but by 1989 the annual report of the Chief Medical Officer was already noting "the importance of health in childhood as a determinant of subsequent health in adult life",[4] while in 1992 the Department of Health strategy document *The health of the nation* made reference to the "increasing evidence to suggest that there is a relationship between growth and development starting from before birth and during childhood, and risk in later life of CHD (coronary heart disease)".[5]

Barker argues that maternal, foetal and infant nutrition are important early-life influences which affect later adult health.[6] In a review entitled 'Nutrition in early life and later outcome', one of the

In D. Smith (ed) (1996) *The history of nutrition in Britain in the twentieth century: Science, scientists and politics*, London: Routledge, pp 214-37

Southampton researchers comments that "There have been few studies in humans of the long-term effects of nutrition in early life....This is not because the possibility of long-term effects of diet has not been considered, but reflects the extreme difficulty in carrying out such studies in humans".[7] Barker's team have drawn attention to the possible role of early nutrition by studying adults in middle and old age whose early growth and development had been recorded. Those whose early growth had been impaired *in utero* or in early post-natal life experienced an increased risk of a number of adult chronic diseases, most notably cardiovascular disease, diabetes and chronic bronchitis. From this evidence Barker hypothesised that impaired growth during critical periods of early life permanently affects or 'programmes' the structure and physiology of a range of organs and tissues.

The notion that adult health is determined by experiences in early life, in particular by nutrition, was accepted wisdom in pre-Second World War public health – a view which many practitioners considered to be supported by the empirical evidence.[8] The decline in the influence of this view after the war occurred while increased attention was being paid to adult life-style in both epidemiological research and public health practice. In this chapter we examine the shifting fortune of ideas linking early nutrition to health in adulthood, relating such shifts to the type of data available during each period, the styles of public health research, the response of the scientific and policy making communities, and the broader social setting.

Latour has illustrated how scientific controversies and the emergence of scientific 'facts' can be seen as social processes.[9] He argues that the construction of scientific facts is a collective process, the fate of a scientific statement depending on its use and adoption by others. Latour details his 'translation model' of the strategies by which the scientist or research team try to mobilise allies and to develop networks and alliances advancing their scientific claim to the status of having established a scientific fact. The response of scientists, policy makers and the general public to research into nutrition and health in the 1930s and 1980s clearly owes much to the assembly of such networks, as we hope to demonstrate.

Heredity or nutrition?

The Inter-Departmental Committee on Physical Deterioration, set up in 1903 in response to the high proportion of men found to be unfit for military service in the Boer War, highlighted the need to understand the origins of the poor state of health of the British working class.[10] Much of the Committee's report was devoted to "conditions affecting the life of the juvenile population", reflecting the generally held belief that the source of adult health problems lay in childhood. Those giving evidence to the committee recognised the importance of nutrition:

> With the exception of Mr Edward Rees, whose panacea is fresh air, all the witnesses concurred in claiming the first place for food. 'Food', says Dr Eicholz, 'is the point about which turns the whole problem of degeneracy. There is, first, the want of food, second the irregularity in the way in which children get their meals, and, thirdly, the non-suitability of the food when they get it; and these three circumstances, want of food, irregularly and unsuitability of food, taken together, are, in his opinion, the determining cause of degeneracy in children.[11]

An editorial in 1904 in the *British Medical Journal* commented that:

> It cannot too often be repeated that a child wisely fed for the first two or three years of its life has every chance of growing up into a strong man or woman; a child rendered rickety and puny by ignorant feeding will in all probability never make up the ground it has lost.[12]

In contrast, social biologists of a hereditarian persuasion, such as Karl Pearson, argued that death in early life had an important role in the process of natural selection, since "a heavy death-rate does mean the elimination of the weaklings".[13] This assertion was supported by the demonstration that between 1838 and 1900 the infant mortality rates correlated negatively with mortality rates for children aged one to five years. Improvements in mortality rates for those aged one to five years were seen to be dependent on rising infant mortality rates, since these were assumed to selectively remove the hereditarily unfit from the population.

For these reasons Pearson viewed the decline in the infant death rate in the early years of the 20th century, coupled with the low birth rate and differential fertility in favour of the lower classes, as "nothing short of calamitous".[14] Since death was seen as a method of removing hereditary inadequacies, to "check Nature's effective and roughshod methods of race betterment", by adapting the environment to man would be to produce a race of degenerate and feeble stock. Pearson considered that the influence of heredity on health was much greater than the influence of the environment: "health is a real hereditary characteristic and the health of the parents is far more important than the question of back-to-back houses, one-apartment tenements, the employment of mothers or breast feeding...".[15]

It was fortunate for Pearson's hypothesis that his analysis stopped in 1900, since from the turn of the century infant and childhood mortality rates began to fall in concert; the negative correlation he identified would no longer have been evident. Arthur Newsholme, the medical officer to the Local Government Board and public health activist, directly challenged Pearson's analysis, by demonstrating that those districts with high infant mortality rates were also the districts with the highest rates of child and adolescent mortality.[16] Newsholme and others maintained that environmental conditions underlay the unfavourable health status of the children of the poor, and that improvements in these conditions led to increased survival and better child health. At this time the link between the health of infants and children and later adult health was, apparently, self-evident. Thus George Newman, Chief Medical Officer to the Board of Education, wrote the following in his 1913 report:

> Recent progress has shown a) that the health of the adult is dependent upon the health of the child, that to grow healthy men we must first grow healthy children; that sickness and disease of children lead to disability and disablement among adolescents and adults; and that the State cannot effectually insure itself against physical disease unless it begins with children; b) that the health of the child is dependent upon the health of the infant and mother.[17]

Later eugenicists, such as Dr Frank White, came to accept a limited role for environmental influences, including diet, in improving survival. However, he questioned the healthiness of the survivors, and feared they would lower the general health of the population. Writing in 1928, White remarked that:

> ...a careful study of the official volumes relating to the health of our nation leaves one with a feeling of disappointment and oppression a falling death rate may be altogether deceptive as indicative of improvement in inherent healthfulness, since the life of a wretchedly-endowed or even mortally-afflicted infant can be amazingly prolonged by a sedulous system of nursing and dietary.[18]

According to White the survivors were "for the most part physical and mental defectives who, under a sterner regime, would unquestionably have been eliminated soon after birth by natural selection. And, unhappily, the more of such we save the worse becomes the outlook for the state".

In the late 1920s and early 1930s, analysis of mortality trends provided evidence to support this emphasis on the early-life origins of health in adulthood. It was suggested by the actuary V.P.A. Derrick that year of birth rather than year of death was the important parameter determining mortality risk: successive cohorts born after the middle of the 19th century experienced decreasing mortality risk at all ages.[19] Derrick interpreted this as indicating improved inherited characteristics of succeeding birth cohorts, but others considered that environmental factors acting in early life were important.[20] W.O. Kermack, of the laboratory of the Royal College of Physicians of Edinburgh, published a paper with A.G. McKendrick and P.L. McKinlay which used a different method from that of Derrick to examine the extent to which death rates were a function of year of health and year of birth. They noted that the data behaved as if "the expectation of life was determined by the conditions which existed during the child's earlier years", and concluded:

> ... the health of the child is determined by the environmental
> conditions existing during the years 0-15, and ... the health
> of the man is determined preponderantly by the physical
> constitution which the child has built up.[21]

The exception to the general pattern detected by Kermack and colleagues was mortality under one year of age (infant mortality), which only started to decline after the turn of the century, well after mortality at later ages. They suggested that infant mortality was dependent on the health of the mother, and thus improvement in infant mortality followed the generational improvement in the vitality of women of childbearing age.

The role of nutrition

While Kermack and colleagues discussed 'environmental influences' acting during childhood in general, inter-war developments in nutrition science led to a greater recognition of the vital role of nutrition in health and a major shift in definitions of dietary quality. According to Celia Petty, "Whereas the 1904 Committee on Physical Deterioration had argued that the diets of the poor were deficient in protein and fat, during the 1920s and 1930s vitamin and mineral deficiencies were widely believed to be the chief nutritional causes of ill health and inferior physique".[22]

Reports of public health officials such as Nesholme and Newman,[23] and of nutritional surveys carried out under the MRC by D. Noël Paton, Leonard Findlay and Edward Cathcart of Glasgow University, claimed that poor diets were the result of maternal habits and ignorance.[24] However, dietary guidelines issued by the British Medical Association in 1933, as well as earlier recommendations by the Advisory Committee on Nutrition of the Ministry of Health, made it increasingly difficult to justify the view that families on low income could secure an adequate diet "simply by improving budgetary efficiency".[25] Nutritional surveys carried out by more radical social reformers, such as John Boyd Orr, were influential in establishing the connection between nutrition and health, and relating malnutrition to poverty and low incomes. Orr's survey of over 1,000 family budgets and food expenditure, first published in 1936, showed that at least half the country's children lived in families whose income was too low to secure a diet which met the nutritional standards for optimum health.[26]

New political lobby groups (such as the Children's Minimum Council, the Committee against Malnutrition and the National Unemployed Workers' Movement), social commentators and public health activists were quick to incorporate the new findings from nutritional and epidemiological research into their activities to promote better child nutrition. Dr G.C.M. M'Gonigle, Medical Officer of Health for Stockton-on-Tees, had worked on surveys of child health and nutrition with Kermack's co-author, P.L. McKinlay, a medical officer of the Scottish Department of Health. In *Poverty and public health*, published in 1936 by Victor Gollancz, M'Gonigle and the public analyst J. Kirby wrote of the overriding importance of child nutrition:

> Children may, and in fact not infrequently do, grow up healthily in spite of a bad material environment. They may avoid clinical illness due to infections, though exposed to the infections; they may survive, undamaged, illnesses resulting from the invasion of their tissues by pathogenic micro-organisms, but they cannot survive unscathed prolonged deprivations or deficiencies of certain essentials for normal nutrition.[27]

Wal Hannington, leader of the National Unemployed Workers' Movement, utilised the same kinds of evidence in his overtly activist Left Book Club volume *The problem of the distressed areas*, published in 1937. In a chapter headed 'Scientists, diets and realities', Hannington stated that he could "lay no claim to a sufficient knowledge of medical science to entitle me to embark upon scientific polemics with the wise men of the BMA and the experts of the Ministry of Health", but added that his "common and everyday experiences of the way the low paid and unemployed workers live" allowed him to judge that "continuous under-feeding of working-class families through long unemployment and insufficient income has so reduced their stamina that they fall easy victims to physical ailments and disease".[28]

The under-nourishment of children, Hannington continued, interfered with their education and produced a body of youth prone to illness and of such poor physical condition that work and playing football were beyond the scope of many. He approvingly quoted the

Chief Medical Officer of the Board of Education as saying that "Medical science has proved that disease and incapacity in adolescence and adult life find their source all too often in the seed-time of childhood". Hannington maintained that "unemployment has existed for so long in the Distressed Areas that many of the youths who are today leaving school were probably handicapped from the moment of their birth as the result of under-nourishment of the mothers during pregnancy". He agreed with Sir Malcolm Stewart, the Commissioner for the Special Areas of England and Wales, that more medical attention was required for such youth, but thought it "callous and brutal, to allow conditions to exist in childhood which produce unhealthy youth, and, when the damage is done, to suggest that efforts be made to repair it by medical treatment".[29]

Ideas regarding the importance of early nutrition to later health influenced an authority with a rather different perspective from those of Hannington and M'Gonigle. H.M. Vernon, investigator for the Industrial Health Research Board, began *Health in relation to occupation*, a book published in 1939 which summarised his understanding of the science of public health, with a discussion of the findings of Kermack, McKendrick and McKinlay. Vernon thought that the first of the "remedial measures that ought to be undertaken to reduce ill health" was the improved distribution of food:

> With the provision of adequate nourishment at all stages of human existence, we should find a further diminution of infant mortality, which has already improved so remarkably in recent years, and ... we should find considerable improvement in the health and physique of the children. Such improvement would certainly lead to a healthier adult life.[30]

When considering the relative importance of different influences on health, Vernon stated that nutrition was:

> ... by far the most important of all the factors, broadly classed as environmental, which influence the health of the human organism ... adequate nutrition is specially important, not only for children but for expectant and nursing mothers, if good physique coupled with good health, is to be attained when the children reach adult life.

For adults other than expectant and nursing mothers, Vernon continued, nutrition was "not so important ... as for children", although it should be adequate "if the maximum degree of health and efficiency is desired".[31]

In *The condition of Britain*, published in 1937, G.D.H. Cole and M. Cole commented at length on the increased attention being paid to nutrition:

> This question of adequate nutrition has, owing to a combination of circumstances, been forced very much on the public attention during the past few years; and the new importance assigned to it is even now revolutionising popular conceptions of what an efficient public health service needs to be.[32]

The Coles attributed this emphasis on nutrition to four factors. There were longstanding concerns about the poor national physique as a consequence of the results of medical examinations of recruits for the First World War. Second, there were concerns about the falling birth rate, leading to "more anxious care about human life as such". Third, there were advances in knowledge, such that "we are now far better informed about the kinds of ill health which arise from defects of diet than we have ever been before". Finally, the Coles noted:

> It is, however, doubtful whether the research workers would have been able to direct nearly so much attention to their discoveries had not these been accompanied by a world-wide 'glut' of food, in the sense of a supply larger than the farmers and middlemen have been able to dispose of at a profit. This 'glut' set the statesmen of those countries in which large surpluses of foodstuffs were produced thinking and talking hard about the means of increasing the consumption of food; and the research workers and social reformers promptly seized their chance of putting their scientific conclusions before a public which was readier to listen because a higher food consumption looked like being 'good for trade'.[33]

The threat of war in 1938-39 was a further stimulus to the development of a national nutritional policy based on advances in scientific knowledge. After the war the Chief Medical Officer of the Ministry of Health felt able to report that "the national provision of milk and vitamin supplements ... has done more than any other factor to promote the health of expectant mothers and young children".[34] However, wartime policies which linked nutrition, poverty and health collapsed in the postwar period. Health policy became dominated by curative medical services; agricultural policy by economic self-interest.[35] Epidemiological research, in its search for the causes of specific chronic disease in later life, shifted its focus to adult life-styles.

The rise of 'life-styles'

As we have seen, during the first four decades of the century there was much public health interest in nutrition in early life as a determinant of susceptibility to disease, interest which dissipated over a relatively short period. One reason for this was that the central finding upon which it rested – the mortality regularities displayed by Derrick, Kermack and others – ceased to obtain, even while these authors were producing their papers.[36] Examination of age-specific mortality trends in Britain over this period shows why the predictions made by Derrick failed to be confirmed. Over the 1920s and 1930s, death rates for adults stopped declining, or increased slightly, as mortality from cardiovascular causes and cancers replaced death from infectious diseases. The increase in cancer mortality could be attributed to a rise in lung cancer.[37] Regarding cardiovascular disease mortality there was much speculation, a suggestion by Morris being the prevailing view: "the principal factor in [the] recent, very unsatisfactory, trend of mortality in middle-aged men [is] ... an increase in ischaemic heart disease".[38]

In the 1930s some commentators suggested that increases in lung cancer followed from increases in cigarette smoking.[39] During the 1950s evidence from studies of lung cancer cases and controls was complemented by the use of more formal cohort analysis techniques, which implicated smoking as the aetiological agent responsible for the dramatic rise in lung cancer mortality.[40] The concentration on nurture in early life as a determinant of susceptibility to illness in general gave way to a focus on environmental factors in adult life which increased the risk of particular causes of death, in particular from lung cancer and coronary heart disease (CHD). Epidemiological research proceeded through ecological comparisons and through prospective studies. The former related the 'life-styles' of adults: dietary habits, smoking, and physical activity, plus factors seen to be related to life-style, such as blood pressure and serum cholesterol – to the large international differences in CHD rates.[41] In 1948 the first major prospective study of CHD was initiated in Framingham, Massachusetts.[42] Middle-aged men were recruited and followed to see how those who died from heart disease differed from the survivors. The aetiological factors studied were generally the same as those examined in the ecological studies.

The pre-war pronouncements regarding the importance of childhood environment and adult health had usually been primarily concerned with health in general, and all-cause mortality as a particular indicator of this, rather than with specific illnesses. The postwar shift towards adult environment, on the other hand, was concerned with particular health problems. Official pronouncements reflected a preoccupation with the apparent increase in CHD. Thus the Registrar General wrote in 1954:

> We must try to determine the factors responsible for the occurrence of the disease at the present time – among which diet, mental stress and lack of physical exercise have come under suspicion – and judge whether the varying influence of the causative factors can have produced a rising incidence of disease.[43]

From the mid-1950s Thomas McKeown began to attribute the dramatic fall in mortality since the mid-19th century mainly to better nutrition, which he argued had improved host resistance to infectious disease,[44] a view which has only recently been challenged.[45] In contrast, when considering mortality rates from non-infective conditions such as cardiovascular disease, which had yet to show signs of decline, McKeown argued, as did other epidemiologists, that 'personal behaviour' was a more important influence than 'food deficiency'.[46]

The rediscovery of childhood

In the tradition of postwar epidemiology, the major concern with regard to the nutrition of infants and children related to the possible effects of over-nutrition. Thus, when it was suggested that "adult coronary disease is really a major paediatric problem", this referred to the need for:

> ... cardiovascular health promotion and the encouragement of healthy lifestyles in childhood. Diet, exercise, and the prevention of unhealthy lifestyles and behaviours, eg cigarette smoking, consumption of alcohol and harmful drugs, are the main areas for intervention.[47]

A few researchers and practitioners, generally coming from outside of the field of epidemiology or public health, took a different view of the relationship between nutrition in early life and risk of coronary disease. The starting point for the investigations of Osborn in the 1960s was the state of the coronary arteries of decedents who came to autopsy. He noted that normal coronary arteries were often found among older people who, according to relatives, took little exercise, ate high-fat diets and smoked. Furthermore, fit young men with exemplary life-styles were being killed by their extensive coronary atherosclerosis. Osborn turned to infant feeding as a possible explanation. He interviewed the mothers of 109 people who died under the age of 20 and found that coronary atherosclerosis was worse among those who had been bottle fed, rather than breast fed, as infants. The questions distressed the mothers of the decedents, however, which made Osborn suspend his enquiries, with the observation that in "20 or more years a satisfactory answer to this question could be obtained if the mothers of entrants into the armed services were questioned, this enquiry would be similar to that of the doctors and their smoking habits". Osborn noted that "the high incidence of coronary diseases in the most civilised countries is commonly ascribed to this or that dietetic habit in its cultivated citizens", but asked:

> Is it not more likely to be due to the fact that as civilisation advances breast feeding becomes increasingly inconvenient and so declines? Unfortunately this is a subject which is apt to arouse unscientific emotions even in medical men; the subject is too important to pay any attention to these.... The greatest problem facing us must be how to raise our children so that they do not eventually share our great liability to untimely death from coronary disease.[48]

While a couple of studies were carried out to examine Osborn's hypothesis,[49] with equivocal results, and the occasional claim was made that "breast is best for coronary protection"[50] this line of research was not taken further. However, theories of the aetiology of CHD were developed which rejected the overriding importance of unhealthy adult life-styles, in part in response to the observation that the major risk factors – high-fat diet, high blood pressure, smoking and elevated blood cholesterol – failed to account for the social, geographical and temporal variations in CHD rates. Thus an ecological study carried out by A. Forsdahl in Norway demonstrated geographical correlations between past infant mortality rates and current adult mortality rates.[51] This was considered to provide evidence of the persistent effects of conditions in childhood. Children born in areas with high infant mortality rates were taken to have experienced greater levels of deprivation than those born in areas with lower infant mortality rates. Forsdahl considered that nutritional deficit in childhood, followed by relative affluence, could increase the risk of CHD in adult life.[52]

In Britain Barker and his colleagues entered the debate regarding the validity of the 1984 recommendations produced by the Committee on Medical Aspects of Food Policy (COMA).[53] Reducing fat and increasing fibre consumption were advocated by COMA as ways of reducing population CHD rates. Favourable trends in CHD during the war had been widely taken to be evidence in favour of the COMA recommendations, since wartime food policy produced dietary changes in the advised direction. A re-analysis of the data by Barker's team suggested that no such favourable CHD trends actually occurred, and hence that there was no support for "the view that compliance with the COMA recommendations on fat, fibre, and sugar consumption will lead, by itself, to an appreciable fall in coronary heart disease mortality in middle aged men".[54]

The alternative notion, that development in early life underlay the risk of CHD, was put forward in the paper 'Infant mortality, childhood nutrition, and ischaemic heart disease in England and Wales', published in 1986.[55] Essentially, this paper reported on an extended analysis of British data along the lines of Forsdahl's study in Norway. Using 212 local authority areas as the unit of analysis, Barker and Osmond found that adult mortality from stroke was most strongly correlated with neonatal mortality, adult mortality from CHD was strongly correlated with both neonatal and post-neonatal mortality, and adult mortality from chronic bronchitis was associated with post-neonatal mortality only. They suggested that "the geographical distribution of ischaemic heart disease in England and Wales reflects variations in nutrition in early life, which are expressed pathologically on exposure to later dietary influences". A second study using the same methods showed that adult mortality from stroke was strongly correlated with maternal mortality, which Barker and Osmond argued reflected the dominant influence of maternal physique and health.[56] Similar conclusions were drawn from a study comparing the current mortality rates in three neighbouring northern English towns. Disparities between the towns, in mortality from CHD, stroke and bronchitis appeared to be more closely related to differences which existed when the older (and now dying) residents were children than to present-day differences.[57] Factors such as maternal health and physique, infant feeding, housing and overcrowding were advanced as possible determinants of current variations in adult mortality.

This line of investigation was developed through studies of reconstructed cohorts of individuals born earlier this century. The detailed records kept by midwives and health visitors in east Hertfordshire between 1911 and 1930 allowed for the examination of the association of birth weight, growth in the first year of life and mode of infant feeding, with CHD risk in later life. Babies who were born with a low birth weight and male infants who grew poorly during the first year of life were at increased risk of dying of a heart attack as adults.[58] By studying survivors from this cohort, and from similar 'catch-up' studies, Barker and his colleagues showed that different patterns of impaired foetal growth (characterised by low birthweight, or low birthweight relative to placental weight, or thinness at birth, or shortness at birth with subsequent failure of infant growth) were associated with different adult risk factors for cardiovascular disease.[59] These included blood pressure, glucose tolerance, cholesterol and apolipoprotein B, fibrinogen and factor VII. This evidence, it was argued, suggested that differences in the timing of under-nutrition in pregnancy had different effects on organs and tissues according to their stage of development.[60] Their interpretation of the findings was guided by earlier animal studies of programming, in particular those that examined the effect of nutritional deficiencies before birth, or immediately preceding birth, on subsequent growth and development.[61]

While the proposal that forces acting during infancy and childhood influenced later health was considered largely uncontroversial during the decades before the Second World War,[62] the later championing of this view with respect to the aetiology of CHD, stroke and diabetes has initiated much debate. The conventional wisdom, against which these hypotheses were pitted, was that overnutrition was one of the root causes of such chronic diseases. Thus the suggestion that their origin lay in malnutrition – albeit malnutrition occurring during early development – ran directly counter to the bulk of both cardiovascular research and health policy. The stream of publications from the Southampton group continued, and the ideas were supported by the MRC,[63] by editorials in the *British Medical Journal*,[64] and by the findings of other research teams.[65] In contrast, those with a long-term investment in cardiovascular epidemiology have tended to criticise[66] or, more usually, to ignore Barker's research.

The critical response to Barker's studies have focused on the difficulties involved in interpreting the observed associations between early-life experiences and health in adulthood when nothing was known about the period in between.[67] It has been argued that it is likely that children born into poor socioeconomic circumstances will, on average, tend to experience retarded growth, compared with those born into a more favourable environment. Indeed, studies carried out in the 1930s had demonstrated this:

> The rate of growth of infants is found to depend to some extent on the economic resources of the family. When a group of working-class families at Birmingham was divided into three, according to wages per head, it was found that there was no characteristic difference in the weight of the infants for the first three weeks, but after thirteen weeks a distinction was quite evident and it persisted throughout the first year. Observations made at Glasgow showed this divergence from the age of 2 till the age of 10 years, and at Stuttgart it has been noted up to the age of 19 years.[68]

Isabella Leitch, who in the mid-1930s had been centrally involved in planning the Carnegie nutrition and health survey with Boyd Orr, considered, in 1951, whether good nutrition and growth in early life influenced later health. She cautioned that:

> Since all the social circumstances, housing, sanitation, spacing of population and hence exposure to infection, as well as education and, on the whole, facilities for prompt medical attention, improve with, and at about the same rate as, growth, it is difficult to judge whether inhibition of growth itself has any effect on morbidity.[69]

These comments suggested that there was a need to examine whether it was possible that aspects of later childhood, adolescence and adulthood could account for the association of early growth with adult disease. In epidemiological parlance, the issue is that of confounding.[70] Catch-up studies such as those conducted by Barker's team have not had the prospective data needed to examine how poor nutrition, overcrowding and other forms social disadvantage in childhood may affect the relationship between early growth and cardiovascular disease. They argue that the specific nature of the relationships between early growth and cardiovascular disease, the strong and graded dose response, and the continued importance of the associations after adjusting for adult social class, smoking and body weight are indicative of causal relationships. However, many commentators consider that further research involving long-term prospective data throughout the lifecourse is needed, if this issue is to be resolved.[71]

Early nutrition and later health: the contexts of the 1930s and the 1980s

In the first four decades of the century, childhood nutrition was firmly established as a factor underlying health in adulthood, a position which was undermined as poor child health lost importance as a social problem. Over the last decade, the resurgence of interest in the early-life origins of adult disease has also been concerned with childhood nutrition, but as the theories have developed, greater emphasis has been placed on nutrition during foetal and infant development rather than on nutrition during later childhood. This reflects the different strengths of the various networks which worked to keep childhood nutrition as an important issue. In the 1930s the suggestion that there were crucial forces during childhood which determined later health was quickly translated into a consideration of nutrition. To develop the explanation of Cole and Cole: the combination of the activities of food producers and distributors, nutritional experts armed with 'newer knowledge', public health doctors increasingly freed from the burden of infectious disease control, political activists, and the state functionaries charged with restraining such activism, ensured that nutrition remained a key social problem of the period.

Throughout the 1930s infant mortality rates in Britain fell,[72] although some economically depressed regions proved to be exceptions to this rule.[73] Similarly, the evidence of sharp decline in nutritional status or health during the Depression is lacking.[74] The Ministry of Health claimed that "the evil effects had been so small as to be barely noticeable".[75] This was rejected by the Coles, M'Gonigle, Hannington and other contemporary observers. The Coles considered that it was fully possible for "a rapid fall in infant deaths to occur, even while the health of the survivors is getting worse".[76] The vital role of good nutrition in guaranteeing the health of the future generation was a part of accepted wisdom that was not dependent on verified statistics.

An illustration of the resilience of the notion that poor early nutrition impairs later health is provided by the manner in which a classic experiment in animal nutrition was reported in 1935. C.M. McCay and colleagues carried out a four-year study in which food restriction was applied after weaning to one group of rats, while others were allowed to feed as desired.[77] The result of this study, which has been replicated many times since, was that the longevity of male rats was greater if their feeding was restricted. This finding would, on the face of it, run counter to the expectations of researchers such as Kermack and colleagues, who saw poor material circumstances in early life as a cause of increased mortality risk in adulthood.[78] Nevertheless, the work of Kermack et al was quoted by McCay et al in a way which suggested that the two sets of findings were complementary.

The nutrition of children was one of the major social problems of the years leading up to the Second World War. Such was not the case in the mid-1980s, the time when the Southampton group were publishing their first papers on the topic. The attitude to the optimal nutrition of children had greatly changed. In *The schoolboy: A study of his nutrition, physical development and health*, published in 1935, Dr G.E. Friend, medical officer of Christ's Hospital, was much concerned with adequate calorie intake and considered that "25-30 per cent of the total daily calories should be derived from fat and as much of this as possible should be derived from certain animal fats".[79] Similarly, M'Gonigle and Kirby thought that there was "no limit to the proportions of animal proteins and fat which the human can eat over prolonged periods without physical injury".[80] Their table of 'highly protective foods' featured milk, eggs, cheese and butter; wholemeal bread, root vegetables and margarine, were consigned to be the "less protective and non-protective foods". By the 1980s, on the other hand, recommendations regarding the diet of children were pointing in almost exactly the opposite direction. The prevention of obesity through limiting calorie intake and the avoidance of foods high in fat – and high in animal fat in particular – had become the target.

Rather than screening children for health problems caused by under-nutrition, screening is now advocated for elevated blood cholesterol levels which, in part, are taken to reflect dietary excess. In keeping with these changed circumstances, childhood under-nutrition featured only briefly as a key component of the current interest in early-life experiences and later health.

Several research networks have been involved in the development and maintenance of the recent early-life origins model of adult disease. Prominent research groups investigating the role of mechanisms of disease production which are not automatically associated with adult environment, such as processes of blood clotting,[81] and impaired glucose metabolism,[82] have engaged in collaborative projects with the Southampton team and have thereby come to have a shared interest in this model. Funding agencies such as the MRC, the Wellcome Trust and the British Heart Foundation have been keen to support research into the early-life origins of disease, seeing this as an exciting area of research with which they want to be associated. Other funding agencies which have supported the work, for example the Milk Marketing Board,[83] have their own particular interest in moving the focus of aetiological research from adult life-styles to early development.

Barker's theories of the origins of cardiovascular disease have attracted considerable television coverage and positive feedback from the 'quality' press. Groups such as Maternity Alliance, whose interests straddle the academic and policy debates, have shown interest in the relevance of these emerging scientific facts for questions of policy. Their own study in 1988 showed that an adequate diet in pregnancy is beyond the means of women on low incomes,[84] and a recent study of low-income families by the National Children's Home showed that 10% of children under five had gone without food at some time during the previous month because of insufficient household income.[85] However, alliances between Barker's team and children's organisations today are unlikely to be as strong as those that developed between researchers and children's organisations in the 1930s. This is because Barker argues that, in order to ensure appropriate levels of foetal and infant nutrition, preventative strategies should focus on improving the health and nutrition of girls and young women, and mothers during pregnancy and lactation, even at the expense of improvements in the nutrition of children.[86] Furthermore, rising public concern about the state of the nation's children today does not focus so much on nutrition but rather on what is seen as the sorry state of contemporary family life and the unprecedented strains under which families live.[87]

The context in which the recent studies of the late effects of early development have occurred is one in which considerations regarding genetic influences on health are again coming to the fore. The subject of genetic influences on health and behaviour has been a strongly contested one.[88] Although genetic explanations could be advanced for the reported associations between patterns of foetal and infant development and later health outcomes, the Southampton group have emphasised environmental factors – in particular maternal nutrition during pregnancy – as being key. Furthermore, a co-worker with the Southampton group has suggested that their findings present a serious challenge to the validity of the twin studies which are used to investigate the genetic influences on health,[89] a claim which has been strongly contested by advocates of major genetic component in disease aetiology.[90]

In 1927, at a time when the relative importance of natural selection and environment was being actively debated, Derrick interpreted the evidence that mortality risk was determined early in life as indicating the predominantly hereditary character of generational robustness. This interpretation was rejected by most of the authorities who developed these ideas through a period when childhood nutrition was a central concern of public health and social policy. Whether the interests of researchers now investigating the early-life origins of adult disease and the interests of those involved in the rapidly developing genetics programme in medical research will continue to be opposed, or will become integrated in a mutually supportive network, remains to be seen.

References

[1] Robinson, R.J. (1992) 'Is the child father of the man?', *British Medical Journal*, vol 304, pp 789-90.

[2] Barker, D.J.P. and Osmond, C. (1986) 'Infant mortality, childhood nutrition, and ischaemic heart disease in England and Wales', *Lancet*, no 1, pp 1077-81.

[3] Barker, D.J.P. (1992) *Fetal and infant origins of adult disease*, London: BMJ Books.

[4] Department of Health (1990) *On the state of public health for the year 1989*, London: DoH, p 7.

[5] Department of Health (1992) *The health of the nation: A strategy for health in England*, London: DoH.

[6] Barker, D.J.P., Gluckman, P.D., Godfrey, K.M., Harding, J.E., Owens, J.A. and Robinson, J.S. (1993) 'Fetal nutrition and cardiovascular disease in adult life', *Lancet*, no 341, pp 938-41; Osmond, C., Barker, D.J.P., Winter, P.D., Fall, C.H.D. and Simmonds, S.J. (1993) 'Early growth and death from cardiovascular disease in women'. *British Medical Journal*, vol 307, pp 1519-24.

[7] Fall, C. (1992) 'Nutrition in early life and later outcome', *European Journal of Clinical Nutrition*, vol 46, suppl 4, pp 57-63.

[8] Kuh, D. and Davey Smith, G. (1993) 'When is mortality risk determined? Historical insights into a current debate', *Social History of Medicine*, vol 6, pp 101-23.

[9] Latour, B. (1987) *Science in action*, Buckingham/Cambridge, MA: Open University Press/Harvard University Press.

[10] For an account of the origins of the Inter-Departmental Committee see Harris, B. (1995) *The health of the schoolchild: A history of the school medical service in England and Wales*, Buckingham: Open University Press, pp 18-20.

[11] *Parliamentary Papers* (1904) Vol 32, Report of the Inter-Departmental Committee on Physical Deterioration, vol 1, pp 56-7.

[12] Quoted in Dwork, D. (1987) *War is good for babies and other young children: A history of the infant and child welfare movement in England 1898-1918*, London: Tavistock, p 20.

[13] Pearson, K. (1912) 'The intensity of natural selection in man', *Proceedings of the Royal Society of London*, Series B, vol 85, pp 469-76.

[14] Quoted in Semmel, B. (1958) 'Karl Pearson: socialist and Darwinist', *British Journal of Sociology*, vol 9, pp 111-25.

[15] Pearson, K. (1912) *Eugenics and public health: Questions of the day and of the fray, No VI*, London: Dulau and Company Ltd, pp 32-3.

[16] Newsholme, A. (1910) *Report on infant and child mortality: Supplement to the Thirty-ninth Annual Report of the Medical Officer of the Local Government Board*, London: HMSO.

[17] Board of Education (1914) *Annual report for 1913 of Chief Medical Officer of the Board of Education*, London: HMSO, pp 16-17.

[18] White, F.W. (1928) 'Natural and social selection: a "blue-book" analysis', *Eugenics Review*, vol 20, pp 98-104.

[19] Derrick, V.P.A. (1927) 'Observations on (1) errors on age on the population statistics of England and Wales and (2) the changes in mortality indicated by the national records', *Journal of the Institute of Actuaries*, vol 58, pp 117-59.

[20] Heron, D. (1927) 'Discussion', *Journal of the Institute of Actuaries*, vol 58, pp 151-3.

[21] Kermack, W.O., McKendrick, A.G. and McKinlay, P.L. (1934) 'Death rates in Great Britain and Sweden: some general regularities and their significance', *Lancet*, vol 226, pp 698-703. (Reprinted in *International Journal of Epidemiology*, 2001, vol 30, pp 678-83; see also Davey Smith, G., Kuh, D.W.O. [2001] 'Kermack and the childhood origins of adult health and disease', *International Journal of Epidemiology*, vol 30, pp 696-703.)

[22] Petty, C. (1989) 'Primary research and public health: the prioritization of nutrition research in inter-war Britain', in J. Austoker and L. Bryder (eds) *Historical perspectives in the role of the Medical Research Council*, Oxford: Oxford University Press, pp 83-4.

[23] Newsholme, A. (1910) *Report on infant and child mortality: Supplement to the Thirty-ninth Annual Report of the Medical Officer of the Local Government Board*, London: HMSO; Newman, G. (1906) *Infant mortality: A social problem*, London: HMSO; Board of Education (1914) *Annual report for 1913 of Chief Medical Officer of the Board of Education*, London: HMSO.

[24] Paton, D.N. and Findlay, L. (1926) *Child life investigations: Poverty nutrition and growth: Studies of child life in cities and rural districts in Scotland*, Medical Research Council Special Report Series No 101; Cathcart, E.P. and Murray, A.M.J. (1931) *A study in nutrition: 154 St Andrews Families*, Medical Research Council Special Report Series No 151.

[25] Petty, C. (1989) 'Primary research and public health: the prioritization of nutrition research in inter-war Britain', in J. Austoker and L. Bryder (eds) *Historical perspectives in the role of the Medical Research Council*, Oxford: Oxford University Press, p 97.

[26] Boyd Orr, J. *(1936) Food health and income*, London: Macmillan.

[27] M'Gonigle, G.C.M. and Kirby, J. (1936) *Poverty and public health*, London: Victor Gollancz, p 148.

[28] Hannington, W. (1937) *The problem of the distressed areas*, London: Victor Gollancz, pp 58-62.

[29] Hannington, W. (1937) *The problem of the distressed areas*, London: Victor Gollancz, pp 78-81.

[30] Vernon, H.M. (1939) *Health in relation to occupation*, London: Oxford University Press, p 9.

[31] Vernon, H.M. (1939) *Health in relation to occupation*, London: Oxford University Press, p 97.

[32] Cole, G.D.H. and Cole, M.I. (1937) *The condition of Britain*, London: Victor Gollancz, p 88.

[33] Cole, G.D.H. and Cole, M.I. (1937) *The condition of Britain*, London: Victor Gollancz, p 88.

[34] Ministry of Health (1946) *On the state of the public health during six years of war*, Report of the Chief Medical Officer of the Ministry of Health, 1939-45, London: HMSO, p 93.

[35] Thomson, A.M. (1978) 'Problems and politics in nutritional surveillance: fourth Boyd Orr Memorial Lecture', *Proceedings of the Nutrition Society*, vol 37, pp 317-33.

[36] Kuh, D. and Davey Smith, G. (1993) 'When is mortality risk determined? Historical insights into a current debate', *Social History of Medicine*, vol 6, pp 101-23.

[37] Case, R.A.M. (1956) 'Cohort analysis and cancer mortality in England and Wales, 1911-1954 by site and sex', *British Journal of Preventative Social Medicine*, vol 10, pp 172-99.

[38] Morris, J.N. (1960) 'Epidemiology and cardiovascular disease of middle age', *Modern Concepts of Cardiovascular Disease*, vol 29, pp 625-32.

[39] Lickint, F. (1935) 'Der Bronchialkrebs der Raucher', *Münchener Medizinische Wochenschrift*, vol 82, pp 1232-4; see also Davey Smith, G., Ströbele, S. and Egger, M. (1994) 'Smoking and health promotion in Nazi Germany', *Journal of Epidemiology and Community Health*, no 48, pp 220-3.

[40] Clemmesen, J. (ed) 'Symposium: cancer of the lung epidemiology', *Acta-Unio Internationalis Contra Cancrum*, vol 9, pp 426-635; Haenszel, W. and Shimkin, M.B. (1956) 'Smoking patterns and epidemiology of lung cancer in the US: are they compatible?', *Journal of the National Cancer Institute,* vol 16, pp 1417-41; the major early case-control studies were: Schairer, E. and Schöniger, E. (1943) 'Lungenkrebs und Tabakverbrauch', *Zeitschrift für Krebsforschung,* vol 54, pp 261-9 (translated in *International Journal of Epidemiology,* 2001, vol 30, pp 24-7); Wynder, E.L. and Graham, E.A. (1950) 'Tobacco smoking as a possible etiologic factor in bronchiogenic carcinoma', *Journal of the American Medical Association,* vol 143, pp 329-36; Doll, R. and Hill, A.B. (1950) 'Smoking and carcinoma of the lung'. *British Medical Journal,* vol 2, pp 739-48.

[41] See, for example, Keys, A. (1953) 'Prediction and possible prevention of coronary disease', *American Journal of Public Health,* vol 43, pp 1399-407.

[42] Dawber, T.R., Meadors, G.F. and Moore, F.J. (1951) 'Epidemiological approaches to heart disease: the Framingham study', *American Journal of Public Health,* vol 41, pp 279-86.

[43] Quoted in Bartley, M. (1985) 'Coronary heart disease and the public health 1850-1983', *Sociology of Health and Illness,* no 7, pp 289-313.

[44] The most complete statement of T. McKeown's views is to be found in his (1976) *The modern rise of population,* London: Arnold.

[45] Szreter, S. (1988) 'The importance of social intervention in Britain's mortality decline 1850-1914: a reinterpretation of the role of public health', *Social History of Medicine,* vol 1, pp 1-37.

[46] McKeown, T. (1979) *The role of medicine: Dream, mirage or nemesis?,* Oxford: Basil Blackwell.

[47] Berenson, G.S., Srinivasan, S.R., Freedman, D.S., Radhakrishnamurthy, B. and Dalferes Jr, E.R. (1987) 'Atherosclerosis and its evolution in childhood', *American Journal of Medical Science,* vol 294, pp 429-40.

[48] Osborn, G.R. (1967) 'Stages in development of coronary disease observed from 1,500 young subjects: relationship of hypotension and infant feeding to aetiology', *Colloques Internationaux du Centre National de la Recherche Scientifique,* vol 169, pp 93-139.

[49] Cowen, D.D. (1973) 'Myocardial infarction and infant feeding', *Practitioner*, vol 210, pp 661-3; Burr, M.L., Beasley, W.H. and Fisher, C.B. (1984) 'Breast feeding, maternal smoking and early atheroma', *European Heart Journal*, no 5, pp 588-91.

[50] Turner, R.W.D. (1976) 'Breast is best for coronary protection', *Lancet*, no II, pp 693-4.

[51] Forsdahl, A. (1977) 'Are poor living conditions in childhood and adolescence an important risk factor for arteriosclerotic heart disease?', *British Journal of Preventative Social Medicine*, vol 31, pp 91-5.

[52] Forsdahl, A. (1978) 'Living conditions in childhood and subsequent development of risk factors for arteriosclerotic heart disease: the cardiovascular survey in Finnmark 1974-75', *Journal of Epidemiology and Community Health*, vol 32, pp 34-7.

[53] Department of Health and Social Security (1984) *Diet and cardiovascular disease*, Report on Health and Social Subjects No 28, London: DHSS.

[54] Barker, D.J.P. and Osmond, C. (1986) 'Diet and coronary heart disease in England and Wales during and after the Second World War', *Journal of Epidemiology and Community Health*, vol 40, pp 37-44.

[55] Barker, D.J.P. and Osmond, C. (1986) 'Infant mortality, childhood nutrition, and ischaemic heart disease in England and Wales', *Lancet*, vol 1, pp 1077-81.

[56] Barker, D.J.P. and Osmond, C. (1987) 'Death rates from stroke in England and Wales predicted from past maternal mortality', *British Medical Journal*, vol 295, pp 83-6.

[57] Barker, D.J.P. and Osmond, C. (1987) 'Inequalities in health in Britain: specific explanations in three Lancashire towns', *British Medical Journal*, vol 294, pp 749-52.

[58] Barker, D.J.P., Winter, P.D., Osmond, C., Margetts, B. and Simmonds, S.J. (1989) 'Weight in infancy and death from ischaemic heart disease', *Lancet*, vol 2, pp 577-80.

[59] Barker, D.J.P., Gluckman, P.D., Godfrey, K.M., Harding, J.E., Owens, J.A. and Robinson, J.S. (1993) 'Fetal nutrition and cardiovascular disease in adult life', *Lancet*, vol 341, pp 938-41.

[60] Barker, D.J.P. (1998) *Mothers, babies, and disease in later life*, Edinburgh: Churchill Livingstone.

[61] McCance, R.A. and Widdowson, E.M. (1962) 'Nutrition and growth', *Proceedings of the Royal Society of London, Series B*, vol 156, pp 326-37; McCance, R.A. and Widdowson, E.M. (1974) 'The determinants of growth and form', *Proceedings of the Royal Society of London, Series B*, vol 185, pp 1-17.

[62] Kuh, D. and Davey Smith, G. (1993) 'When is mortality risk determined? Historical insights into a current debate', *Social History of Medicine*, vol 6, pp 101-23.

[63] Medical Research Council (1992) *Medical Research Council Corporate Plan*, London: MRC.

[64] Robinson, R.J. (1992) 'Is the child father of the man?', *British Medical Journal*, vol 304, pp 789-90.

[65] As discussed in Barker, D.J.P. (1992) *Fetal and infant origins of adult disease*, London: BMJ Publications, and Barker, D.J.P. (1995) 'Fetal origins of coronary heart disease', *British Medical Journal*, vol 311, pp 171-4.

[66] Elford, J., Whincup, P. and Shaper, A.G. (1991) 'Early life experience and adult cardiovascular disease: longitudinal and case control studies', *International Journal of Epidemiology*, vol 20, pp 833-44; Elford, J., Shaper, A.G. and Whincup, P. (1992) 'Early life experiences and adult cardiovascular disease: ecological studies', *Journal of Epidemiological Community Health*, vol 46, pp 1-11.

[67] Ben-Shlomo, Y. and Davey Smith, G. (1991) 'Deprivation in infancy or adult life: which is more important for mortality risk', *Lancet*, vol 337, pp 530-4; Baker, D., Illsley, R. and Vagero, D. (1993) 'Today or in the past? The origins of ischaemic heart disease', *Journal of Public Health Medicine*, vol 15, pp 243-8; Elford, J., Shaper, A.G. and Whincup, P. (1992) 'Early life experiences and adult cardiovascular disease: ecological studies', *Journal of Epidemiological Community Health*, vol 46, pp 1-11; Paneth, N. and Susser, M. (1995) 'Early origins of coronary heart disease', *British Medical Journal*, vol 310, pp 411-12.

[68] Vernon, H.M. (1939) *Health in relation to occupation*, London: Oxford University Press, p 129.

[69] Leitch, I. (1951) 'Growth and health', *British Journal of Nutrition*, vol 5, pp 142-51. (Reprinted in *International Journal of Epidemiology*, 2001, vol 30, pp 212-15.)

[70] Davey Smith, G. and Phillips, A.N. (1992) 'Confounding in epidemiological studies: why "independent" effects may not be all they seem', *British Medical Journal*, vol 305, pp 757-9.

[71] Paneth, N. and Susser, M. (1995) 'Early origins of coronary heart disease', *British Medical Journal*, vol 310, pp 411-12; Bartley, M., Power, C., Blane, D., Davey Smith, G. and Shipley, M.J. (1994) 'Birthweight and later socioeconomic disadvantage: evidence from the 1958 British cohort study', *British Medical Journal*, vol 309, pp 1475-8; Barker D.J.P. (1990) 'The fetal and infant origins of adult disease', *British Medical Journal*, vol 301, p 1111.

[72] Winter, J.M. (1984) 'Unemployment, nutrition and infant mortality in Britain 1920-1950', in J.M.Winter (ed) *The working class in modern British history*, Cambridge: Cambridge University Press.

[73] Webster, C. (1982) 'Healthy or hungry thirties?', *History of Workshop Journal*, vol 13, pp 110-29.

[74] Winter, J.M. (1984) 'Unemployment, nutrition and infant mortality in Britain 1920-1950', in J.M.Winter (ed) *The working class in modern British history*, Cambridge: Cambridge University Press.

[75] Cole, G.D.H. and Cole, M.I. (1937) *The condition of Britain*, London: Victor Gollancz, p 99.

[76] Cole, G.D.H. and Cole, M.I. (1937) *The condition of Britain*, London: Victor Gollancz, p 100.

[77] McCay, C.M., Crowell, M.F. and Maynard, L.A. (1935) 'The effect of retarded growth upon the length of life span and upon the ultimate body size', *Journal of Nutrition*, vol 10, pp 63-79.

[78] Kermack, W.O., McKendrick, A.G. and McKinlay, P.L. (1934) 'Death rates in Great Britain and Sweden: some general regularities and their significance', *Lancet*, vol 226, pp 698-703.

[79] Friend, G.E. (1935) *The schoolboy: A study of his nutrition, physical development and health*, Cambridge: Heffer and Sons, p 4.

[80] M'Gonigle, G.C.M. and Kirby, J. (1936) *Poverty and public health*, London: Victor Gollancz, p 150.

[81] Barker, D.J.P., Meade, T.W., Fall, C.H.D., Lee, A., Osmond, C., Phipps, K. and Stirling, Y. (1992) 'Relation of fetal and infant growth to plasma fibrinogen and factor VII concentrations in adult life', *British Medical Journal*, vol 304, pp 148-52.

[82] Hales, C.N., Barker, D.J.P., Clark, P.M.S., Fox, L.J., Fall, C., Osmond, C. and Winter, P.D. (1991) 'Fetal and infant growth and impaired glucose tolerance at age 64', *British Medical Journal*, vol 303, pp 1019-22.

[83] Barker, D.J.P., Winter, P.D., Osmond, C., Margetts, B. and Simmonds, S.J. (1989) 'Weight in infancy and death from ischaemic heart disease', *Lancet*, no II, pp 577-80.

[84] Durward, L. (1988) *Poverty in pregnancy: The cost of an adequate diet for expectant mothers*, London: Maternity Alliance.

[85] National Children's Home (1992) *Poverty and nutrition survey*, London: National Children's Home.

[86] Barker, D.J.P. (1998) *Mothers, babies, and disease in later life*, Edinburgh: Churchill Livingstone.

[87] National Children's Bureau (1987) *Investing in the future: Child health ten years after the Court Report*, London: Policy and Practice Review Group; Cornia, G.A. (1990) *Child poverty and deprivation in industrialised countries: Recent trends and policy options*, Innocenti Occasional Papers No 2, Florence; Fuchs, V.R. and Reklis, D.M. (1992) 'America's children: economic perspectives and policy options', *Science*, vol 255, pp 41-6; Spock, B. (1992) *Baby and child care* (6th edn), London: W.H. Allen.

[88] Rose, S., Kamin, L.J. and Lewontin, R.C. (1984) *Not in our genes: Biology, ideology and human nature*, Harmondsworth: Penguin.

[89] Phillips, D.I.W. (1993) 'Twin studies in medical research: can they tell us whether diseases are genetically determined?', *Lancet*, vol 341, pp 1008-9.

[90] Leslie, R.D.G. and Pyke, D.A. (1993) 'Twin studies in medical research', *Lancet*, vol 341, p 1418; Duffy, D.L. (1993) 'Twin studies in medical research', *Lancet*, vol 341, pp 1418-19.

Section IX
Social inequality and
population health

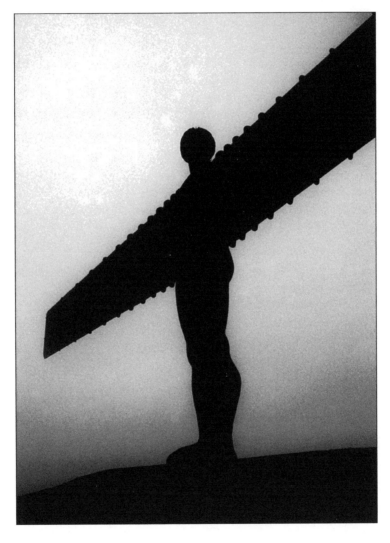

The Angel of the North, Gateshead – a celebration of the mining
industry built on the site of a former colliery pit head baths,
by Anthony Gormley. Photograph: Mary Shaw.

34

Income inequality and mortality: why are they related?

Income inequality goes hand in hand with underinvestment in human resources

George Davey Smith

The long-held belief that household income is an important indicator of risk of death has recently received strong support from a series of large prospective studies.[1,2] Income inequality within a population has also been suggested to be an important determinant of population mortality. In a cross-national comparison, Rodgers found associations between income inequality and three mortality indicators – infant mortality, life expectancy at birth, and life expectancy at age five – after taking overall gross national product into account.[3] Several replications of this, across both a wide range of countries and within industrialised nations alone, using a variety of health indicators, have appeared.[4-7] These studies have related income inequality to infant mortality,[4] life expectancy,[5] height,[6] and morbidity,[7] with a consistent finding that the less equitable the income distribution in a country, the less favourable the health outcome.

Two studies have related income inequality between states in the US to mortality rates within these states. Kennedy and colleagues find that greater income inequality is associated with higher mortality from several broad causes of death, although taking levels of poverty and smoking prevalence into account attenuates these associations.[8] Kaplan et al find associations between level of inequality and mortality in both 1980 and 1990, with trends in mortality differences between states over this decade being inconsistently related to changes in income inequality.[9]

British Medical Journal, 1996, vol 312, pp 987-8

In Britain, reliable data on income inequality by area are not readily available. However, Ben-Shlomo et al have used the variation in small area deprivation scores within local authority areas in Britain as their indicator of socioeconomic inequality[10] and have demonstrated that both overall level of deprivation and variation in deprivation contribute to an area's mortality experience, with overall level of deprivation being of somewhat greater explanatory power.

The existence of these associations seems secure, but what do they mean? They seem to show that inequality per se is bad for national health, whatever the absolute material standards of living within a country. The reasons for this have been framed by the leading proponent of the income inequality hypothesis in explicitly psychological terms: "the evidence strongly suggests that the health effects of income distribution involve comparative social and cognitive processes, rather than the direct effects of material standards."[5] The implication is that the psychological effects of being low down the social ladder have detrimental health effects, whatever the actual material conditions of life. Biological plausibility can be sought in human and animal psychoneuroendo crinological studies, but this rarely goes beyond analogy. When the major causes of death are considered – cardiovascular diseases and cancers – it seems odd to find apparently instantaneous changes in mortality in response to changes in income inequality,[5,9] since these diseases are ones in which causal exposures are thought to act for many years before death. Studies based on individuals have borne out the expectation that cumulative measures of lifetime social circumstances – such as wealth,[11] family assets,[12] lifetime earnings,[1] and occupational careers[13] – are the crucial socioeconomic predictors of longevity. Short-term changes in income inequality will have only a moderate influence on such lifetime exposure.

Changes in absolute income levels and changes in mortality over time have not been strongly associated,[14] in part because material factors will produce changes in mortality with very different latency periods depending on the cause of death. This makes interpreting changes in all-cause mortality problematic. Increases in permanent but not transitory income are associated with declines in relative mortality,[15] in keeping with the evidence on the importance of cumulative socioenvironmental insults.

Early exposures will have long-lasting effects

In general, however, secular declines in mortality have been remarkably resistant to the influence of even dramatic social changes. This reflects the fact that such changes cannot retrospectively alter what has gone before, so the influence of such social assets as education, welfare coverage, and infrastructural improvement are not reversed in the short term. The well established benefits of preschool programmes in deprived areas on the social and personal functioning of the recipients of these programmes when they are adults[16] would not be expected to disappear instantly when the socially progressive administrations which established them are replaced. Similarly, there are likely to be long-lasting biological assets, reflected in secular increases in height together with the improvements in health during youth and early adulthood that were seen for the cohorts who are now elderly. These assets, too, are not lost during periods of increasing social polarisation.

Considering time trends in mortality provides a framework for viewing the effects of income inequality. In Britain and the US, the continuing secular decline in mortality was not reversed by increases in income inequality seen earlier in this century[17,18] and more recently.[19] This is well illustrated by the analysis of Kaplan et al, in which income inequality in the US increased from 1980 to 1990 while overall mortality fell.[9] The only group for which the continued fall in mortality does not survive increases in inequality is the young adults, for whom recent trends in mortality have not been favourable,[5] particularly for residents of deprived areas.[20] It is, of course, the people within this age group who die of causes – in particular, accidents and violence – which are not the outcome of long-term biological processes and which will plausibly respond rapidly to increasing social disruption. Indeed, homicide is the cause of death found to be most strongly related to both income inequality indices used by Kennedy et al.[8] Similarly, more rapid responses to increasing inequality and social polarisation may be expected for psychological distress, general well-being, and morbidity than for chronic disease mortality. The finding of a relative deterioration in health status of civil servants anticipating job change and non-employment in comparison with those remaining in stable employment[21] provides an example of this. Inequality may make people miserable long before it kills them.

The apparently overly rapid response of mortality to changes in income distribution may have various explanations. First, relatively small absolute changes in mortality are involved, with increases in life expectancy of about two years being seen in the period covered by the analyses of Wilkinson[5] and Kaplan,[9] while 30-year increases, unrelated to any systematic change in income distribution,[17,18] have been seen over the century. Major determinants of variations in mortality between countries or between areas within countries need not be the same as the major determinants of overall population mortality. Second, those countries that are now experiencing the largest increases in income inequality are precisely those that have systematically underinvested in human resources for many years. The countries and governmental units which are currently those experiencing the greatest increases in inequality will contain the populations whose social and biological assets have been most undermined.

Increases in income inequality go hand in hand with underinvestment, which will reap poor health outcomes in the future. In the US, poor investment in education and low expenditure on medical care is seen in the states with the most unequal income distribution.[9] Similarly, low birth weight is commoner in the states with the greatest inequalities, with the possible long-term detrimental influences on adult health that go with this. Cross-nationally, higher levels of both social expenditure and taxation as a proportion of gross domestic product are associated with longer life expectancy, lower maternal mortality, and a smaller proportion of low birthweight deliveries.[22] The relative and even absolute deterioration in social and biological assets that is occurring in increasingly unequal societies can be expected to produce poor health outcomes in the future.

The only coherent argument against redistributive social policies is that they hinder overall economic growth. Here it is supposed that the greater rewards offered to the entrepreneurially successful makes them even more successful and in turn drives overall economic growth, which, through the 'trickle down' effect, ultimately benefits the poor. Cross-national comparisons, however, show the reverse: if anything, countries with greater income inequalities have shown lower levels of economic growth.[23]

The current [Conservative] government, however, continues to pay no heed to the growing evidence[5,18,20,21] that increasing income inequality is bad for the economy, bad for crime rates, bad for people's working lives, bad for infrastructural development, and bad for health – in both the short and long term.

References

[1] Wolfson, M., Rowe, G., Gentleman, J.F. and Tomiak, M. (1993) 'Career earnings and death: a longitudinal analysis of older Canadian men', *Journals of Gerontology, Series B, Psychological Sciences and Social Sciences*, vol 48, pp S167-79.

[2] **Davey Smith, G., Neaton, J.D., Wentworth, D., Stamler, R. and Stamler, J. (1996) 'Socioeconomic differentials in mortality risk among men screened for the MRFIT: Part I – results for 300,685 white men', *American Journal of Public Health*, vol 86, pp 486-96.**

[3] Rodgers, G.B. (1979) 'Income and inequality as determinants of mortality: an international cross-sectional analysis', *Population Studies*, vol 33, pp 343-51.

[4]   Waldman, R.J. (1992) 'Income distribution and infant mortality', *Quarterly Journal of Economics*, vol 107, pp 1283-302.

[5]   Wilkinson, R.G. (1994) *Unfair shares*, Ilford: Barnardo's.

[6]   Steckel, R.H. (1995) 'Stature and the standard of living', *Journal of Economic Literature*, vol 33, pp 1903-40.

[7]   van Doorslaer, E., Wagstaff, A., Bleichrodt, H., Calonge, S., Gerdtham, U.-G., Gerfin, M., Geurts, J. Gross, L., Hakkinen, U., Leu, R.E., O'Donnell, O., Propper, C., Puffer, F., Rodriguez, M., Sundberg, G. and Winkelhake, O. (1997) 'Income-related inequalities in health: some international comparisons', *Journal of Health Economics*, vol 16, pp 93-112.

[8]   Kennedy, B.P., Kawachi, I. and Prothrow-Stith, D. (1996) 'Income distribution and mortality: cross sectional ecological study of the Robin Hood index in the US', *British Medical Journal*, vol 312, pp 1004-7.

[9]   Kaplan, G.A., Pamuk, E.R., Lynch, J.W., Cohen, R.D. and Balfour, J.L. (1996) 'Inequality in income and mortality in the US: analysis of mortality and potential pathways', *British Medical Journal*, vol 312, pp 999-1003.

[10]   Ben-Shlomo, Y., White, I.R. and Marmot, M. (1996) 'Does the variation in the socioeconomic characteristics of an area affect mortality?', *British Medical Journal*, vol 312, p 1013.

[11]   Menchik, P.L. (1993) 'Economic status as a determinant of mortality among black and white older men: does poverty kill?', *Population Studies*, vol 47, pp 427-36.

[12]   Mare, R.D. (1990) 'Socioeconomic careers and differential mortality among older men in the US', in J. Vallin, S. D'Souza and A. Palloni (eds) *Measurement and analysis of mortality: New approaches*, Oxford: Clarendon Press, pp 362-87.

[13]   Hart, C., Davey Smith, G., Blane, D., Gillis, C. and Hawthorne, V. (1995) 'Social mobility, health and cardiovascular mortality', *Journal of Epidemiology and Community Health*, vol 49, pp 552-3.

[14]   Kunitz, S.J. and Engerman, S.L. (1992) 'The ranks of death: secular trends in income and mortality', *Health Transition Review*, vol 2, suppl, pp 29-46.

[15] Graham, J.D., Chang, B.-H. and Evans, J.S. (1992) 'Poorer is riskier', *Risk Analysis*, vol 12, pp 333-7.

[16] Schweinhart, L.J., Barnes, H.V. and Weikart, D.P. (1993) *Significant benefits: The High / Scope Perry preschool study through age 27*, Ypsilanti, MI: High/Scope Press.

[17] Routh, G. (1980) *Occupation and pay in Great Britain 1906-79*, London: Macmillan.

[18] Williamson, J.G. and Lindert, P.H. (1980) *American inequality: A macroeconomic history*, New York, NY: Academic Press.

[19] Atkinson, A.B., Rainwater, L. and Smeeding, T.M. (1995) *Income distribution in OECD countries*, Paris: Organisation for Economic Cooperation and Development.

[20] McCarron, P.G., Davey Smith, G. and Womersley, J. (1994) 'Deprivation and mortality: increasing differentials in Glasgow 1979-1992', *British Medical Journal*, vol 309, pp 1481-2.

[21] Ferrie, J.E., Shipley, M.J., Marmot, M.G., Stansfeld, S. and Davey Smith, G. (1995) 'Health effects of anticipation of job change and non-employment: longitudinal data from the Whitehall II Study', *British Medical Journal*, vol 311, pp 1264-9.

[22] Gough, I. and Thomas, T. (1994) 'Why do levels of human welfare vary among nations?', *International Journal of Health Services*, vol 24, pp 715-48.

[23] Glyn, A. and Miliband, D. (eds) (1994) *Paying for inequality: The economic cost of social injustice*, London: Rivers Oram Press.

35

Understanding it all: health, meta-theories, and mortality trends

George Davey Smith and Matthias Egger

Investigations into the determinants of health within and between countries contribute to a generally slow, but incremental, process. Leaping forward to the big picture of how it all fits together represents an attractive alternative to merely continuing with this laborious spadework. An example of such 'big picture' thinking is the suggestion by Bunker and colleagues[1] that bounded freedom is the key to health and wellbeing, a viewpoint which shares some characteristics with others who consider embeddedness within strong social networks as being the important determinant of population health.[2] The positive benefits of strong social ties seem self-evident, but "the plausible role of biological pathways leading from social disconnection to disease" that Bunker and colleagues evoke has not been satisfactorily elucidated. Indeed, degree of social support may be influenced by health rather than the reverse. The supposedly protective influence of social support has been shown among the majority populations of the US, UK, and Scandinavia, but in groups that have different connotations for such networks social ties can appear detrimental, rather than beneficial, to health.[3]

One theory of population health that has received considerable attention is the income inequality perspective of Richard Wilkinson, recently elegantly summarised in his book *Unhealthy societies*.[4] This view, which incorporates explanations relating to social networks, considers that the psychological consequences of living in an unequal society are the primary determinants of overall state of health. Several alternative models of the important determinants of population health to these essentially psychosocial accounts exist. The high profile of the human genome project has certainly led to the revival of primarily genetic accounts of the distribution of sickness. Conversely, the importance of life-style factors and their concomitants – for example,

British Medical Journal, 1996, vol 313, pp 1584-5

smoking, alcohol consumption, cholesterol concentrations, and blood pressure – may have been underestimated because only one measurement is used in epidemiological studies. Thus some contend that if proper account is taken of their importance there might be little left to explain,[5,6] within developed countries at least. An almost diametrically opposed view took its lead from the failure of such life-style factors to account for the geographical and social distribution of many diseases.[7,8] The hypothesis that influences from early life, particularly intrauterine and infant growth, influence long-term health was advanced and has now been tested in an impressive array of ecological and prospective studies.[9] The arrival of a new paradigm of the determinants of adult health was announced.[10]

These, then, are some of the meta-theories of population health: social cohesion and the psychological consequences of inequality; genes; life-style factors; and long-term effects of suboptimal early development. It would be worth considering how they fare in accounting for the important population differences in health: the large time trends in life expectancy and the unequal distribution of mortality risk between and within countries. Let us briefly consider one issue that has generated a great deal of interest – the relative (and in some cases absolute) deterioration in state of health in Eastern Europe.[11-13]

The data seem to provide strong support for the income inequality hypothesis since life expectancy and income inequality (measured by the Gini coefficient) are inversely correlated[14] (Figure 1). Changes in income inequality and changes in life expectancy between 1987 and 1993 also show a sizeable correlation ($r=-0.62$). These countries have undergone a transformation from Stalinist pseudosocialism to the vagaries of the free market, and even the chief cheerleader for unfettered free market capitalism, the World Bank, was forced to ask: "Is transition a killer?"[14] The growth of capitalism in Britain after the industrial revolution was associated with unfavourable mortality trends[15] and a growth in inequalities in health,[16] and the same now seems to be happening as capitalism penetrates the final frontier.

With the exception of genetic accounts, the various explanatory categories have been proposed as major contributors to the unfavourable mortality trends in Eastern Europe. Thus in discussing the potential contribution of psychosocial stress Bobak and Marmot suggest that 30% of the excess mortality can be accounted for by a sense of pessimism.[12] The unfavourable mortality trends in Russia have been attributed to alcohol misuse, with the improvements in mortality during Gorbachev's anti-alcohol campaign being cited in support of this.[14] Smoking and nutritional factors have also been considered important.[13] Much of Eastern Europe suffered greatly during the Second World War, and unfavourable mortality trends have been attributed to the long-term effects of people living through

Figure 1: Life expectancy and income inequality in post-transition Eastern Europe

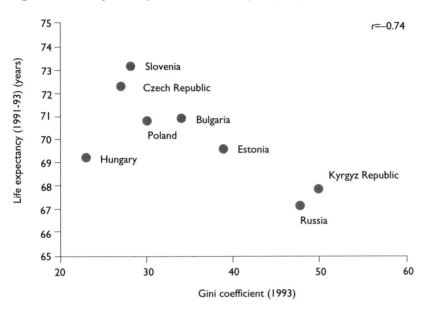

these times.[17] Indeed, mortality rates of men and women who were born or were children in the most affected parts of the former Soviet Union during the war show just such an effect,[18] although the overall contribution to changing life expectancy seems to be comparatively small.

Taken together, the mechanisms that have been advanced could account for greater mortality changes than have actually happened. This is probably because we are in some cases double counting – for example, the psychosocial effects of social disintegration will be expressed in increased alcohol and tobacco consumption and decreased self-care. Direct psychological mechanisms, are, indeed, unlikely causes of mortality trends: the reduction in mortality in Britain since the late 19th century has hardly been accompanied by improved social support and social networks. Happiness, life satisfaction, and job satisfaction in Britain have changed little over the past 30 years, while death rates have continued to plummet.[19,20] The causes of death responsible for rising mortality in Eastern Europe – coronary heart disease, lung cancer, and accidents[15] – are those that increased during a period of generally declining mortality in Western Europe and the US. As these diseases can increase while overall mortality is falling and economic progress is being made, their accompaniment by a general worsening of health or increasing social disintegration is not inevitable. A mainly psychological attribution may be as one-sided as earlier attempts to consider these conditions, which affect poor people, as diseases of affluence. Coronary heart disease was considered by many to be caused by type A behaviour – the rushed, time-pressured businessman was the paradigmatic coronary case. This association, which soon stopped being apparent, was generated by socially conditioned perceptions of associations, which were then reified into pathophysiological mechanisms. As many plausible biological pathways between type A behaviour and coronary heart disease were produced as is now the case for the currently fashionable psychosocial factors.

The problems that psychosocial explanations have with accounting for trends and geographical differences in mortality are also seen with respect to the other categories of explanation. Consider (among many others) these paradoxes: low overall and cardiovascular disease mortality in Japan, a country with high smoking rates; the decreasing overall death rates during increases in smoking and dietary fat intake that occurred in many countries; and the low international correlations between past infant mortality rates or current birth weight and mortality from coronary heart disease. For different causes of death, and in different temporal and geographical situations, the determinants of mortality patterns will be distinct. Extrapolating from the past to the present and from one place to another is necessary for broad theorising on the underlying determinants of mortality trends but, in the end, this can only be the start of the more difficult empirical task of understanding the particular factors which act together to produce the patterns seen in any one specific instance.[21]

References

[1] Bunker, J.P., Stansfeld, S. and Potter, J. (1996) 'Freedom, responsibility and health', *British Medical Journal*, vol 313, pp 1582-4.

[2] Judge, K. (1994) 'Beyond health care', *British Medical Journal*, vol 309, pp 1454-5.

[3] Kunitz, S.J. (1994) *Diseases and social diversity*, Oxford: Oxford University Press.

[4] Wilkinson, R.G. (1996) *Unhealthy societies: The afflictions of inequality*, London: Routledge.

[5] Peto, R. (1994) 'Smoking and death: the past 40 years and the next 40', *British Medical Journal*, vol 309, pp 937-9.

[6] Peto, R. (1993) 'Epidemiology of blood cholesterol', in M. Laker, A. Neil, and C. Wood (eds) *Cholesterol-lowering trials: Advice for the British physician*, London: Royal College of Physicians.

7   Barker, D.J.P. and Osmond, C. (1986) 'Infant mortality, childhood nutrition, and ischaemic heart disease in England and Wales', *Lancet*, vol 1, pp 1077-81.

8   Barker, D.J.P. (1989) 'Rise and fall of Western diseases', *Nature*, vol 338, pp 371-2.

9   Barker, D.J.P. (1994) *Mothers, babies, and disease in later life*, London: British Medical Journal Publishing Group.

10 Robinson, R.J. (1992) 'Is the child father of the man?', *British Medical Journal*, vol 304, pp 789-90.

11 Watson, P. (1995) 'Explaining rising mortality among men in Eastern Europe', *Social Science and Medicine*, vol 41, pp 923-34.

12 Bobak, M. and Marmot, M.G. (1995) 'East-West mortality divide and its potential explanations: proposed research agenda', *British Medical Journal*, vol 312, pp 421-5.

13 Chenet, L., McKee, M., Fulop, N., Bojan, F., Brand, H., Hort, A. et al (1996) 'Changing life expectancy in central Europe: is there a single reason?', *Journal of Public Health Medicine*, vol 18, pp 329-36.

14 World Bank (1996) *From plan to market: World development report*, New York, NY: Oxford University Press.

15 Floud, R., Wachter, K. and Gregory, A. (1990) *Height, health and history*, Cambridge: Cambridge University Press.

16 Woods, R. and Williams, N. (1995) 'Must the gap widen before it can be narrowed? Long-term trends in social class mortality differentials', *Continuity and Change*, vol 10, pp 105-37.

17 Dinkel, R.H. (1985) 'The seeming paradox of increasing mortality in a highly industrialised nation: the example of the Soviet Union', *Population Studies*, vol 39, pp 87-97.

18 Anderson, B.A. and Silver, B.D. (1989) 'Patterns of cohort mortality in the Soviet population', *Population and Development Review*, vol 15, pp 471-501.

19 Clark, A.E. and Oswald, A.J. (1994) 'Unhappiness and unemployment', *Economic Journal*, vol 104, pp 648-59.

[20] Clark, A.E., Oswald, A.J. and Warr, P.B. (1996) 'Is job satisfaction U-shaped in age?', *Journal of Occupational Psychology*, vol 69, pp 57-81.

[21] Kunitz, S.J. (1994) 'The value of particularism in the study of the cultural, social, and behavioral determinants of mortality', in L.C. Chen, A. Kleinman and N.C. Ware (eds) *Health and social change in international perspective*, Boston, MA: Harvard University Press.

Section X
Reducing health inequalities, now and in the future

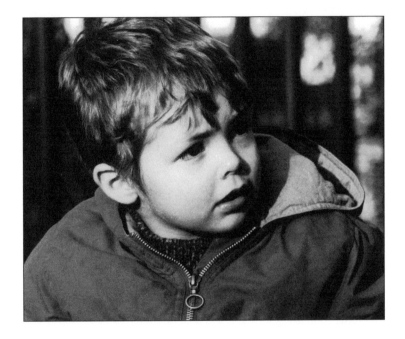

Photograph: Mary Shaw.

36

The widening health gap: what are the solutions?

George Davey Smith, Daniel Dorling, David Gordon and Mary Shaw

Introduction

Throughout the long 18 years of Conservative government the Labour Party referred to the issue of increasing social inequalities in health as an area of particular concern. Before the May 1997 General Election, Labour announced that it would launch an Independent Inquiry into Inequalities in Health. The Inquiry was launched in July 1997, and at the launch Tessa Jowell, the Minister for Public Health, criticised the health strategy of the previous administration for "its excessive emphasis on life-style issues" which "cast the responsibility back on to the individual".[1] Tessa Jowell gave a commitment regarding the Independent Inquiry's findings that these "conclusions, based on evidence, will contribute to the development of a new strategy for health".[1]

The Independent Inquiry report appeared in 1998.[2] It presents a wealth of evidence on the extent and trends of inequalities in health. Together with a large body of other evidence, the new report demonstrates clearly that the last two decades have seen large and growing inequalities in income in Britain, and that these have been accompanied by equally stark increasing inequalities in health and in life chances more generally.

The main task of the Independent Inquiry was to produce recommendations for policies that could alleviate inequalities in health. In fact 39 recommendations, many with sets of sub-recommendations, are given. While these contain some focused policies, the overall force of the recommendations is considerably weakened by a lack of prioritisation; by being inadequately concrete; and by being uncosted.[3]

Critical Public Health, 1999, vol 9, pp 151-70

No prioritisation: The recommendations are not presented in any hierarchy and the essential fact that inequalities in health follow closely on inequalities in wealth is underemphasised. The one (of 39) sets of recommendations on the necessity to reduce poverty and income inequalities thus appears to have the same status as those regarding reducing traffic speed, or offering concessionary fares to pensioners. The fundamental role of inequalities in material circumstances in producing the inequalities in other exposures is therefore missed and it is possible that many of the recommendations could be adopted – at least nominally – without addressing the underlying determinants of health inequalities.

Inadequately concrete: Many of the sets of recommendations are too vague to be useful. Recommending "measures to prevent suicide among young people, especially among young men and seriously mentally ill people" or "the development of policies to reduce the fear of crime and violence, and to create a safe environment for people to live in" would receive universal support, but they are of little use if it is not specified how these things are to be brought about. For example, the report advocates the development of a high quality public transport system which is affordable to the user and specifically refers to the large relative increases in rail fares compared to motoring costs, but fails to make the obvious link with the privatisation of the railways.

No costings: As the recommendations are not costed it is impossible to evaluate the relative costs of their implementation, the predicted social benefits which would follow and the opportunity costs of not investing in other areas. This lack of costing will allow the recommendations to be side-stepped by declaring that they are unrealistic and cannot be implemented in the current economic climate.

The last major report on inequalities in health was that of the committee chaired by Sir Douglas Black (which produced the Black Report[4]), commissioned by the last Labour government in 1977 and reporting to the then new Conservative administration in 1980. The Black Report discussed the inequalities in health and in income that existed at the time and made a series of policy recommendations. These were rejected by Patrick Jenkin (the then Secretary of State for Social Services) as being unrealistic and the report was deliberately released before a national holiday, with no press release or press conference and with only 260 copies produced.

For 17 of the 18 years of Conservative government the Labour Party made political capital out of the non-implementation of the recommendations of the Black Report. Indeed the enthusiasm for addressing inequalities in health was one element which survived the transformation from old to new Labour. A few weeks before the May 1997 Labour election victory, Baroness Jay – now Leader of the House of Lords and Minister for Women – stated that the Black Report "provided the essential base and policy guide to any responsible government wanting to take action" on inequalities in health.[5] She committed the incoming Labour government to a health strategy in which the distribution of economic resources would be a key element.[5] In the same debate another Labour peer stated that the "failure since 1980 to implement any of the Black Report recommendations has caused disappointment to many and must have caused a great deal of needless suffering on the part of many of the poorest families".[5]

In the light of Labour's long-term declared policy on inequalities in health it is very disappointing that a major limitation on the Independent Inquiry was its brief from the government which stated that it had to be carried out "within the broad framework of the Government's overall financial strategy". This constrained the Inquiry from proposing markedly redistributive fiscal policies, given some of the commitments on taxation made by Labour before the 1997 Election.

In this chapter we consider the current evidence on increasing inequalities in health, in many cases using data which are more recent than those available to the Independent Inquiry. Our focus is on socioeconomic differentials, not only the important differences in health status and health service access which are seen between ethnic groups or according to gender or sexuality. When reading the information contained in our report it is worth remembering that the Black Report was commissioned in 1977, when inequalities in income were at a historic low point. In 1977, 7% of the population were on incomes below half of the average after housing costs; in 1995/96 this had more than trebled to 24%.[6] The increasing inequalities in income – which have resulted in the UK leading the developed world in income inequality and child poverty[7] – started under the last Labour government, in 1977. Tony Blair has declared that "I believe in greater equality. If the Labour government has not raised the living standards of the poorest by the end of its time in office it will have failed".[8] To ensure it does not fail the government should take the Independent Inquiry's evidence seriously and reconsider its stance of distancing itself yet further from redistributive social policies.

Inequalities in health in Britain

Mortality rates in different communities

The widening health gap in Britain can be seen when considering the difference in mortality rates between communities living in different parts of Britain. Table 1 lists the 20 areas (county boroughs

Table 1: Ranked SMRs for deaths under 65 for the 20 areas with the highest mortality in 1990-92, with SMRs for 1993-95

Rank	Area (1993-95)	SMR<65 (1990-92)	SMR <65 (1993-95)
1	Glasgow	179	196
2	Shoreditch	169	166
3	Greenock Burgh	168	189
4	Salford	166	163
5	Port-Glasgow Burgh	166	180
6	Clydebank Burgh	163	154
7	Oldham	157	149
8	Southwark	155	151
9	Middlesbrough	154	145
10	Coatbridge Burgh	153	161
11	Dumbarton Burgh	148	152
12	Manchester	147	158
13	Lambeth	147	149
14	Hammersmith	147	154
15	Preston	146	149
16	Bermondsey	144	169
17	Hamilton Burgh	143	154
18	Rutherglen Burgh	141	158
19	Poplar	141	146
20	Warrington	141	146
Overall in these areas		158	167
England and Wales		100	100

and urban and rural remainders of counties) which were reported as having the highest standardised mortality ratios (SMRs[9]) in 1990-92.[10] In nearly all of these 20 areas the SMRs increased between the early 1990s (1990-92) and the mid-1990s (1993-95).

In the period 1993-95 the same areas that had high SMRs in 1990-92 have even higher SMRs. This demonstrates the importance of structural factors in determining life chances. A person's likelihood of dying young is not a matter of chance, since their social position and their life trajectory are conditioned by the social circumstances of the community in which they live.

If we consider the SMRs for all 292 of these areas in Britain, grouped according to deciles ('tenths') of the population (Table 2), then we can see that the gap in deaths between the best tenth and worst tenth of the British population had grown wider by the mid-1990s (1993-95) than at any time since the 1950s. The SMR of the decile with the highest mortality in 1990-92 (SMR=142) is even higher in 1993-95 (SMR=147). In terms of absolute numbers of deaths, 45,095 people died in the 10% of areas with the highest mortality in 1993-95 compared to 27,738 in the 10% of areas with the lowest mortality. The ratio of the death rates in the worst and best

Table 2: Age-gender SMRs for deaths under 65 in Britain by deciles of population

Decile	1950-53	1959-63	1969-73	1981-85	1986-89	1990-92	1993-95
1	131.0	135.5	131.2	135.0	139.2	142.3	147.4
2	118.1	123.0	115.6	118.6	120.9	121.4	120.9
3	112.1	116.5	112.0	114.2	113.9	111.3	112.7
4	109.0	110.7	108.1	109.8	106.9	104.9	106.7
5	102.5	104.5	103.0	102.1	102.2	99.0	98.5
6	98.6	97.4	96.9	95.7	95.6	93.5	94.6
7	93.1	90.9	91.8	91.6	91.9	90.9	91.7
8	88.7	87.6	88.9	89.3	89.1	86.5	86.6
9	85.7	83.1	87.0	84.3	83.0	80.4	80.2
10	81.8	77.1	83.0	79.2	78.1	76.2	74.5
Ratio of worst tenth:best tenth							
	1.6	1.8	1.6	1.7	1.8	1.91.	2.0

10% areas has been increasing since the late 1960s/early 1970s, but increased most rapidly during the 1980s.

It could be argued that the polarisation of mortality ratios shown in Table 2 is an artefact of the method used to rank areas by mortality ratios and is not indicative of a polarisation of health inequalities by poverty, income and wealth. To counter this possibility we have recalculated the SMRs for people in Britain according to the average incomes of people in the workforce in the areas in which they live estimated from 1991 Census data by parliamentary constituency. From Table 3 it can be seen that the poorest 10% of the population, with average incomes for those in the workforce of £9,785, saw mortality ratios rise from 127 to 134 over the last 10 years, whereas the richest 10% saw mortality ratios fall over this period. We can only calculate these ratios by income for the 1980s and 1990s, but it is apparent that

Table 3: SMRs for deaths under 65, by area and average income (1981-95)

SMR <65 all	Average income	SMR 1981-85	SMR 1986-90	SMR 1991-95	% change
1	9,785	127	131	134	8
2	10,508	118	119	120	2
3	10,904	110	110	108	−2
4	11,200	103	104	101	−2
5	11,446	101	100	100	−1
6	11,728	99	99	97	−2
7	12,039	94	93	90	−4
8	12,330	89	87	84	−4
9	12,744	87	86	83	−4
10	13,485	84	81	80	−4

the polarisation in mortality has followed the polarisation of incomes geographically.

Infant mortality

The widening gap in health by social class can be seen not only in the mortality rates of adults. In his last report as Chief Medical Officer[11] Sir Kenneth Calman highlighted in his introduction a number of overall improvements in health, including the fact that infant mortality had reached its lowest recorded rate, of 5.9 deaths per 1,000 live births. However, a closer inspection of these rates reveals that when these rates are considered by social class (of father) there are growing differences between the death rates of babies with social class I fathers (professional occupations) and babies with social class V fathers (unskilled manual workers) – babies of unskilled manual workers are 2.2 times more likely to die than babies with fathers in professional occupations (Figure 1).[12] For every 1,000 babies born whose father is social class V, eight babies have died within their first year.

These trends are based on only a few years – because of changes in how data are reported – and a relatively small number of deaths. Therefore, it is important to monitor the infant mortality rate by social class over the coming years to see if this worrying trend continues.

Mortality and social class

While life expectancy has been rising for both men and women throughout the [20th] century not all social groups have enjoyed the

Figure 1: Infant mortality by social class (1993-96)

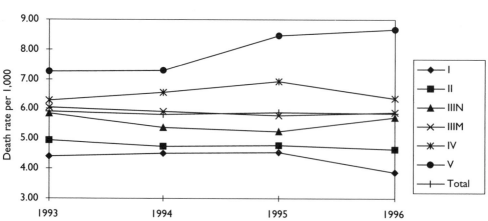

Table 4: SMRs for men under 65, by social class (1921-93[a])

	I	II	IV	V	Ratio class V:I
1921-23	82	94	101	125	1.5
1930-32	90	94	102	111	1.2
1949-53	96	92	104	118	1.4
1959-63	76	81	103	143	1.9
1970-72	44	91	114	137	1.8
1979-83	66	76	116	165	2.5
1991-93	66	72	116	189	2.9

[a] Social class III was divided into two groups – III non-manual and III manual – from 1970 onwards and so has been omitted from the table.

same improvements. The difference in life expectancy between social classes has widened such that on average a man from a professional or managerial occupation (classes I and II, such as a doctor or lawyer), can expect to live 5.2 years longer than a man who works in a semi- or unskilled manual job (classes IV and V). For women, the difference is 3.4 years.[13] This difference means that a male labourer was 2.9 times more likely to die at any time before retirement than a doctor or a lawyer. This is the widest gap reported since 1921, when the government first reported figures in this way, and it continues to grow.

Table 4 shows SMRs for men of working age by social class,[14] from 1921 to 1993. From this it can be seen that the mortality gap between classes V (unskilled manual jobs) and I (professional occupations) has been growing since the 1930s.[15]

We can also see the widening gap in health by social class in terms of 'years of potential life lost'. While SMRs have the advantage of taking into account the different age structures of the social class groups, they are heavily influenced by the deaths occurring in the oldest age category. However, the largest relative class differences in absolute mortality are at younger ages, and so it is also worth considering the relative number of years of productive life which are lost through premature mortality. As Table 5 shows, the ratio of years of life lost for social class V as compared to social class I between the early 1970s and early 1990s rose from 2.1 to 3.3.[16]

Increases in poverty and inequality

Poverty and income inequality in Britain are now greater than at any time since the 1930s. Poverty and inequality have increased particularly rapidly since 1979. This alarming increase was a direct result of successive Conservative government economic and social policies that were designed to promote efficiency and reduce inflation.

Table 5: Annual age-adjusted rate of years of potential life lost per 1,000 of the population (data refer to males age 20-64, all-causes of death, England and Wales)[16]

Social class	1970-72	1979-80, 1982-83	1991-93
I	49	37	28
II	52	42	32
III non-manual	65	54	46
III manual	66	58	51
IV	76	68	53
V	103	106	93
Ratio V:I	2.1	2.9	3.3

These had the effect of increasing unemployment, increasing indirect taxes that effect the poorest most and reducing the adequacy of welfare benefits.

Inequality and poverty have increased much faster in Britain over the past 20 years than in almost any over country. For example, Bradshaw and Chen[17] looked at levels of poverty in Australia, Canada, Germany, Israel, the Netherlands, Norway, Sweden, Taiwan, UK, and USA in circa 1979, 1985 and 1990. Poverty was defined as households below half (50%) average income after social security benefits and direct taxes. They conclude: "There has been an increase in poverty in all countries except Israel and Canada over this period between 1979 and 1990 but by far the sharpest increase in poverty has occurred in the UK where between 1979 and 1990 the poverty rate more than doubled".[17]

Other evidence suggests that income inequality – the inequitable distribution of income in the population – increased faster in Britain over the period 1967-92 than in comparable countries (Table 6).[7]

As shown in Table 7, over the same period the child poverty rate has also increased at a faster rate in Britain than in other comparable countries (many of which saw a reduction in the rate).[7]

The rapid growth of inequality and poverty in Britain can be clearly seen from official statistics on the percentage of the population living in households with incomes of less than half the average after allowing for differences in housing costs. This is the poverty/income inequality measure that is currently favoured by both the British government and the European Statistical Office (Eurostat). Figure 2 shows that during the 1960s the amount of income inequality in Britain remained fairly constant, with around 11% of the population living on incomes below half of the average. The recession and stagflation of the early 1970s caused by the OPEC oil price increases lead to the numbers living on less than half average incomes to rise to a peak of just over 13%. The relatively progressive government social and economic

Table 6: Increases in income inequality (1967-92)[7]

Increase (%)	Country
More than 30	UK
16-29	US, Sweden
10-15	Australia, Denmark
5-10	Norway, Netherlands, Belgium
Around 0	Spain, France, Finland, Canada, Germany
Decreases	Italy

Table 7: Increases in child poverty (1967-92)[7]

Increase (%)	Country
More than 30	UK, US
10-15	Norway
5-10	Netherlands, Belgium, Germany
Around 0	Australia, Spain, France
Decreases	Sweden, Denmark, Finland, Canada, Italy

Figure 2: Percentage of the population with below half average incomes after housing costs (1961-96)

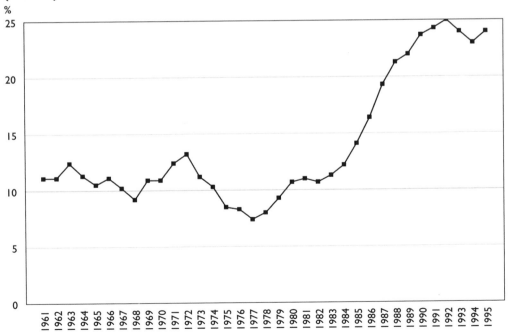

Source: DSS[6]; Hills[18].

policies until the mid-1970s resulted in poverty and inequality falling rapidly to a low of under 8% of the population in 1977/78.[18] From this point a rise in income inequality occurred. The 1979 Election victory of the Conservative Party under Margaret Thatcher's leadership caused a rapid growth in poverty and inequality which increased throughout the 1980s and early 1990s. By 1995-96, almost a quarter (24%) of the British population were living on incomes that were so low that they were below half the average income.

Similarly studies that examine poverty in terms of both low income and low standard of living (high deprivation) have shown that poverty increased by almost 50% between 1983 and 1990. In 1983, 14% of households (approximately 7.5 million people) were living in poverty and, by 1990, 20% of households (approximately 11 million people) were living in poverty.

Table 8 shows that, after housing costs, the richest 10% of the population have 27% of total income, whereas the poorest 10% have only 2.2% of total income. This compares with 20.9% and 4%, respectively, in 1979.[6,18]

Britain is now a country where the richest 50 people in 1996 had income and wealth of over £34 billion,[19] which is far in excess of the wealth and incomes of the 'poorest' 5.5 million Britons.

Table 9 shows the changes in incomes of the poorest and richest 10% of families between 1979 and 1995-96. The poorest 10% of single adult households received, on average, £208 less in 1995-96 than

Table 8: Distribution of income: households below average income series (1979 to 1994-95)[a,6,18]

	Poorest	2	3	4	5	6	7	8	9	Richest
(a) before housing costs										
1979	4.3	5.7	6.6	7.6	8.5	9.5	10.7	12.2	14.2	20.6
1981	4.0	5.6	6.5	7.4	8.4	9.5	10.7	12.2	14.5	21.1
1987	3.6	5.0	5.9	6.9	8.0	9.1	10.4	12.2	14.9	24.2
1990/91	2.9	4.5	6.0	6.0	8.0	9.0	11.0	12.0	15.0	26.0
1992/93	2.9	4.6	6.0	6.0	8.0	9.0	10.0	13.0	15.0	26.0
1994/95	3.2	4.7	6.0	6.0	8.0	9.0	10.0	12.0	15.0	26.0
(b) after housing costs										
1979	4.0	5.6	6.6	7.5	8.5	9.5	10.8	12.3	14.3	20.9
1981	3.7	5.4	6.3	7.3	8.3	9.5	10.7	12.3	14.7	21.8
1987	2.9	4.6	5.6	6.7	7.6	9.1	10.6	12.3	15.1	25.0
1990/91	2.1	4.1	5.0	7.0	7.0	10.0	10.0	12.0	16.0	27.0
1992/93	1.9	4.1	5.0	6.0	8.0	9.0	10.0	13.0	15.0	28.0
1994/95	2.2	4.1	6.0	6.0	8.0	9.0	10.0	12.0	16.0	27.0
1995/96	2.2	4.1	5.0	7.0	7.0	9.0	11.0	12.0	16.0	27.0

[a] Share of total income received by individuals by tenths of of the income distribution including self-employed (income after housing costs).

they did in 1979 – they were absolutely poorer. By comparison the richest 10% of single adult households were £6,968 richer in 1995-96 than in 1979. The situation was even worse for large families with three children where the poorest 10% were on average £624 poorer in 1995-96 compared with 1979 and the richest 10% were over £21,000 richer.[6]

Hills points to various factors driving the growth in inequality during the 1980s and 1990s:

- The gap between low and high pay grew, linked to the declining importance of unions and of minimum wage protection.
- The number of workless households rose faster than overall official unemployment, with more 'no-earner' and 'two-earner' households.
- Price-linking of benefits meant that benefit levels fell further behind the rest of the population when overall incomes rose.

The European context

Table 10 shows the numbers and proportions of the populations of 14 European countries living on incomes below half of the average in their countries after allowing for differences in the purchasing power of the different currencies. In absolute terms, Britain has more people living on incomes below half the average than any other country in Europe (11.4 million people) and the third highest percentage of population living on below average incomes (20% of the population) after Ireland and Portugal.

The impact of growing inequalities on health

Inequalities between communities

It is not surprising that the health gap between different communities grew during the 1980s and continued to grow into the 1990s. Inequalities in many other areas of life grew first and are reflected by

Table 9: Change in incomes (after housing costs) of the richest and poorest 10% of different types of families between 1979 and 1995-96 (in April 1998 prices)[6]

Family type	Poorest 10%	Richest 10%
Single adult	−£208	+ £6,968
Couple with no children	−£364	+ £12,688
Couple with 3 children aged 3, 8 and 11	−£624	+ £21,164

Table 10: Number and percentage of the population living on incomes below half of the average in 1994 in 14 European countries

Country	Number of people below 50% of average income	% of the population below 50% of average income
UK	11,426,766	20
Germany	11,327,673	14
Italy	9,321,853	17
France	7,949,907	14
Spain	7,196,406	19
Portugal	2,424,533	25
Greece	2,041,923	20
Belgium	1,474,158	15
Netherlands	1,275,048	8
Austria	1,108,082	14
Ireland	837,490	23
Denmark	386,015	7
Finland	192,153	4
Luxembourg	56,734	14

the growing inequalities in health. For instance, unemployment rose at different rates in different places in Britain at the start of the 1980s and many areas continue to be blighted by very high unemployment rates. The government has, so far, introduced no new policies designed to narrow the gap in unemployment rates between local areas. Many new jobs that are created in inner cities go to people who commute into these areas. A more focused set of policies is needed which do not simply concentrate on 'problem estates' but which look at the wider range of differences in opportunities found between areas. The children living in the richest quarter of areas in Britain have a 50% chance of going to university. Those in the poorest quarter have a 10% chance. Ways of narrowing community inequalities such as these are available to the government.

Inequalities between regions

For similar reasons it is not surprising that regional inequalities in health in Britain are among the widest in Europe. The recent rise in branch plant closures in peripheral regions suggests that the current and limited policies of what used to be called regional assistance are not working. New industries are unlikely to emerge in poorer areas without greater government assistance – whereas the Home Counties of England benefit from the indirect advantages of being near the seat of government. Greater regional autonomy should reduce this inequality, but so far this has only been suggested for London within England.

The North of England, Wales, the far South West and much of Scotland suffer from their remoteness from power in the capital. It remains to be seen how much devolution will change this picture.

Inequalities between children

Similarly it would not be surprising to find that the mortality rates of children born to the poorest families in Britain continue to rise when the government has implemented policies such as reducing the single parent premium which will have had the greatest damaging effect on the poorest of children. Encouraging mothers to work will not reverse the rise in inequalities in mortality for children aged under one, most of whose mothers do not and cannot work. Improving the material living standards of their families would have a direct effect on the health of these children.

Inequalities between families

It is not surprising that inequalities in the health of adults in different social groups continue to grow when we know that the inequality in the incomes of their families has risen over this period and remains at very high levels. Most importantly inequalities in wealth are higher than those of income. If these inequalities are not reduced then we should not expect to see reductions in the health inequalities between families in different social locations. The government's unwillingness to reverse the regressive taxation changes of the 1980s and its reluctance to increase inheritance tax will help to maintain these inequalities and to ensure that the gap between the health of different families in Britain continues to grow.

Reducing inequalities in health

The Independent Inquiry into Inequalities in Health reviewed the evidence on inequalities in health and presented a number of policy recommendations. However, the 39 sets of recommendations are not adequately prioritised. We consider that in order to reduce health inequalities, as the government has pledged in a Green Paper,[20] policies must be aimed at their underlying cause. There is *one central and fundamental policy* that should be pursued: the reduction of income inequality and consequently the elimination of poverty. Ending poverty is the key to ending inequalities in health. Any child can tell you how this can be achieved: the poor have too little money so the solution to ending their poverty is to give them more money. Poverty reduction really is something that can be achieved by 'throwing money at the problem'.

Social policy researchers and economists have proposed a range of affordable and cost-effective anti-poverty policies. Policies aimed at increasing the standard of living and incomes of poor families with children, disabled people and older people will have the greatest impact on reducing inequalities in health. The quickest and most cost-effective method of alleviating poverty is to increase the value of welfare benefits (especially for families with children) and pensions and to improve public services and social housing. A powerful case for introducing a number of specific policies, by building on existing schemes, will be discussed in the next section.

Economists have also designed and costed a number of 'affordable' basic income schemes that if properly implemented would effectively end poverty in Britain.[21] A Basic Income is a payment received by every person or household, which provides a minimum income and the amount is based only on age and family status, but is otherwise unconditional.

There are three main advantages claimed for Basic Income schemes.

1. They should plug the gaps and loopholes in social security and reduce the number of people living in poverty.
2. They should remove unemployment and poverty traps that result from the high rates of benefit withdrawal when unemployed people obtain work, or people with low incomes move up the earnings ladder.
3. They are desirable because people should have a source of subsistence independent of needs and not dependent on complicated contribution records or intrusive scrutiny of personal means.

Most existing social security benefits in industrialised countries are contingent. That means that they are related to misfortune or conditions such as age, sickness or unemployment. By contrast, a basic income depends only on very general characteristics such as number of dependants. There are no questions or conditions relating to effort to find work, state of health, contribution records or capital holdings. Basic Incomes could replace many existing specific social security benefits. There would always be people with special needs requiring extra sums on a conditional or discretionary basis, but fewer cases than at present.

Some advocates believe that Basic Income payments should take the form of a tax credit to be set off against tax but received as a positive payment from the state by those with insufficient tax liabilities.

The government proposed implementing legislation to provide a guaranteed minimum income for working families with children of £180 per week from April 1999, increasing to £190 per week in October 1999. Pensioners will also have guaranteed minimum income of £75 for single people and £117 for couples from April 1999. Similarly, severely disabled people who are unable to work will be guaranteed a minimum income of £128 per week. However, these proposals do not go much beyond existing levels of income support and family credit and, like all existing means-tested benefits, will fail to reach large numbers of those legally entitled to those benefits. In practice, the proposals will make little difference to existing living standards especially when, as in the case of Incapacity Benefit, the government is proposing to save more money in cuts than it is prepared to spend on additions to selected means-tested benefits for severely disabled adults and young children.

The political will does not presently exist to implement a broad-based Minimum Income Guarantee for the whole population at a sufficient level to end poverty. In the absence of this, a number of specific targeted policies could be implemented that would reduce poverty among older people, sick and disabled people and families with children. These would have the effect of also reducing inequalities in health.

Child poverty and health

The experience of poverty and deprivation during childhood can have life-long consequences on health. One of the most worrying aspects of the growth in poverty and inequality over the past 20 years has been the very high rates of poverty experienced by lone-parent families, families with young children and large families.[22]

The government's increases in Child Benefit are welcome but do not cover all children, and are in large measure a catching-up exercise because of the fall in the real value of this benefit in recent years. Child Benefit is the key factor in any policy designed to raise family living standards. The Black Report recommended that Child Benefit should be fixed at 5.5% of average gross earning and this policy should be implemented.

It is essential for reducing inequalities in child health that all pregnant women are able to afford an adequate diet. Budget standards research at the Universities of York and Loughborough indicates that the current maternity allowance is insufficient to achieve this aim. The abolition of the universal maternity allowance was a retrograde step.

Maternity entitlements need to be increased, particularly for women dependent on Income Support and/or in low-paid jobs.

A third of all children live in families dependent on Income Support and a third of all children are born into families that are dependent on Income Support. The scale rates are therefore one of the most crucial factors that determine the amount of child poverty in Britain. These are currently so low that families with children will eventually sink into poverty if they become dependent on Income Support for any length of time. Additional benefits are required to support families with children.

Approximately, a quarter of all children are born to mothers under 25 years old. Therefore, the supposition that people aged less than 25 require less benefit than those over 25 needs to be re-examined urgently.

Adequate additional benefits are needed by lone parents following the abolition of the Lone Parent premium. Lone-parent families face additional financial and time costs compared with two-parent households and the level of benefits available to lone-parent families needs to adequately reflect these additional costs.

Means-tested benefits are a costly and inefficient method of alleviating poverty as they can rarely achieve better than 80% take-up rate.

Although increasing the value of benefits available to families with children is the most important social policy for reducing poverty and inequalities in health, there are also a number of specific policies of secondary importance which will also help reduce child poverty.

The rent limit on Housing Benefit needs to be removed for families with children and increased building of social housing is required to end the need for Bed & Breakfast accommodation. Subsidies for social housing would also enable real rent levels to be reduced.

The essential policy aim needs to be the reduction of child poverty, as indicated by our suggestions above. There are other policy recommendations which deserve consideration. We list some of these below:

- The mortality rate of pedestrians in road traffic accidents (RTAs) in Britain is one of the highest in the industrialised world. Pedestrian child deaths and injury due to RTAs have a steep poverty gradient. An immediate and rigid enforcement of the speed limits in residential areas would be a rapid and inexpensive means of reducing inequalities in health. The law needs to be enforced and the technology to achieve this (traffic calming measures, speed cameras, and so on) is both readily available and relatively cheap. Speed traps might well prove to be income generating.
- Nutritional standards for school meals have now been reintroduced but new technology (eg smart cards) needs to be employed to

remove the stigma attached to free school meals. Free school meals entitlement should be extended to families receiving Family Credit and free school milk provision should be made mandatory. School breakfast schemes should be examined, and where successful be extended.

- An effective educational campaign needs to be introduced to reduce teenage pregnancies.
- The imprisonment and criminalisation of parents for non-payment of debt (particularly TV licence offences) needs to be stopped.
- Subsidised childcare and after-school care places are needed to enable parents to take up paid work. Progress is currently being made in this area.

Old age and ill health

Older people are more likely to die or be ill than any other group. Poverty in old age exacerbates this situation; poor pensioners are more likely to become sick or disabled than richer pensioners and if they become ill, poor pensioners are more likely to die younger. The most effective way of alleviating poverty among older people is through pensions policy, and Barbara Castle and others proposed that:

> The government should fulfil its Manifesto commitment to make the basic state pension the foundation of its pension's policy by immediately restoring the earnings link.

The current level of the state pension is too low and needs to be increased to an adequate level by a one-off topping up exercise along the lines advocated by John Smith in 1992. The government should be aiming at reducing means testing, not extending it.

The government should ensure that everyone makes an adequate minimal provision for their retirement by compelling them to contribute to a second-tier pension sufficient to lift them out of dependency on means-tested benefits. The Conservative governments of 1979 to 1997 slashed the State Earnings Related Pension Scheme (SERPs) which had been introduced with all-party support in the 1970s. A modernised version of SERPs would be comprehensive and meet the needs of people on low incomes, unlike the stakeholder pension alternative proposed by the government. A return to the "twenty best years formula when pensions reflect the peak earnings of people during their working lives" is important for manual and part-time workers and women whose working lives are interrupted by family responsibilities.

Good quality occupational pensions need to be encouraged and tighter regulation of personal pensions is required to prevent miss-selling.

Disability, long-term illness and poverty

Poverty and lack of adequate income are among the main reasons why disabled people can often become ill and why ill health can often persist. It is self-evident that inequalities in health can be reduced if the standard of living of long-term sick and disabled people can be improved. Yet welfare and benefits policy towards this group throughout much of the 20th century can best be described as "irrational, inequitable and inadequate". Policy development was plagued by "haphazard and piecemeal incrementalism ... when money was available or pressure strong, and have been grafted onto existing systems. Nothing has been jettisoned and nothing rethought from first principles".[23] The 1980s were described as "disastrous for disabled people, involving threats to opportunities, living standards, independence and choice".[24]

It is therefore unsurprising that analysis of government surveys has shown that 60% of disabled people have to claim safety-net benefits and 47% of them did not have enough to meet their minimum costs.[25] Independent surveys of families with disabled children have also shown that "For many, their greatest need was for more financial assistance.... Most parents felt higher weekly disability benefits would be the best way to provide further financial assistance".[26]

This is a clear message that requires specific policies:

- The levels of disability benefits are too low to prevent poverty and they need to be increased, substantially in some cases, to meet the additional costs of disability and ill health. This applies in particular to Disability Living Allowance and Incapacity Benefit.
- The rates of long-term disability benefits should be linked to earnings, not prices.
- There is a need for mental health component criteria to be introduced into the assessment for Disability Living Allowance.
- Any test for claimants of Incapacity Benefit must take account of fluctuating health conditions as well as the continuum for capacity to work.
- A Disability Earnings Concession (DEC) should be introduced which allows people in receipt of disability benefits to work and earn as and when their health allows it, without any risk to benefit entitlement, work thus having no effect on benefits. But a higher tax code for DEC earners will deduct the usual tax and National Insurance, plus a reasonable percentage towards Department of Social Security, Council Tax and Housing Benefits when that person does work (Disability Living Allowance would be excluded from this consideration).
- The cuts in funding and eligibility criteria of the Access to Work Scheme need to be restored. Finally, a fully inclusive educational

system is needed that delivers the same standard of education to both disabled and non-disabled children alike.

However, the exclusion experienced by sick and disabled people will not end while discrimination on the grounds of health is still acceptable and legal.[27] Merely implementing the remaining provisions of the Disability Discrimination Act (DDA) and increasing welfare benefits and services will not introduce effective civil rights for disabled people. The DDA as it stands is flawed in its acceptance of "justifiable discrimination", its exemptions and its omission of crucial areas such as education and transport. Wholesale amending or repealing the DDA is necessary in order that it be replaced with legislation similar to that suggested in the Berry and Barnes Private Members Bills. Only then can the Disability Rights Commission work fully to protect, enforce and promote the rights of disabled people.[28]

What is required are more comprehensive, legally enforceable anti-discrimination policies and adequate income guarantees, which are relevant to all sick and disabled people including disabled children and their families.

Conclusions

The report of the Independent Inquiry into Inequalities in Health points out, albeit in one sentence:

> We consider that without a shift of resources to the less well off, both in and out of work, little will be accomplished in terms of a reduction of health inequalities by interventions addressing particular 'downstream' influences.[2]

Inequalities in health can only be effectively tackled by policies that reduce poverty and income inequality. Adequate living standards and protection against income insecurity are basic human rights enshrined in the Universal Declaration of Human Rights (Article 25) and the International Covenant on Economic, Social and Cultural Rights (Articles 7 and 9). Everybody should be entitled to a sufficient income to allow them to participate in the economic, social, cultural and political life of the country.

Acknowledgements

This chapter is adapted from a report from the Townsend Centre for International Poverty Research at the University of Bristol, which was released in response to the Acheson Report of the Independent Inquiry into Inequalities in Health.

References

[1] Department of Health (1997) 'Public health strategy launched to tackle the root causes of ill health', Press release, 7 July.

[2] Independent Inquiry into Inequalities in Health (1998) *Report*, London: The Stationery Office.

[3] Davey Smith, G., Morris, J. and Shaw, M. (1998) 'The Independent Inquiry into Inequalities in Health: a worthy successor to the Black Report?', *British Medical Journal*, vol 317, pp 1465-6.

[4] Department of Health and Social Security (1980) *Inequalities in health: Report of a research working group (The Black Report)*, London: DHSS.

[5] *Lords Hansard* (1997) 12 February, cols 248-9.

[6] Department of Social Security (1998) *Households below average income 1979-1996/7*, London: The Stationery Office.

[7] Lynch, J.W. and Kaplan, G.A. (1997) 'Understanding how inequality in the distribution of income affects health', *Journal of Health Psychology*, vol 2, pp 297-314.

[8] Howarth, C., Kenway, P., Palmer, G. and Street, C. (1998) *Key indicators of poverty and social exclusion*, York: Joseph Rowntree Foundation.

[9] Standardised mortality ratios: the ratio of the number of deaths observed in the study population to the number that would be expected if the study population had the same specific rates as the standard population, multiplied by 100.

[10] Dorling, D. (1997) *Death in Britain: How local mortality rates have changed: 1950s-1990s*, York: Joseph Rowntree Foundation.

[11] *On the state of the Public Health 1997: The annual report of the Chief Medical Officer of the Department of Health for the year 1997*, London: The Stationery Office.

[12] Infant mortality rates cannot meaningfully be considered by social class before 1993 due to the exclusion of births/deaths outside marriage.

[13] Hattersley, L. (1997) 'Expectation of life by social class', in F. Drever and M. Whitehead (eds) *Health inequalities*, London: The Stationery Office.

[14] Social class I includes professional occupations (eg accountants, electronic engineers); social class II includes managerial and technical/intermediate occupations (eg proprietors and managers – sales, production, works and maintenance managers); social class III non-manual includes skilled non-manual (eg clerks and cashiers – not retail) occupations; social class III manual includes skilled manual (eg drivers of road goods vehicles, metal working production fitters) occupations; social class IV includes partly skilled (eg storekeepers and warehousemen, machine tool operators) occupations; social class V includes unskilled (eg building and civil engineering labourers, cleaners etc) occupations.

[15] 1921-23, 1930-32, 1949-53, 1959-63, 1970-72 from Lawton, R. (1982) 'People and work', in J.W. House (ed) *The UK space: Resources, environment and the future*, London: Weidenfeld and Nicolson. 1981-83 from Blaxter, M. (1991) 'Fifty years on – inequalities in health', in M. Murphy and J. Hobcraft (eds) *Population research in Britain: A supplement to Population Studies*, vol 45, Cambridge: Cambridge University Press. 1991-93 from 'Appendix', in F. Drever and M. Whitehead (eds) (1997) *Health inequalities*, London: The Stationery Office.

[16] Blane, D. and Drever, F. (1998) 'Inequality among men in standardised years of potential life lost, 1970-73', *British Medical Journal*, vol 317, p 255. Years of potential life lost are the average number of years that people who have died have lost – the years of working life that they would have had if they had lived.

[17] Bradshaw, J. and Chen, J.R. (1997) 'Poverty in the UK: a comparison with nineteen other countries', *Benefits*, vol 18, pp 13-17.

[18] Hills, J. (1998) *Income and wealth: The latest evidence*, York: Joseph Rowntree Foundation.

[19] *Sunday Times* (1996) 14 April.

[20] Department of Health (1997) *Our healthier nation*, Green Paper, London: The Stationery Office.

[21] Brittan, S. and Webb, S. (1990) *Beyond the welfare state: An examination of basic incomes in a market economy*, The David Hume Institute, Aberdeen: Aberdeen University Press.

[22] Adelman, L. and Bradshaw, J. (1998) 'Children in poverty in Britain: an analysis of the Family Resources Survey 1994/95', Paper prepared as part of the ESRC project 'Poverty: the outcomes for children in the Children 5-16 Programme', York: Social Policy Research Unit, University of York.

[23] Baldwin, S., Bradshaw, J., Cooke, K. and Glendinning, C. (1981) 'The disabled person and cash benefits', in D. Guthrie (ed) *Disability: Legislation and practice*, London: Macmillan.

[24] Glendinning, C. (1991) 'Losing ground: social policy and disabled people in Great Britain 1980-1990', *Disability, Handicap and Society*, vol 6, no 1, pp 3-19.

[25] Berthoud, R., Lakey, J. and McKay, S. (1993) *The economic problems of disabled people*, London: Policy Studies Institute.

[26] Beresford, B. (1995) *Expert opinions: A national survey of parents caring for a severely disabled child*, Bristol/York: The Policy Press/Joseph Rowntree Foundation.

[27] Gordon, D. and Heslop, P. (1998) 'Poverty and disabled children', in D. Dorling and S. Simpson (eds) *Statistics in society: The arithmetic of politics*, London: Arnold.

[28] Heslop, P. (1999) 'Response to the government Green Paper on welfare reform', *Radical Statistics*, vol 70, pp 70-4.

37

Inequalities in health: what is happening and what can be done?

George Davey Smith and Yoav Ben-Shlomo

Introduction

Mortality differentials according to socioeconomic group have long been recognised in the UK. In 1845, Engels reproduced such data, using both area-based and individual indicators of socioeconomic status (Table 1).[1] Engels went on to quote from the *Report on the sanitary conditions of the working class*:

> In Liverpool in 1840 the average life-span of the upper classes, gentry, professional men, etc, was thirty-five years; that of the business men and better-placed handicraftsmen,

Table 1: Mortality ratios (number of living people for each death) in Chorlton-on-Medlock, Manchester[1]

	Class of house		
	1st (best)	2nd	3rd (worst)
Class of street			
1st (best)	51	45	36
2nd	55	38	35
3rd (worst)	a	35	25

a No data.

In G. Scally (ed) (1997) *Progress in public health*, London: RSM Press, pp 73-100 twenty-two years; and that of the operatives, day-labourers, and serviceable class in general, but fifteen years.[1]

Socioeconomic differentials in mortality appear to have persisted from the time of Engels' description of early Victorian conditions until the present day.[2,3] The best longitudinal series of such data available internationally comes from statistics on social class mortality differences produced around each British Census. Figure 1 presents mortality rates for middle-aged men from the years around the 1921 Census to the years around the 1991 Census. Dramatic declines in mortality are seen for social classes I and II, while for social classes IV and V small and inconsistent decreases in mortality are seen.[4] Increases in both the relative and absolute differentials in mortality between the social class groups have occurred since the early 1950s;[5] a pattern which recent data demonstrate has continued throughout the 1980s.[6,7] The most recent analysis, for the years around the 1991 Census (Figure 2), demonstrates substantial social class differences in all-cause mortality for men, while data for women have yet to appear. For males of working ages, the relative differentials in mortality for all-causes, stroke, ischaemic heart disease, lung cancer and suicide have continued to increase.[6] While a decline in mortality rate for social class V men

Figure 1: Death rates (all-causes) per 100,000 men aged 55-64, by social class, in England and Wales (1921-81)[4]

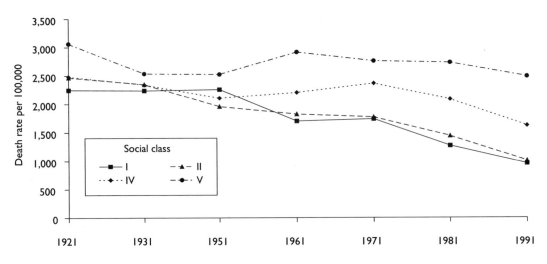

Source: Decennial Supplements on Occupational Mortality

Figure 2: Death rates per 100,000 men aged 20-64 according to social class (1992-93)[7]

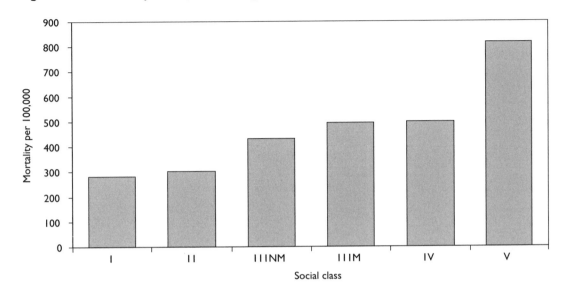

occurred between 1981 and 1991, mortality in 1991 is still higher than in 1971 for this group.

Morbidity data according to social position are more difficult to locate than mortality data. A series of recent studies have demonstrated that common forms of morbidity demonstrate the same socioeconomic patterning as does mortality and limiting long-term illness.[8,9]

Table 2 displays the differing prevalences of various chronic conditions according to the socioeconomic characteristics of area of residence in a sample of more than 20,000 men and women in Somerset and Avon. The introduction of a question regarding 'limiting long-term illness' in the 1991 Census has allowed the strong and consistent associations of chronic morbidity with deprivation to be demonstrated.[10] Reliable data on trends in socioeconomic differentials in morbidity from particular causes are not available, however.

Investigating the origins of socioeconomic differentials in health

Several reviews of the contribution of different sets of factors to socioeconomic differentials in health have appeared recently.[11-13] They have extensively considered the degree to which observed inequalities in health may be artefactual, that is, produced by the ways in which data are collected and analysed. Such processes appear, if anything, to lead to underestimation, rather than overestimation, of the magnitude

Table 2: Age-standarised prevalence per 100 of self-reported diseases, by deprivation category[9]

	1st fifth	2nd fifth	3rd fifth	4th fifth	5th fifth	*p* value
Men						
Musculoskeletal diseases	14.1	15.1	16.1	16.1	17.7	<0.001
Angina	4.4	5.5	5.5	5.5	6.9	<0.001
Myocardial infarction	3.2	3.7	4.0	4.5	4.8	<0.001
Asthma	5.6	6.1	6.2	6.4	6.4	0.18
Bronchitis	5.2	6.3	7.3	7.7	9.1	<0.001
Depression	3.9	4.8	5.9	6.2	6.9	<0.001
Stroke	2.0	1.8	1.3	2.3	2.6	0.03
Diabetes	2.4	2.5	3.7	2.7	2.1	0.83
Diabetic eye disease	0.5	0.6	0.9	1.0	0.7	0.05
Women						
Musculoskeletal diseases	27.3	28.6	30.6	30.5	34.5	<0.001
Angina	3.8	4.4	4.6	4.4	5.8	<0.002
Myocardial infarction	1.5	1.9	1.7	1.8	2.5	0.03
Asthma	6.4	6.2	7.5	7.0	9.8	<0.001
Bronchitis	7.5	8.1	9.0	10.2	13.2	<0.001
Depression	10.1	10.5	11.4	12.5	12.7	<0.001
Stroke	1.6	2.0	2.1	2.2	2.4	0.04
Diabetes	2.6	2.4	2.1	2.1	2.4	0.56
Diabetic eye disease	0.6	0.5	0.6	0.7	1.5	<0.001

of health inequalities. This relates both to measurement of socioeconomic position and the measurement of health. Conventional measures of socioeconomic position suffer from a lack of discriminatory power and the use of enriched indicators leads to the demonstration of greater mortality and morbidity gradients.[12] Differences in the way in which social groups report ill health may also dilute associations between social position and serious morbidity.[14,15] Furthermore the notion that health determines social position through health-related social mobility, rather than poor health being produced by adverse socioeconomic circumstances, is also not supported in any simple way by the available data.[16]

Several studies have investigated the contribution of particular health-related behaviours and physiological risk factors to mortality differentials. In the first Whitehall Study, considerable differences in mortality risk were demonstrated according to two socioeconomic indicators – employment grade in the civil service and car ownership (Figure 3).[17] While the lower grade and non-car owning civil servants were more likely to smoke than the higher grade and car owning ones, the pattern of mortality differentials was identical among men who had never smoked (Figure 4).[12,18]

Cholesterol levels were higher among high rather than low grade

Figure 3: Mortality by employment grade and car ownership in the Whitehall Study[17]

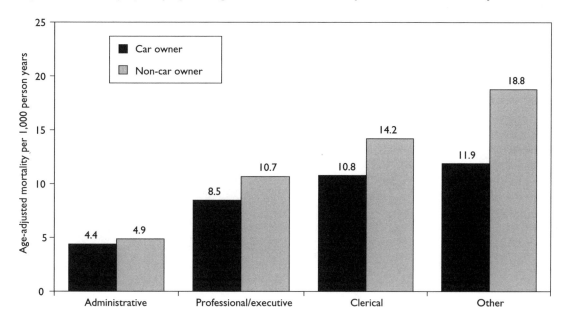

civil servants in the late 1960s, when this study was established. Differences in cholesterol levels could not, therefore, account for the higher rates of coronary heart disease (CHD) among the lower grade employees. This can be taken to suggest that differences in dietary fat intake between grades in this cohort were not responsible for the CHD mortality differentials. Indeed simultaneous consideration of a range of risk factors (including smoking, blood pressure, cholesterol levels and prevalent cardio-respiratory disease) failed to account for the grade differences in cardiovascular and non-cardiovascular mortality.[17]

Similar findings have emerged from a study in the west of Scotland established around the same time as the first Whitehall study.[19,20] Large differentials in cardiovascular disease mortality according to both educational attainment and social class existed at a time when blood cholesterol levels were highest in those with the most education and in the professional and managerial classes. Adjustments for a wide range of risk factors failed to explain the considerable mortality differentials from major causes of death in this study.

As a result of findings suggesting that conventional risk factors could not explain socioeconomic differentials in health, the Whitehall II cohort was established in 1985 to investigate additional factors which might contribute to the social gradients.[8] The Whitehall II Study found differentials in prevalent ECG abnormalities in both sexes at baseline, which paralleled the findings in the original cohort.

Figure 4: Mortality by employment grade and car ownership in the Whitehall Study among men who had never smoked[17]

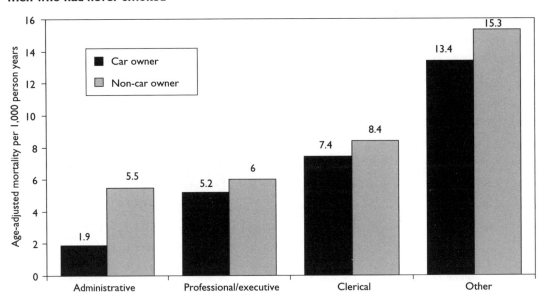

In this more recent study, mean total cholesterol levels again appeared not to contribute to the occupational gradient in CHD risk, as in both sexes the mean cholesterol level at baseline was similar in each grade.

Concentrations of serum apolipoprotein AI, the main structural protein of HDL cholesterol, did show an association with grade[21] and suggested that characteristic disturbances of metabolism associated with lower occupational status were potentially identifiable.

Central, or male-type, obesity, which has long been recognised as a factor predisposing to diabetes and coronary disease,[22] is in both sexes more prevalent among the lower grade civil servants. The related components of the metabolic, or insulin resistance syndrome, of elevated triglycerides and a higher prevalence of impaired glucose tolerance are also found more commonly among the lower grade civil servants.[23]

Low level of control over the nature of one's work – that is, little ability to decide what one does, and when – has emerged as a potential CHD risk factor. In the Whitehall II study, low level of job control is associated with an increased risk of CHD among both men and women, whether measured by self-reports or by external assessments of job characteristics.[24] It is, however, difficult to separate low control over work from other aspects of the socioeconomic environment.[25] Indeed certain aspects of work relations may be considered a fundamental complement of social stratification in capitalist economies.[26]

A study of Finnish men constitutes the most detailed prospective investigation of factors contributing to the socioeconomic gradient in cardiovascular mortality undertaken to date.[27] The risk of all-cause and cardiovascular disease mortality across quintiles of adulthood income showed two to threefold differences. It was possible to adjust for 22 risk factors – plasma fibrinogen, serum HDL cholesterol, serum apolipoprotein B, blood leukocytes, serum copper, mercury in hair, serum ferritin, blood haemoglobin, serum triglycerides, systolic blood pressure, body mass index, height, cardio-respiratory fitness, cigarette smoking, alcohol consumption, leisure time physical activity, depression, hopelessness, cynical hostility, participation in organisations, quality of social support and marital status.[27]

On adjustment for all these factors the association between social position and cardiovascular disease mortality was greatly attenuated, while the associations between social positions and all (fatal and non-fatal) CHD incidence remained substantial. As the authors acknowledge, it is difficult to interpret such analyses, for several reasons. First, some of the factors adjusted for may be markers of disease presence (for example, blood leukocytes, fibrinogen), and statistical adjustment for these could, in essence, be adjusting for the presence of cardiovascular disease, which is itself produced by social factors. The reduction in relative risks in the lower income groups which occurs on adjustment for these factors cannot be taken as demonstrating the 'explanation' of why the social distribution of cardiovascular mortality exists. Second, some factors – for example, height, body mass index, serum triglycerides – may be the outcome of socioeconomic processes, which act in early life. Adjusting for these factors similarly fails to account for the reasons for the social distribution in cardiovascular mortality, since it automatically leads to questions as to how childhood social conditions may influence growth, insulin resistance syndrome and thus coronary disease risk. Finally, the reasons for the social distribution of certain behaviour – for example, smoking and exercise – itself should become a target for explanation.[3]

Lifecourse influences on health inequalities

Until recently debates regarding inequalities in health generally related to the relationship between socioeconomic circumstances in adulthood and poor health. There has recently been a revival of interest in the effects of poor social circumstances in early life on health in adulthood.[28] The UK Department of Health report *Variations in health*[29] has recognised the importance of a lifecourse perspective on inequalities in health. It concluded that it:

... is likely that cumulative differential lifetime exposure to health-damaging or health-promoting physical and social environments is the main explanation for observed variations in health and life expectancy.

Few empirical data regarding such cumulative effects exist, however. In a cohort study in which men have been followed for over 20 years in the West of Scotland[19] it was possible to relate mortality experience to the social class of the fathers of the study participants; to the social class of their first occupation on entering the labour market; and to the social class of their occupation at the time of screening, when aged 35-64. In Table 3 it is demonstrated that cumulative social class, together with indicators of socioeconomic position at the time of screening, are strongly associated with mortality risk. When social class locations at different periods of the lifecourse are related to mortality from specific causes, it is seen that the social class of the fathers of the men and their own social class at the time of screening independently contribute to all-cause mortality (Table 4). This suggests that there are some long-lasting influences of socioeconomic circumstances in childhood on mortality in adulthood. With respect to particular causes of death, childhood socioeconomic conditions have particular importance for cardiovascular disease, but are related less strongly to cancer and other mortality. The suggestion that mortality risk reflects the accumulation of environmental insults or the cumulative effects of unfavourable behavioural or psychological factors which progressively increase susceptibility to disease[30,31] is supported by a study based on record linkage of the 1960, 1970 and 1980 Census records for Norway, in which particularly high mortality

Table 3: All-cause mortality by cumulative social class, car driving, and deprivation category of area of residence[a]

		Cumulative social class		
	All three non-manual	Two non-manual, one manual	Two manual, one non-manual	All three manual
Regular car driver				
Yes	1	1.28 (1.01-1.63)	1.36 (1.08 -1.73)	1.57 (1.27-1.95)
No	1.22 (0.91-1.64)	1.52 (1.19-1.95)	1.76 (1.40-2.21)	2.00 (1.64-2.44)
Deprivation category of area of residence				
1-4	1	1.25 (1.01-1.56)	1.37 (1.09-1.72)	1.70 (1.39-2.09)
5-7	1.06 (0.74-1.52)	1.41 (1.10-1.82)	1.54 (1.25-1.90)	1.74 (1.45-2.09)

[a] Values are age-adjusted relative rates (with 95% CI).

Table 4: Mortality by social class at three different stages of life, manual versus non-manual relative rates[a]

	Father's social class	First social class	Current social class
All-causes			
Individual	1.44 (1.27-1.64)	1.29 (1.16-1.43)	1.40 (1.27-1.55)
Simultaneous	1.28 (1.11-1.47)	1.01 (0.89-1.16)	1.29 (1.14-1.47)
Cardiovascular causes			
Individual	1.58 (1.32-1.89)	1.35 (1.16-1.56)	1.38 (1.20-1.59)
Simultaneous	1.41 (1.15-1.72)	1.08 (0.90-1.30)	1.20 (1.01-1.43)
Cancer			
Individual	1.26 (1.02-1.56)	1.25 (1.04-1.50)	1.35 (1.13-1.61)
Simultaneous	1.11 (0.87-1.41)	1.04 (0.82-1.31)	1.28 (1.03-1.60)
Non cardiovascular non cancer causes			
Individual	1.45 (1.07-1.98)	1.18 (0.92-1.53)	1.59 (1.24-2.03)
Simultaneous	1.28 (0.91-1.80)	0.80 (0.58-1.10)	1.67 (1.22-2.28)

[a] Values are age-adjusted relative rates (with 95% CI), with individual and simultaneous adjustment for each social class indicator.

risks are seen among men who obtain limited education and then go on to work in manual occupations and live in poor housing.[32] Similar findings have come from the US national longitudinal study of older men.[33] The particular dependence of cardiovascular disease risk on childhood socioeconomic circumstances in comparison to other causes of death has been observed in area-based studies from Finland.[34,35]

Of particular current research interest are the long-term effects of development during foetal and early infant life on disease risk in adulthood. A series of ecological and prospective studies have demonstrated that birth weight and weight at one year of age are inversely related to cardiovascular disease risk, diabetes risk and blood pressure in later life.[36] While it is difficult to separate out the effects of such early life exposures from later experiences,[37,38] these findings are strongly suggestive of important persisting influences from early life into adulthood.

In a study from South Wales, men with low birth weight were at a particularly elevated risk of CHD if they became obese in adulthood (Figure 5).[39] Thus the socially patterned exposure of sub-optimal intrauterine development, indexed by low birth weight, interacts with the socially patterned exposure of obesity in adulthood to generate elevated disease risk.

Less research has been carried out recently on the effects of childhood nutrition on later disease, although earlier in the 20th century it was considered unproblematically obvious that such effects did exist.[40] Preliminary data are now available from a mortality follow-up of the children included in surveys of poverty, nutrition and child health carried out under the auspices of John Boyd Orr in the immediate pre-Second World War period.[41] At the time this survey was carried out it was recognised by one of the investigators that leg length was a particularly good indicator of childhood socioeconomic and nutritional circumstances:

> When the Carnegie UK Dietary and Clinical Survey was planned at the Rowett Research Institute in 1937, cristal height as a measure of leg length was included in the measurements ... it was found that cristal height was consistently better than total height for indicating expenditure group ... we find the longer-legged children suffered less bronchitis than the short at all ages. Since there is neither complicating immunity mechanism nor specific cure for bronchitis, we might argue that constitution built up when the complete harmonious pattern of growth is unfolded is, in some way, superior to that associated with inhibition of growth, however slight.[42]

A re-analysis of these data clearly demonstrates this to be the case as age-standardised indicators of total height, leg length and trunk length reveal differential associations with nutritional and socioeconomic factors (Table 5).[43,44] In particular, it is noticeable that the negative correlations between overcrowding and social class of head of

Figure 5: CHD incidence by birthweight and body mass index in the Caerphilly Study[39]

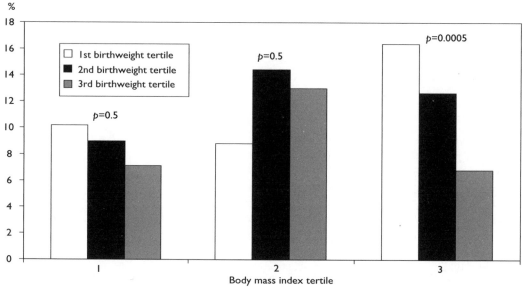

household (scored from 1 for professional groups to 5 for unskilled manual workers) are considerably stronger for leg length than for trunk length, while the positive correlations between weighted per capita food expenditure and relative family per capita calorie consumption are similarly stronger for leg length than trunk length. Results for females are similar to those for males.

Leg length in childhood is associated with mortality over the subsequent 60 years (Table 6). These data suggest that there may be important long-term consequences of childhood nutrition on health

Table 5: Pearson's correlation coefficients between anthropmetry, childhood dietary and socioeconomic variables and adult socioeconomic status (males)[43]

Anthropmetric, dietary or socioeconomic index (*n*)	'z' score for height	'z' score for leg length	'z' score for trunk length
Birth order (1,397)	−0.14	−0.14	−0.06
Number of children (1,394)	−0.25	−0.24	−0.15
Weighted per capita food expenditure (1,394)	0.28	0.28	0.15
Social class of head of household (1,287)	−0.18	−0.21	−0.05*
Overcrowding (1,220)	−0.19	−0.20	−0.08
Relative family per capita calorie consumption (1,394)	0.23	0.26	0.08

Note: all *p* <0.05 except*.

Table 6: Leg length and mortality: Carnegie survey follow-up[44]

Quintile	CHD mortality Fully adjusted relative risk ([a]95% CI)	Cancer mortality Fully adjusted relative risk ([a]95% CI)
Males		
1 (shortest)	2.5 (1.0-6.2)	0.5 (0.2-1.5)
2	2.3 (0.9-5.6)	0.5 (0.2-1.3)
3	2.0 (0.9-4.9)	0.8 (0.3-1.9)
4	2.4 (1.1-5.4)	0.9 (0.4-1.9)
5 (tallest)	1.0	1.0
Linear trend test	*p*=0.14	*p*=0.22
Females		
1 (shortest)	3.9 (0.8-19.0)	0.9 (0.4-2.1)
2	3.4 (0.7-16.7)	1.0 (0.4-2.2)
3	1.9 (0.3-10.5)	0.9 (0.4-2.1)
4	0.9 (0.1-6.6)	0.8 (0.3-1.9)
5 (tallest)	1.0	1.0
Linear trend *test*	*p*=0.006	*p*=0.56

[a] Adjusted for age and indices of childhood and adult socioeconomic circumstances, calorie consumption, and birth order.

in later life. They do not, however, paint a one-sided view of rapid growth in childhood. In line with evidence from animal studies and some epidemiological findings,[45,46] cancer risk may be increased by greater calorie intake and growth in early life. Thus reductions in cardiovascular disease mortality in response to socioeconomic and nutritional conditions which encourage growth in childhood may, in part, be counterbalanced by increases in cancer mortality. Studies which obtain data over the lifecourse of participants are required to untangle the relative contributions of factors acting at different stages of life (and the importance of interactions between such factors across the lifecourse) to further understand their role in generating disease risk in adulthood.

Health-related behaviours: are they life-style choices?

Writing in 1845, Engels considered that nutritional deficiencies contributed to the poor health of the labouring classes. Rather than take this to indicate poor health-related behaviours among this deprived group, he realised that the dependence of dietary adequacy on financial wherewithal was clear:

> The better paid workers, especially those in whose families every member is able to earn something, have good food as long as this state of things lasts; meat daily and bacon and cheese for supper. Where wages are less, meat is used only two or three times a week, and the proportion of bread and potatoes increases. Descending gradually, we find the animal food reduced to a small piece of bacon cut up with the potatoes; lower still, even this disappears, and there remain only bread, cheese, porridge, and potatoes, until on the lowest rung of the ladder, among the Irish, potatoes form the sole food.[1]

Engels recognised that the financial disadvantages of poor people were compounded by other social factors in determining their poor diet. The payment of wages on Saturday evening meant that workers could only buy their food after the middle class had been given first choice during Saturday morning.

When the workers reached the market,

> ... the best has vanished, and, if it was still there, they would probably not be able to buy it. The potatoes which the workers buy are usually poor, the vegetables wilted, the cheese old and of poor quality, the bacon rancid, the meat lean,

tough, taken from old, often diseased, cattle, or such as have
died a natural death, and not fresh even then, often half
decayed.

The working classes were also more liable to be sold adulterated
food, because while the rich developed sensitive palates through
habitual good eating and could detect adulteration, the poor had
little opportunity to cultivate their taste and were unable to detect
adulteration. They also had to deal with small retailers who could
not sell:

> ... even the same quality of goods so cheaply as the largest
> retailers, because of their small capital and the large
> proportional expenses of their business, ... [and] must
> knowingly or unknowingly buy adulterated goods in order
> to sell at the lower prices required, and to meet the
> competition of the others.

The capitalist class, naturally, failed to acknowledge the poor health
generated by the inadequate diet of the working class. Indeed, the
philosopher of industrialisation, Andrew Ure, was quoted by Engels
as suggesting that the workers pampered themselves into nervous
ailments "by a diet too rich and exciting for their indoor
employments".

Several studies have demonstrated that Engels' conclusions remain
applicable today: those least able to purchase a healthy diet, due to
financial constraints are those most likely to be disadvantaged with
regard to access to healthy micronutrient-dense food. Thus a shopping
basket survey in Glasgow demonstrated that households in a less
economically favoured area paid more for a healthy basket of food
than households in a more favoured area, while there was no difference
in the cost of an unhealthy basket of food. It was also noted that
several items of the healthy food basket were simply not available in
the less favoured area.[47] A similar survey was carried out in London
in 1988 and repeated in 1995. At both times, healthy food was more
expensive in the deprived area while unhealthy food was slightly
cheaper in the deprived area.[48] This study suggested that the situation
for those living in the deprived area had become relatively worse
between 1988 and 1995.

Poorer families have been disadvantaged by changes in food retailing.
Between 1980 and 1992 the number of food retail outlets decreased
by 35%.[49] This reflects a decline in the number of small grocery
retailers and specialist shops, including butchers and greengrocers,
and an increase in large supermarkets. Such large retailers tend to be
based outside of towns and customers require transport to them. The
low rate of car ownership among poorer households makes it difficult

for them to utilise these generally cheaper outlets. In essence, the transfer of food retailing from smaller local retailers to large out-of-town superstores represents a transfer of costs from the food wholesaler, who is required to transport food to fewer outlets, to the customer, who must travel further to purchase food. This transfer represents a disproportionate burden to poorer households and contributes to widening inequalities in material circumstances.

Low-income households, residing in less affluent areas, are disadvantaged in other ways with respect to food, diet and nutrition. Such households may especially value the social resource represented by the personal nature of local shopping more, given fewer alternative social opportunities. Shopping can become a demoralising experience for those whose choice is constrained by a lack of income.[50] The costs of cooking and of stocking essential items required for food preparation represent additional expenditure which may not be available in less well-off households. Thus the use of convenience foods or items such as sandwiches which require no cooking is encouraged.

In a detailed ethnographic study of the social organisation of nutritional inequities,[51] concluded that:

> The public discourse most consistent with the findings and experience of this research was apparently informed by an individualistic ideology. Individualism assumes that the current social system provides sufficient and equal opportunity for individuals to move within the social system according to their abilities. Within this ideological construct, poverty results from the individual's failure to seize the opportunity or to work sufficiently hard within the current social structure; it is not a reflection of inadequacies and inequities within that social order.

This need not go unchallenged, however. The women in Travers' study were aware that inequitable pricing policies existed, such that the more expensive food stores are located in the inner city, closer to the areas of residence of socially and economically disadvantaged households. The women initiated a letter-writing campaign to supermarket managers which resulted in a reduction in the pricing differentials between inner city and suburban stores.

Other health-related behaviours – such as smoking, leisure time physical activity and excessive alcohol consumption – have been shown to be constrained by the material and psychosocial conditions of life in similar ways to diet.[52,53] The need for health promotion approaches, which recognise that such practices are not simple life-style choices, are required if the components of the overall pattern of health inequalities which are produced by differential adoption of such behaviours are to be addressed.

Influences outside the individual: the importance of residential area

It is difficult to define the concept of 'community' and this varies depending on the discipline or theorist.[54] However, independent of the particular theoretical framework, there is now a growing body of research which demonstrates that characteristics of areas and communities, as well as individuals, have an impact on health. Many previous ecological studies have shown strong relationships between area deprivation and mortality.[55,56] Some have suggested that these relationships simply reflect an increased mortality risk for individuals of lower socioeconomic position who reside in such areas and do not reflect any additional area effect.[57] However, this conflicts with findings from other studies. The Alameda county study examined the nine-year mortality rates of residents in Oakland, California. Those subjects living in a federally designated poverty area had around 70% higher all-cause mortality.[58] This persisted after adjustment for a wide array of potentially confounding variables, including individual socioeconomic position, health practices, social networks and psychological factors.

The development of multi-level modelling techniques now allow more formal empirical testing of area or 'contextual' effects. Results confirm that area characteristics such as deprivation, enable better prediction of physiological measures such as lung function,[59] long-term illness[60] and suicide,[61] than does the use of individual risk factors alone. For example, evidence from a recent multi-level analysis of data from the Scottish Heart Health Study illustrates the relative importance of area effects.[62] This study was set up, in part, to examine geographical variations in cardiovascular disease risk factors. Significant area effects were found for diastolic blood pressure, cholesterol, and alcohol consumption, although not for smoking, after individual characteristics had been taken into account. The magnitude of the area effects were, however, relatively small compared to the effect of the individual factors. In general, developmental and other lifecourse experiences or exposures may act more directly at an individual level and have a greater impact than do indirect contextual effects, which must be mediated through other pathways. However, the above studies have simply modelled the effect of current area of residence and have therefore assumed both non-migration as well as the temporal constancy of area effects. If full residential histories were available on subjects and both temporal as well as geographical effects were modelled, it is likely that the proportion of variance explained by area would be greater.

Influences outside the individual: the importance of community cohesiveness

Valuable epidemiological insights can sometimes be gained through 'natural experiments'. One such example is the so-called 'Roseto-effect'. In the 1960s, it was noted that the town of Roseto, Pennsylvania, which contained an Italian American community, had a strikingly low rate of CHD mortality compared to several neighbouring communities with similar socioeconomic characteristics. Investigation ruled out the possible role of differential medical services or confounding by conventional risk factors such as smoking. However, it was clear that this close immigrant community had a particularly stable social structure, strong family cohesion and provided a supportive environment. Among the younger generation, acculturation towards aspects of the generic US experience was evident and hence it was hypothesised that breakdown of traditional values would be accompanied by an increase in mortality.

Recent temporal data provide support for this hypothesis. Over a 40-year period the protective effect of residing in Roseto has disappeared, so that mortality from CHD is now no different from its neighbours.[63] It is unlikely that the original low rate of CHD mortality in this community can be explained by any simple genetic model as this would not explain the subsequent rapid convergence in mortality experience. However, it only provides indirect evidence on the role of community solidarity.

More general attitudes to the local area and community of residence have been found to be related to measures of anxiety and health. In a Scottish study an area assessment score based on residents' opinions on amenities, problems with the area, poor reputation, neighbourliness, fear of crime, and area satisfaction significantly predicted both anxiety and self-assessed health after adjustment for individual socioeconomic position.[64]

It is difficult to know exactly what sort of policies would enhance local community cohesion and satisfaction. Local empowerment is one method which forms an underlying principle behind the *Healthy cities* movement.[65] While engaging all the population is a difficult endeavour, measuring and promoting 'civic' communities is possible.[66] A sociopolitical study in Italy set out to understand why local regional governments in the north of Italy were more responsive to local needs than those based in the south. To measure the degree of local 'civicness', community participation in local elections, football matches attendance, membership of clubs and readership of local papers were used as measures of an engaged community. Not surprisingly areas with more civic engagement also had more responsive institutional structures, although it was not clear that this was directly as a result of local involvement. A re-analysis of these data show that enhanced community participation was associated with lower rates of infant mortality.[67] It was not, however, associated with premature mortality in middle-aged men, highlighting either the inadequacies of this measure or its more complex inter-relationship with individual-based characteristics.

It is interesting that politicians of all complexions tend to advocate decentralisation and communitarianism, although this usually remains at a rhetorical level rather than contributing to the provision of infrastructure and financial support to enable local communities to experience a real sense of empowerment. The latter approach may, however, both enhance the democratic process and have a beneficial impact on health variations.

Education and health

Many studies have shown a clear linear relationship between educational achievement and mortality from a wide variety of conditions.[68,69] US studies often use education as an indication of socioeconomic position instead of income or occupation. It is clear that both education and socioeconomic position are usually closely related as occupation and hence income is often determined by educational achievement. However, the sociocultural implications of each measure may have a different meaning, for example, in the Diez-Roux et al study, white men showed a bigger social differential for prevalent CHD by education (odds ratio 3.8) while for black men income was a better discriminator (odds ratio 3.4).[69] Education may directly influence knowledge about health-protective behaviours, accessing of health services and psychosocial mechanisms such as engagement in social networks and the ability to cope with life stressors. This may explain why some studies find an independent effect of education after adjustment for either income[70] or other markers of socioeconomic status.[71] The most detailed study of this issue in the UK[20] finds little residual influence of education after taking adult occupation into account, however, indicating that education may influence health through the better opportunities it creates with respect to the type of employment people get, the income they earn, the living conditions they can afford and the area of residence they can live in.

There is evidence that educational interventions targeted at high risk populations may have long-term benefits,[72] although the outcomes for such studies have not usually included specific health measures. One such example is the Perry Preschool study, which was a trial comparing children allocated to either preschool or no preschool interventions. At age 27 those allocated to the active intervention were more likely to be earning more money, be a homeowner, a high school graduate, and less likely to have had contact with social services or have had five or more arrests. Evidence exists that intervention programmes in infancy, preschool and school-age children can have positive impacts on cognitive development, social-emotional development, and coping skills.[72] Several studies have indicated that benefits are not restricted to the school environment but also result in more positive self-perception and family functioning.[72] It is clear that in some cases, with appropriate re-enforcement, such changes in self-attitude can produce dramatic alterations to an individual's life trajectory, both in terms of occupation, psychosocial functioning, adult health behaviours and risk of subsequent disease.

The role of medical and health-related interventions in reducing inequalities

A recent Department of Health commissioned review examined all studies with an experimental design that targeted poorer sections of the population in order to reduce inequalities in health.[73] From a large number of original papers, only 94 studies could be identified that met the inclusion criteria and many were of dubious methodological quality. The characteristics that were found to be associated with greater success were (a) needs assessment and community commitment prior to the intervention, (b) intensive, multidisciplinary, multifaceted, interventions delivered in a variety of settings, and (c) face-to-face, culturally appropriate interventions delivered by an appropriate agent with sufficient training. The authors concluded that:

> It is important that strategies developed to reduce inequalities are not assumed to be having a positive impact simply because the aim is 'progressive' and so rigorous evaluations of promising interventions are important.

The apparent paucity of evidence demonstrating the success of health service interventions in reducing inequalities has led some to take an overly nihilistic view of the possible contribution of such interventions.[74]

While it is generally accepted that medical care has made only a limited contribution to the improvements in mortality rates seen over this century,[75,76] there is now much evidence on the effect of certain medical interventions in reducing mortality and morbidity and improving quality of life. For example, it is estimated that medical services in general may add around five years towards life expectancy.[77] Regarding CHD mortality, all types of cardiac surgery, medical treatments and coronary care units together have been estimated to have prolonged life expectancy by 1.2 years at a population level, as well as resulting in a substantial improvement in quality of life.[77] These estimates must be treated with some caution, but do make the point that the role of medical interventions may be appreciable. Assuming that these benefits apply equally across the socioeconomic spectrum, and that all sections of society access them equitably (but see below), then they may play a role in reducing inequalities in mortality for at least some diseases. On the other hand, they could also contribute to the generation of inequalities in health. A suggestion of this is given by the data in Table 2. While diabetes prevalence was not related to socioeconomic position in this study, the prevalence of diabetic eye disease was higher among men and women residing in more deprived areas. Since good control of diabetes reduces the development of complications like diabetic eye disease, differential experience of medical care for diabetes across socioeconomic groups could contribute to the generation of this important inequity.

Unfortunately most studies, in particularly randomised controlled trials, do not explicitly address the issue of whether medical interventions are of equal benefit regardless of socioeconomic position. In addition, participants in trials are often unrepresentative of the general population. A recent re-analysis of the Multiple Risk Factor Intervention Trial clearly indicated an under-representation of poorer groups.

However, despite the selection biases, limited evidence suggests that improvements in diastolic blood pressure, smoking cessation, and LDL-cholesterol, seen under trial conditions, are very similar for both well educated and less educated subjects; education being used as a marker of socioeconomic position.[78] The Hypertension Detection and Follow-up Program (HDFP) provides more compelling evidence that medical care can help address socioeconomic differences in mortality.[79] Among the group who received conventional medical care (referred care) there was a twofold mortality gradient, according to education level. In contrast, the special (stepped care) group showed almost non-existent gradients among both black and white subjects (see Figure 6). Similarly the Systolic Hypertension in the Elderly Program (SHEP) anti-hypertension trial also found similar reductions in cardiovascular mortality for different educational-level groups, with the less educated group showing, if anything, larger benefits.[79]

These data provide evidence on the efficacy of treatments but do not reflect the reality of day-to-day healthcare provision. Observational data consistently indicate that sociodemographic factors such as socioeconomic position,[80] gender,[81] ethnicity[82] and other factors such as smoking status,[83] have an influence on the likelihood of receiving health interventions. This has been best documented in the US, where the two-tier healthcare system ensures a large vulnerable segment of the population who may not be able to afford major healthcare

Figure 6: Five-year all-cause mortality by educational level, ethnicity and intervention in the HDFP trial[79]

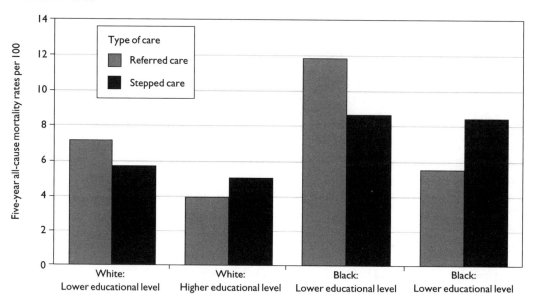

expenditure.[84] In England, it is assumed that a free health care system will not deter poorer individuals from treatment. However, inequities appear to exist both for receiving surgery for heart disease[80] and other common surgical conditions.[85] Men living in more affluent areas were more likely to receive coronary revascularisation surgery (see Figure 7) despite having less need as measured by mortality rates.[80] A more recent study has confirmed these findings with better data, indicating that people living in the most deprived wards had only about half the number of revascularisations per head of population with angina.[86]

In affluent wards individuals with symptoms had almost three times the rate of coronary angiograms than those in poorer wards. Similarly, Asian patients with heart disease appear to wait almost twice as long from symptom onset to being seen by a cardiologist,[82] as well as being less likely to receive thrombolytic therapy.[87] Women are generally less likely to receive surgical intervention for heart disease.[88] This is partially explained by the fact that they are more likely to have non-cardiac chest pain or less severe disease.[89,90] However, among men and women with a past history of myocardial infarction, women still appear to be less likely to receive surgical intervention compared with men[88,91] despite the fact that natural history studies suggest they have the same or worse prognosis as men.[92]

Differences in access are not inevitable and have not always been found. In Northern Ireland, for example, no differences were noted

Figure 7: Male mortality rates for CHD and coronary artery by-pass graft operation rates by deprivation quartiles[80]

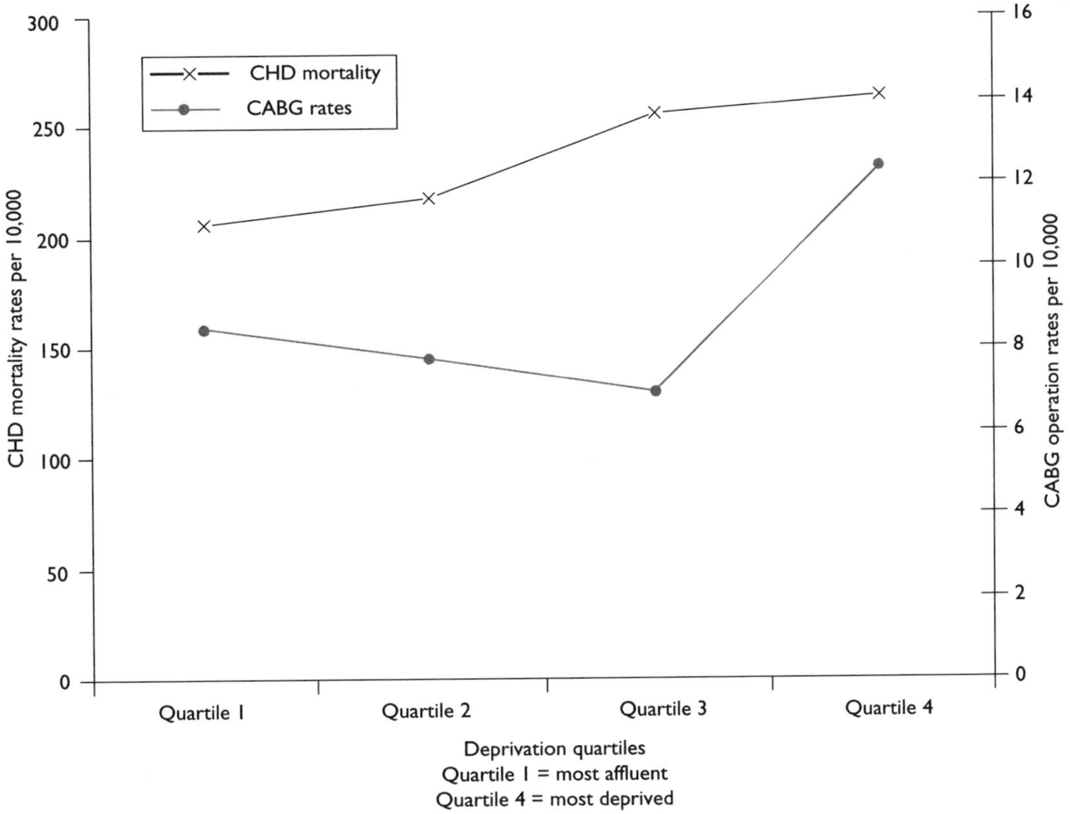

Note: CABG = coronary artery by-pass graft.

in access to coronary revascularisation surgery by area deprivation.[93] A recent report from Finland similarly failed to find differences in the survival of diabetics by socioeconomic position.[94] Equitable health services has been an important goal in Finnish health policy for decades. This suggests that healthcare purchasers must not only explicitly contract for equitable service provision but also take an active role in monitoring this both through routine health services activity data and clinical audit.[95] One obvious and simple way of reducing potential inequities of service delivery is by the use of explicit guidelines. While it is not always easy to get clinicians to apply guidelines, such a method, as in the stepped care approach used by the Hypertension Detection and Follow-up Program trial, may prevent demographic factors influencing the provision of healthcare, particularly if this is audited.

Conclusions

Inequalities in health in the UK are substantial and of increasing magnitude. The main way to address such health differentials is clearly through broader social and political changes leading to a more equitable society. Public health practitioners are failing in achieving their major objective – an improvement in population health status – if they do not become advocates for such changes.

References

[1] Engels, F. (1987, first published 1845) *The condition of the working class in England*, Harmondsworth: Penguin.

[2] **Davey Smith, G., Carroll, D., Rankin, S. and Rowan, D. (1992) 'Socioeconomic differentials in mortality: evidence from Glasgow graveyards', *British Medical Journal*, vol 305, pp 1554-7.**

[3] Davey Smith, G. and Morris, J. (1994) 'Increasing inequalities in the health of the nation' (Editorial), *British Medical Journal*, vol 309, pp 1453-4.

[4] Blane, D., Bartley, M. and Davey Smith, G. (1998) 'Disease aetiology and maternalist explanations of socioeconomic mortality differentials: a research note', *European Journal of Public Health*, vol 8, pp 259-60.

[5] Pamuk, E.R. (1985) 'Social class inequality and mortality from 1921-1971 in England and Wales', *Population Studies*, vol 39, pp 17-31.

[6] Harding, S. (1995) 'Social class differences in mortality of men: recent evidence from the OPCS Longitudinal Study', *Population Trends*, vol 80, pp 31-7.

[7] Drever, F., Whitehead, M. and Roden, M. (1996) 'Current patterns and trends in male mortality by social class (based on occupation)', *Population Trends*, vol 86, pp 15-20.

[8] Marmot, M.G., Davey Smith, G., Stansfeld, S., Patel, C., North, F., Head, J., White, I., Brunner, E. and Feeney, A. (1991) 'Inequalities in health twenty years on: the Whitehall II Study of British civil servants', *Lancet*, vol 337, pp 1387-94.

9   Eachus, J., Williams, M., Chan, P., Davey Smith, G., Grainge, M., Donovan, J. and Frankel, S. (1996) 'Deprivation and cause-specific morbidity: evidence from the Somerset and Avon Survey of Health', *British Medical Journal*, vol 312, pp 287-92.

10   Bentham, G., Eimermann, J., Haynes, R., Lovett, A. and Brainaird, J. (1995) 'Limiting long term illness and its association with mortality and indicators of social deprivation', *Journal of Epidemiology and Community Health*, vol 49, suppl 2, pp S57-S64.

11   Whitehead, M. (1992) 'The health divide', in P. Townsend, N. Davidson and M. Whitehead (eds) *Inequalities in health*, Harmondsworth: Penguin.

12   Davey Smith, G., Bartley, M. and Blane, D. (1994) 'Explanations for socioeconomic differentials in mortality: evidence from Britain and elsewhere', *European Journal of Public Health*, vol 4, pp 131-44.

13   Marmot, M., Bobak, M. and Davey Smith, G. (1995) 'Explanations for social inequalities in health', in B.C. Amick, S. Levine, A. Tarlov and D.C. Walsh (eds) *Society and health*, New York and Oxford: Oxford University Press.

14   Elstad, J.I. (1996) 'How large are the differences really? Self-reported longstanding illness among working class and middle class men', *Sociology of Health and Illness*, vol 18, pp 475-98.

15   Mackenbach, J.P., Looman, C.W.N. and van der Meer, J.B.W. (1996) 'Differences in the misreporting of chronic conditions, by level of education: effect on inequalities in prevalence rates', *American Journal of Public Health*, vol 86, pp 706-11.

16   Blane, D., Davey Smith, G. and Bartley, M. (1993) 'Social selection: what does it contribute to social class differences in health?', *Social Health Illness*, vol 15, pp 1-15.

17   **Davey Smith, G., Shipley, M.J. and Rose, G. (1990b) 'The magnitude and causes of socioeconomic differentials in mortality: further evidence from the Whitehall Study', *Journal of Epidemiology and Community Health*, vol 44, pp 260-5.**

18   **Davey Smith, G. and Shipley, M.J. (1991) 'Confounding of occupation and smoking: its magnitude and consequences', *Social Science and Medicine*, vol 32, pp 1297-300.**

[19] **Davey Smith, G., Hart, C., Blane, D., Gillis, C. and Hawthorne, V. (1997) 'Lifetime socioeconomic position and mortality: prospective observational study',** *British Medical Journal*, **vol 314, pp 547-52.**

[20] **Davey Smith, G., Hart, C., Hole, D., Gillis, C., Watt, G. and Hawthorne, V. (1998) 'Education and occupational social class: which is the more important indicator of mortality risk?',** *Journal of Epidemiology and Community Health*, **vol 52.**

[21] Brunner, E.J., Marmot, M.G., White, I.R., O'Brien, J.R., Etherington, M.D., Slavin, B.M., Kearney, E.M. and Davey Smith, G. (1993) 'Gender and employment grade differences in blood cholesterol, apolipoproteins and haemostatic factors in the Whitehall II Study', *Atherosclerosis*, vol 102, pp 195-207.

[22] Vague, J. (1956) 'The degree of masculine differentiation of obesities', *American Journal of Clinical Nutrition*, vol 4, pp 20-34.

[23] Davey Smith, G. and Brunner, E. (1997) 'Socioeconomic differentials in health: the role of nutrition', *Proceedings of the Nutrition Society*, vol 56, pp 75-90.

[24] Bosma, H., Marmot, M.G., Hemingway, H., Nicholson, A.C., Brunner, E. and Stansfeld, S. (1997) 'Low job control and risk of coronary heart disease: Whitehall II (prospective cohort) Study', *British Medical Journal*, vol 314, pp 558-65.

[25] Carroll, D., Davey Smith, G. and Bennett, P. (1996) 'Some observations on health and socioeconomic status', *Journal of Health Psychology*, vol 1, pp 23-39.

[26] Braverman, H. (1974) *Labor and monopoly capital*, New York, NY: Monthly Review Press.

[27] Lynch, J.W., Kaplan, G.A., Cohen, R.D., Tuomilehto, J. and Salonen, J.T. (1996) 'Do known risk factors explain the relation between socioeconomic status, risk of all-cause mortality, cardiovascular mortality and acute myocardial infarction?', *American Journal of Epidemiology*, vol 144, pp 934-42.

[28] Kuh, D. and Davey Smith, G. (1993) 'When is mortality risk determined? Historical insights into a current debate', *Social History of Medicine*, vol 6, pp 101-23.

[29] DoH (Department of Health) (1995) *Variations in health: What can the Department of Health and the NHS do?*, London: DoH.

[30] Jones, H.B. (1956) 'A special consideration of the ageing process, disease and life-expectancy', *Advances in Biological and Medical Physics*, vol 4, pp 281-337.

[31] Alter, R. and Riley, J. (1989) 'Frailty, sickness and death: models of morbidity and mortality in historical populations', *Population Studies*, vol 43, pp 25-46.

[32] Salhi, M., Caselli, G., Duchêne, J., Egidi, V., Santini, A., Thiltgés, E. and Wunsch, G. (1995) 'Assessing mortality differentials using life histories: a method and applications', in A. Lopez, G. Caselli and T. Valkonen (eds) *Adult mortality in developed countries: From description to explanation*, Oxford: Clarendon Press.

[33] Mare, R.D. (1990) 'Socioeconomic careers and differential mortality among older men in the US', in J. Vallin, S. D'Douza and A. Palloni (eds) *Measurement and analysis of mortality: New approaches*, Oxford: Clarendon Press, pp 362-87.

[34] Valkonen, T. (1987) 'Male mortality from ischaemic heart disease in Finland, relation to region of birth and region of residence', *European Journal of Population*, vol 3, pp 61-83.

[35] Koskinen, S. (1994) 'Origins of regional differences in mortality from ischaemic heart disease in Finland', National Research and Development Centre for Welfare and Health Search Report 41, Helsinki: NAWH.

[36] Barker, D.J.P. (1995) 'Early nutrition and CHD', in D.P. Davies (ed) *Nutrition in child health*, London: Royal College of Physicians.

[37] Ben-Shlomo, Y. and Davey Smith, G. (1991) 'Deprivation in infancy or in adult life: which is more important for mortality risk?', *Lancet*, vol 337, pp 530-4.

[38] Bartley, M., Power, C., Blane, D., Davey Smith, G. and Shipley, M.J. (1994) 'Birthweight and later socioeconomic disadvantage: evidence from the 1958 British cohort study', *British Medical Journal*, vol 309, pp 1475-8.

[39] Frankel, S., Elwood, P., Sweetnam, P., Yarnell, J. and Davey Smith, G. (1996) 'Birthweight, body-mass index in middle age, and incident coronary heart disease', *Lancet*, vol 348, pp 1478-80.

[40] Davey Smith, G. and Kuh, D. (1996) 'Does early nutrition affect later health: views from the 1930s and 1980s', in D. Smith (ed) *The history of nutrition in Britain in the twentieth century: Science, scientists and politics*, London: Routledge.

[41] Rowett Research Institute (1955) *Family diet and health in pre-war Britain*, Dunfermline: Carnegie UK Trust.

[42] Leitch, I. (1951) 'Growth and health', *British Journal of Nutrition*, vol 5, pp 142-51.

[43] Gunnell, D.J., Davey Smith, G., Frankel, S.J., Kemp, M., Peters, T.J. (1998) 'Socioeconomic and dietary influences on leg length and trunk length in childhood: a reanalysis of the Carnegie (Boyd Orr) Survey of diet and growth in pre-war Britain', *Paediatric and Perinatal Epidemiology*, vol 12 (Supplement 1) pp 96-113.

[44] Gunnell, D.J., Davey Smith, G., Frankel, S., Nanchahal, K., Braddon, F.E.M., Pemberton, J. and Peters, T.J. (1998) 'Childhood leg length and adult mortality – follow up of the Carnegie (Boyd Orr) Survey of diet and growth in pre-war Britain', *Journal of Epidemiology and Community Health*, vol 52, pp 142-52.

[45] Tannenbaum, A. (1947) 'Effects of varying caloric intake upon tumor incidence and tumor growth', *Annals of the New York Academy of Sciences*, vol 49, pp 5-18.

[46] Albanes, D., Jones, D.Y., Schatzkin, A., Micozzi, M.S. and Taylor, P.R. (1988) 'Adult stature and risk of cancer', *Cancer Research*, vol 48, pp 1658-62.

[47] Sooman, A., Macintyre, S. and Anderson, A. (1993) 'Scotland's health: a more difficult challenge for some?', *Health Bulletin*, vol 51, pp 276-84.

[48] Lobstein, T. (1995) 'The increasing cost of a healthy diet', *Food Magazine*, vol 31, p 17.

[49] DoH (1996) *Low income, food, nutrition and health: Strategies for improvement*, London: DoH.

[50] Dowler, E. (1996) 'Women and food in poor families: focus for concern?', in J. Buttriss and K. Hyman (eds) *Focus on women: Nutrition and health*, London: National Dairy Council.

[51] Travers, K.D. (1996) 'The social organisation of nutritional inequalities', *Social Science and Medicine*, vol 43, pp 543-53.

[52] Cameron, D. and Jones, I.G. (1985) 'An epidemiological and sociological analysis of the use of alcohol, tobacco, and other drugs of solace', *Community Medicine*, vol 7, pp 18-29.

[53] Graham, H. (1988) 'Women and smoking in the UK', *Health Promotion*, vol 3, pp 371-82.

[54] For a detailed review see Patrick, D. and Wickizer, T.M. (1995) 'Community and health', in B.C. Amick, S. Levine, A.R. Tarlov and D.C. Walsh (eds) *Society and health*, New York, NY: Oxford University Press.

[55] Centrewell, B.S. (1984) 'Race, socioeconomic status, and domestic homicide: Atlanta, 1971-72', *American Journal of Public Health*, vol 74, pp 813-15.

[56] Carstairs, U. and Morris, R. (1991) *Deprivation and health in Scotland*, Aberdeen: Aberdeen University Press.

[57] Sloggett, A. and Joshi, H. (1994) 'Higher mortality in deprived areas: community or personal disadvantage', *British Medical Journal*, vol 309, pp 1470-4.

[58] Haan, M., Kaplan, G.A. and Camacho, T. (1987) 'Poverty and health: prospective evidence from the Alameda County study', *American Journal of Epidemiology*, vol 125, pp 989-98.

[59] Jones, K. and Duncan, C. (1995) 'Individuals and their ecologies: analysing the geography of chronic illness within a multilevel modelling framework', *Health & Place*, vol 1, pp 27-40.

[60] Shouls, S., Congdon, P. and Curtis, S. (1996) 'Modelling inequality in reported long term illness in the UK: combining individual and area characteristics', *Journal of Epidemiology and Community Health*, vol 50, pp 366-76.

[61] Congdon, P. (1996) 'The epidemiology of suicide in London', *Journal of the Royal Statistical Society, Series A: Statistics in Society*, vol 159, pp 515-33.

[62] Hart, C., Ecob, R. and Davey Smith, G. (1997) 'People, places and coronary heart disease risk factors: a multilevel analysis of the Scottish heart health study archive', *Social Science and Medicine*, vol 45, pp 893-902.

[63] Egolf, B., Lasker, J., Wolf, S. and Potvin, L. (1992) 'The Roseto effect: a 50-year comparison of mortality rates', *American Journal of Public Health*, vol 82, pp 1089-92.

[64] Sooman, A., Macintyre, S. and Anderson, A. (1993) 'Scotland's health: a more difficult challenge for some?', *Health Bulletin*, vol 51, pp 276-84.

[65] Ashton, J. (1992) *Healthy cities*, Milton Keynes: Open University Press.

[66] Putnam, R.D., Leonardi, R. and Nanetti, R.Y. (1993) *Making democracy work: Civic traditions in modern Italy*, Princeton, NJ: Princeton University Press.

[67] Hertzman, C. (1996) 'What's been said and what's been hid: population health, global consumption and the role of national health data systems', in D. Blane, E. Brunner and R. Wilkinson (eds) *Health and social organization: Towards a health policy for the 21st century*, London: Routledge.

[68] Tyroler, H.A., Wing, S. and Knowles, M.G. (1993) 'Increasing inequality in coronary heart disease mortality in relation to educational achievement profiles of places of residence, US, 1962 to 1987', *Annals of Epidemiology*, vol 3, suppl, pp S51-S4.

[69] Diez-Roux, A.V., Nieto, F.J., Tyroler, H.A., Crum, L.D. and Szklo, M. (1995) 'Social inequalities and atherosclerosis: the atherosclerosis risk in communities study', *American Journal of Epidemiology*, vol 141, pp 960-72.

[70] Elo, I.T. and Preston, S.H. (1996) 'Educational differentials in mortality: US, 1979-85', *Social Science and Medicine*, vol 42, pp 47-57.

[71] Holme, I., Helgeland, A., Hjermann, I., Leren, P. and Lund-Larsen, P.G. (1980) 'Four-year mortality by some socioeconomic indicators: the Oslo study', *Journal of Epidemiology and Community Health*, vol 34, pp 48-52.

[72] Hertzman, C. and Wiens, M. (1996) 'Child development and long term outcomes: a population health perspective and summary of successful interventions', *Social Science and Medicine*, vol 43, pp 1083-95.

[73] Arblaster, L., Lambert, M., Entwistle, V., Forster, M., Fullerton, D., Sheldon, T. and Watt, I. (1996) 'A systematic review of the effectiveness of health service interventions aimed at reducing inequalities in health', *Journal of Health Services Research and Policy*, vol 1, pp 93-103.

[74] Foster, P. (1996) 'Inequalities in health: what health systems can and cannot do', *Journal of Health Services Research and Policy*, vol 1, pp 179-82.

[75] McKeown, T., Record, R.G. and Turner, R.D. (1975) 'An interpretation of the decline of mortality in England and Wales during the twentieth century', *Population Studies*, vol 29, pp 391-421.

[76] Mackenbach, J.P., Bouvier-Colle, M.H. and Jougla, E. (1990) '"Avoidable" mortality and health services: a review of aggregate data studies', *Journal of Epidemiology and Community Health*, vol 44, pp 106-11.

[77] Bunker, J.P., Frazier, H.S., and Mosteller, F. (1995) 'The role of medical care in determining health: creating an inventory of benefits', in B.C. Amick, S. Levine, A.R. Tarlov and D.C. Walsh (eds) *Society and health*, New York, NY: Oxford University Press.

[78] Cutler, J.A. and Grandits, G. (1995) 'What have we learned about socioeconomic status and cardiovascular disease from large trials?', in J. Stamler and H.P. Hazuda (eds) *Report of the conference on socioeconomic status and cardiovascular health and disease: November 6-7, 1995*, Bethesda, MD: National Institute of Health.

[79] Hypertension Detection and Follow-up Program Cooperative Group (1987) 'Education level and 5-year all-cause mortality in the HDFP', *Hypertension*, vol 9, pp 641-6.

[80] Ben-Shlomo, Y. and Chaturvedi, N. (1995) 'Assessing equity in access to health care provision in the UK: does where you live affect your chances of getting a coronary artery bypass graft?', *Journal of Epidemiology and Community Health*, vol 49, pp 200-4.

[81] Petticrew, M., McKee, M. and Jones, J. (1993) 'Coronary artery surgery: are women discriminated against?', *British Medical Journal*, vol 306, pp 1164-6; Phillmore, P., Beattie, A. and Townsend, P. (1994) 'Widening inequality of health in Northern England, 1981-91', *British Medical Journal*, vol 308, pp 1125-8.

[82] Shaukat, N., de Bono, D.P. and Cruickshank, J.K. (1993) 'Clinical features, risk factors, and referral delay in British patients of Indian and European origin with angina matched for age and extent of coronary atheroma', *British Medical Journal*, vol 307, pp 717-18.

[83] Morris, R.W., McCallum, A.K., Walker, M., Whincup, P.H., Ebrahim, S. and Shaper, A.G. (1996) 'Cigarette smoking in British men and selection for coronary artery bypass surgery', *Heart*, vol 75, pp 557-62.

[84] Hayward, R.A., Shapiro, M.F., Freeman, H.E. and Corey, C.R. (1988) 'Inequities in health services among insured Americans', *The New England Journal of Medicine*, vol 318, pp 1507-12.

[85] Chaturvedi, N. and Ben-Shlomo, Y. (1995) 'From the surgery to the surgeon: does deprivation influence consultation and operation rates', *British Journal of General Practice*, vol 45, pp 127-31; CPAG (Child Poverty Action Group) *Poverty: The facts*, London: CPAG.

[86] Payne, N. and Saul, C. (1997) 'Variations in use of cardiology services in a health authority: comparison of coronary artery revascularisation rates with prevalence of angina and coronary mortality', *British Medical Journal*, vol 314, pp 257-61.

[87] Shaukat, N., Lear, J., Lowy, A., Fletcher, S., de Bono, D.P. and Woods, K.L. (1997) 'First myocardial infarction in patients of Indian subcontinent and European origin: management and long-term outcome', *British Medical Journal*, vol 314, pp 639-42.

[88] Steingart, R.M., Packer, M., Hamm, P. et al (1991) 'Sex differences in the management of coronary artery disease', *The New England Journal of Medicine*, vol 325, pp 226-30.

[89] Harris, R.B. and Weissfeld, L.A. (1991) 'Gender differences in the reliability of reporting symptoms of angina pectoris', *Journal of Clinical Epidemiology*, vol 44, pp 1071-8.

[90] Shaw, L.J., Miller, D.D., Romeis, J.C., Kargl, D., Younis, L.T. and Chaitman, B.R. (1994) 'Gender differences in the noninvasive evaluation and management of patients with suspected coronary artery disease', *Annals of Internal Medicine*, vol 120, pp 559-66.

[91] Dong, W., Colhoun, H., Ben-Shlomo, Y. and Chaturvedi, N. (1996) 'Cardiac surgery in England – do men and women have equal access?', *Journal of Epidemiology and Community Health*, vol 50, pp 590-1.

[92] Weaver, W.D., White, H.D., Wilcox, R.G. et al (1996) 'Comparisons of characteristics and outcomes among women and men with acute myocardial infarction treated with thrombolytic therapy', *Journal of the American Medical Association*, vol 275, pp 777-82.

[93] Kee, F., Gaffney, B., Currie, S. and O'Reilly, D. (1993) 'Access to coronary catheterisation: fair shares for all?', *British Medical Journal*, vol 307, pp 1305-7.

[94] Koskinen, S.V.P., Martelin, T.P. and Valkonen, T. (1996) 'Socioeconomic differences in mortality among diabetic people in Finland: five year follow up', *British Medical Journal*, vol 313, pp 975-8.

[95] Majeed, F.A., Chaturvedi, N., Reading, R. and Ben-Shlomo, Y. (1994) 'Equity in the NHS: monitoring and promoting equity in primary and secondary care', *British Medical Journal*, vol 308, pp 1426-9.

38

How policy informs the evidence – 'evidence-based' thinking can lead to debased policy making

George Davey Smith, Shah Ebrahim and Stephen Frankel

Who would not want health policy to be based on evidence? 'Evidence-based medicine' and 'evidence-based policy' have such reassuring and self-evidently desirable qualities that it may seem contrary to question their legitimacy in relation to reducing health inequalities. However, these terms are now so familiar that it is easy to forget the important question about what sort of data provide appropriate evidence for particular types of decisions. The sort of evidence gathered on the benefits of interventions aimed at individuals may not help in guiding policies directed towards reducing health inequalities.

It is instructive to assess the process leading to the recommendations of the Independent Inquiry into Health Inequalities (the Acheson inquiry),[1] established in 1997 to help the government formulate policy to reduce health inequalities. The inquiry established an evaluation group to report on the quality of the evidence it used to reach its conclusions and support is recommendations.[2] This group critiqued submissions to the Inquiry, and a list of its own remedies for health inequalities – their '10 steps to health equality' – was released before the Acheson Inquiry had itself reported (see Box 1).[3]

The evaluation group appears to have applied evidence-based principles to its consideration of ways to reduce inequalities in health. Essentially it wanted evidence from controlled intervention studies and its main evaluation consisted of checking each recommendation against three earlier reviews (two conducted within an explicit evidence-based framework) and the Cochrane Library.

British Medical Journal, 2001, vol 322, pp 184-5

Box 1: The '10 steps to health equality'[4]

Nicotine gum and patches free on the NHS: double the chances of stopping smoking.

Pre-school education and childcare: strong evidence that it improves long-term prospects for children.

Fluoridation of drinking water: cuts tooth decay.

Accident prevention (for example, fit cars with soft bumpers): accidents are the principal cause of death in young people.

Drugs education in schools: prevents children becoming hooked.

Support round childbirth to promote breastfeeding and mental health: good evidence of long-term benefits.

Improved access to NHS for ethnic minorities (for example, by appointing link workers).

Adding folate to flour: prevents spina bifida in babies, and early evidence suggests it may prevent heart disease and Alzhiemer's Disease.

Free school milk.

Free smoke alarms: good evidence they save lives.

The task of the Acheson Inquiry was to make recommendations that would reduce inequalities in health, not merely have a positive overall health benefit. For most of the evaluation group's suggested interventions there are no high quality controlled studies showing that they would reduce health inequalities – for example, the evidence that fluoridation of drinking water would reduce inequalities in dental health is scanty.[4] Indeed, some of these interventions could increase inequalities. Smoking cessation may be more successful in advantage groups. Drugs education in schools may have less impact on those most at risk, because they are more likely to be truants and thus less exposed to it.

On the general question of what sort of evidence is useful to set policy in the public health domain, it is helpful to think back to earlier eras. In the first half of the 19th century there were no 'evaluation groups' to point out the lack of evidence from controlled intervention studies showing the health benefits of, for example, stopping children under nine from working in cotton mills, fencing off dangerous machinery, or reducing the number of hours children could work to only 10 a day. With an evaluation group, implementation of the Factory Acts could have been resisted. The factory owners were certainly keen on 'evidence': the claim that working-class children aged 5-10 had lower death rates than middle-class children was used to suggest that factory labour was good for the under 10s.[5]

Clearly the situation is now different, but health inequalities are still large and have increased over the past two decades. Premature death rates are over three-and-a-half times higher in Glasgow Shettleston than in Wokingham,[6] and a remarkable three quarters of premature deaths in Glasgow Shettleston would not occur if it had the mortality rates of Wokingham. It is no surprise that in Glasgow Shettleston child poverty rates are over six times, and unemployment rates over five times higher than in Wokingham. Clearly the need is for substantial reductions in socioeconomic inequality, which can follow only from the concerted implementation of policies of progressive taxation and substantial income redistribution.

The evaluation group states that randomised trials of Income Support have been carried out and could, in principle, have examined health outcomes.[7] However, the effects of income redistribution would not be to give a few people a little more money while they remain living in a highly unequal society, but to change the nature of the society. Health is influenced by micro and macro social environments,[8] and societies with high levels of income inequality are characterised by a wide range of social–structural attributes that have a detrimental impact on health.[9]

As Schwartz and Carpenter have pointed out, inappropriately focusing on individual level determinants of health while ignoring more important macro level determinants is tantamount to obtaining the right answer to the wrong question.[10] Consider the situation of examining risk factors for unemployment. Conventional individual-level studies would probably find that low education, not dressing smartly for interviews, being short, being over 50, or being a member of a minority ethnic group predict being unemployed. Indeed these 'risk factors' would probably explain a high percentage of the variance in unemployment. A controlled study finding that counselling on how to dress and behave at job interview increases success in getting a job could be added to the Cochrane Library. The same risk factors may explain a high percentage of inter-individual variance in unemployment, both when unemployment is 1% and when it is 14%.

The big difference for the population – and thus for the individual risk of unemployment – is, however, the 14-fold difference in overall levels of unemployment at times when different fiscal policies are being implemented. High variance apparently 'explained' by individual-level risk indicators (for markers manipulable in a discrete way within populations does not mean that they are important determinants of the population level of any outcome.[11] These are, however, precisely the factors that evidence-based research focuses on. Despite occasional rhetorical interest in wider determinants of health, evidence-based assessments are largely restricted to individualised interventions. The Cochrane Library is unlikely ever to contain systematic reviews or trials of the effects of redistributive national fiscal policies, or of economic investment leading to reductions in unemployment, on health.

The insidious nature of this mismatch between evidence and policy is highlighted by the fact that the evaluation group is, as one would expect of such informed commentators, aware of the problem, while implicitly ignoring it. One of the evaluation group stated when launching the '10 steps to health equality', "Our recommendations are quite medical because those are the sort that tend to have evidence behind them. Health differentials between social groups or between poor and rich countries, are not primarily generated by medical causes and require solutions at a different level".

One source of the scientific innovation that was institutionalised within the Cochrane Collaboration was a powerful critique of a complacent and uncritical form of healthcare delivery.[12] The establishment of the evidence-based medicine movement is a remarkable achievement with an unquestionably favourable influence on the probability that individuals will receive healthcare that benefits them and be protected from interventions that harm them. It would be ironic, and inconsistent with Cochrane's radical instincts, if the inappropriate application of those ideas were to provide a complacent barrier to implementing those measures necessary to redress health inequalities.

References

[1] *Independent Inquiry into Inequalities in Health* (1998) London: The Stationery Office.

[2] Macintyre, S., Chalmers, L., Horton, R. and Smith, R. (2001) 'Using evidence to inform health policy: case study', *British Medical Journal*, vol 322, pp 222-5.

[3] Laurance, J. (1998) 'Experts' 10 steps to health equality', *The Independent*, 12 November, p 14.

[4] NHS Centre for Reviews and Dissemination (2000) *A systematic review of public water fluoridation*, York: University of York.

[5] Bennett, A. (1995) *A working life: Child labour through the nineteenth century* (2nd edn), Launceston: Waterfront Publications.

⁶ Shaw, M., Dorling, D., Gordon, D. and Davey Smith, G. (1999) *The widening gap: Health inequalities and policy in Britain*, Bristol: The Policy Press.

⁷ Connor, J., Rodgers, A. and Priest, P. (1999) 'Randomised studies of income supplementation: a lost opportunity to assess health outcomes', *Journal of Epidemiology and Community Health*, vol 53, pp 725-30.

⁸ Dies Roux, A.V. (1998) 'Bringing context back into epidemiology: variables and fallacies in multilevel analysis', *American Journal of Public Health*, vol 88, pp 216-22.

⁹ Lynch, J., Davey Smith, G., Kaplan, G. and House, J. (2000) 'Income inequality and mortality: importance to health of individual income, psychosocial environment, or material conditions', *British Medical Journal*, vol 320, pp 1200-4.

¹⁰ Schwartz, S. and Carpenter, K.M. (1999) 'The right answer for the wrong question: consequences of type III error for public health research', *American Journal of Public Health*, vol 89, pp 1175-80.

¹¹ Rose, G. (1985) 'Sick individuals and sick populations', *International Journal of Epidemiology*, vol 14, pp 32-8.

¹² Cochrane, A.L. (1972) *Effectiveness and efficiency*, London: Nuffield Provincial Hospitals Trust.

39

Rationing for health equity: is it necessary?

George Davey Smith, Stephen Frankel and Shah Ebrahim

The literature on health inequalities that has emerged from the health economics world has similarities and differences to that produced from within medical sociology, social epidemiology and public health. Here we consider three premises which commonly underlie health economic discussions of the issue.[1] First, health services have relatively little influence on population health and therefore are not a primary focus for those concerned with reducing health inequalities. Second, there are limited health service resources and consequently some form of explicit or implicit rationing is necessary (even if these services have little influence on population health). And, third, manipulating the way in which rationing is carried out can (and should) redress some aspects of inequity of health service access and use. Here we briefly examine these premises to establish grounds for considering the role of health service provision in reducing health inequalities.

Health services: are they marginal to population health?

The widely accepted notion that the quality and quantity of health service provision has little impact on population health is generally the starting point for discussions of the role of the National Health Service in promoting health equity.[2] This view reflects the powerful influence of the historical work of Thomas McKeown,[3] the central claim of which was that long-term declines in mortality in Britain were primarily the outcome of improvements in nutrition and hygiene. The contribution of clinical medicine was viewed as minor, even after the modern era of antibiotics and other effective treatments. While McKeown's work was primarily concerned with historical trends and may be an accurate assessment of what happened in the

Health Economics, 2000, vol 9, pp 575-9

past (but there are dissenters from this view[4,5]), it may not necessarily be of relevance to the present experience of countries undergoing demographic and epidemiologic transitions, or of the determinants of current health trends within economically developed countries. However, McKeown certainly intended his work to be extrapolated to the present: "In order of importance the determinants of health were nutritional, environmental and behavioural in the past, and will probably be behavioural, environmental and nutritional in the future, at least in developed countries".[3]

Estimates of the degree to which medical care has influenced mortality trends have been made by John Bunker,[6] using the most rigorous available data – from randomised trials if possible – as the source of evidence on effectiveness. Grouping effective clinical preventative services (including screening for and treatment of hypertension; immunisation for diphtheria, polio and tetanus; and screening for cervical cancer) and clinical therapies (including appendectomy; insulin for type I diabetes; treatment of kidney failure and ischaemic heart disease) he estimated that in the US medical care had contributed about a fifth to the 30 years of increased life expectancy seen during the 20th century. While improvements in quality of life and reductions in morbidity have been more difficult to identify and evaluate, a meaningful contribution from medical care is also claimed for this domain.[6]

The potential contribution of medical care to mortality has certainly increased over recent decades. The major cause of death in both men (coronary heart disease) and women (breast cancer) were little influenced by treatment after disease onset when McKeown was writing in the mid-1970s; now the introduction of treatments that produce substantial increases in life expectancy following disease development have contributed importantly to the declining levels of mortality from these conditions.[7,8] The inequitable delivery of healthcare for these, and other, conditions could contribute importantly to socioeconomic differentials and the widening mortality gap seen between socioeconomic groups.[9] Realising the potential population health gain due to medical care requires that effective treatments are delivered properly – care should be available, targeted at those in need, providers should maintain high standards of care, and patients should adhere to treatment. Improving these fragile steps in the chain of care delivery are appropriate interventions for reducing socioeconomic inequalities in health.

The rationing non-debate: why does everyone want to ration healthcare?

The second premise, shared by virtually all commentators, is that publicly funded healthcare systems cannot fully meet the population's need for healthcare. Furthermore, the situation is seen to be deteriorating as the population grows older, new technologies appear and expectations rise. The striking point about this generally accepted wisdom is the extremely limited empirical evidence that it is based on. This is seen with respect to several apparent indicators of failure. Thus waiting lists, seen as a ubiquitous problem, are actually concentrated in relatively few parts of the country, while most areas show only small, if any, indications of serious problems (Figure 1). Bed crises during periods of raised demand (in particular during winter 'flu epidemics) are taken to be an indicator of the inevitable outcome of an ageing population and changing strategies within community and primary care.[10] However, the notion that emergency admissions are increasing everywhere and at a rapid rate is supported only by isolated local examples. While increasing in some areas, in others the apparent increases are artefacts of methods of counting and recounting admissions.[11] Rather than being an indicator of the accelerating move towards general chaos, this suggests that there are problems that should be investigated and dealt with locally. In the

Figure 1: Proportions of English NHS trusts with specified numbers of patients waiting for day case surgery

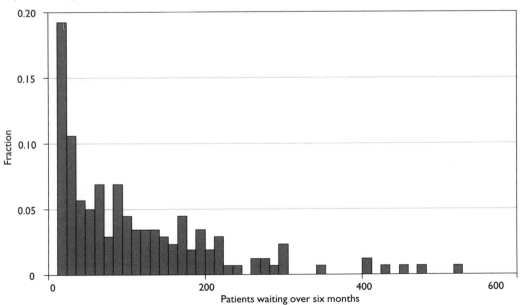

UK, the proportion of the population admitted to hospital each year has remained steady for the last 15 years[12] and in the Oxford area — where this issue can be quantified — there has been a decrease in total ordinary admissions between 1988 and 1993 of 0.3%.[13]

The major academic failure in this area has been to accept certain assumptions and not to engage in empirical investigations of the distribution of need for healthcare in the population and the capacity of services to deal with this need. The starting point is an 'epidemiology of indications',[14] using a case definition comprising of the ability to benefit from medical care if treated, in those whose global health status would allow such treatment to be performed with the benefits outweighing the risks, and who would accept treatment if offered it.

Two classic examples of apparent health service failure are total hip replacement and cataract extraction, with long waiting lists in some places. Population-based studies demonstrate that the imbalance between need and provision is, despite popular belief, relatively easily manageable.[15,16] In the case of cataract surgery, a local intervention in Brighton rapidly reduced waiting lists by temporarily increasing provision,[17] with the clear implication being that maintaining the level of service provision after this could prevent the re-emergence of the waiting list problem. Unfortunately, however, perverse reward mechanisms in the health service give benefit to those who ensure the expansion of waiting lists, which provides a steady flow of patients for lucrative private surgery.

The health economic literature is largely focussed on issues of resource availability and consumption at the macro level. A more intimate analysis reveals that relatively few interventions contribute greatly to elective NHS activity. Thus joint replacement, cataract extraction, prostatectomy, coronary revascularisation, hernia repair and biliary tract surgery constitute a quarter of such NHS activity.[18] Examining the true need for care in the restricted number of cases where treatment produces benefits is the only way of finding out the degree to which rationing is, or is not, necessary. As indicated above, in the cases when this has been done, there is no serious evidence of mismatch.[19]

In many domains of medical care, there is an extensive academic and quasi-academic industry producing guidelines as to how rationing should be carried out. One example of this is the case of the statins — cholesterol lowering drugs.[20] Trials of statin therapy have shown clear reductions in cardiovascular disease mortality, with no evidence of a counterbalancing increase in mortality from other causes (as have been seen with other cholesterol-lowering drugs).[21] Benefits of statin treatment have been recorded in people with low cardiovascular disease risk and with below average values of total and LDL blood cholesterol. Therefore, neither a particular level of cardiovascular disease risk above which clinical benefit in terms of mortality reduction occurs, nor the concentration of total or LDL blood cholesterol, can be used as a threshold for treatment decisions.

Cost-effectiveness is thus a key criterion for deciding on the amount of statin treatment that a population should receive. In many cost-effectiveness analyses drug costs are treated as invariant and in this way seem to give some semblance of objectivity to the assessment. This is not, however, the case. For example, simvastatin treatment at the dose used in the 4S trial costs £1.37 per day – or £500 per year – in the UK. In India, however, the same drug costs only 19p per day or £67 per year.[22] If statin costs were of this order in the UK their cost-effectiveness would be close to that for other secondary prevention interventions.[23]

Clearly the main factor determining such enormous disparities in costs is pharmaceutical industry profits. In the case of another effective class of drugs, serotonin re-uptake inhibitor (SRI) antidepressants, industry profits have been reduced as a result of professional and political concerns. In the case of statins the acceptance of high drug costs – recent reductions in UK costs of some statins were trivial – has resulted in a rationing policy based on an arbitrary level of risk.[24] The costs to society of accepting excessive pharmaceutical profits are substantial. If every person aged 45-74 in the UK with clinical evidence of coronary heart disease were treated with a statin for five years, about 22,000 deaths and major clinical events would be avoided. Currently, the five-year costs of the statins alone would be £1.6 billion but this would fall to £228 million if the costs incurred in India prevailed. The notion that rationing is inevitable – owing to financial constraints – is widespread. A public debate about the value of improved public health relative to high (and highly concentrated) industry profits is needed before the idea that rationing is inevitable is accepted.

The heretical notion that the apparently inexorable under-provision of healthcare is a chimera is indirectly supported by the universality of apparent crises of under-provision – and thus of the need for rationing – across countries which spend vastly different amounts in real or proportional (to GDP) terms.

Similarly, the ubiquitousness of waiting lists over time – during which there have been considerable fluctuations in level of provision and changes in the apparent level of need – suggests that these are not being maintained by the sum of two measurable (and not necessarily correlated) variables: the amount of need within the population and the resources provided to meet this need. The rationing debate (or more properly the rationing non-debate, given the almost universal acceptance of unsupported premises) should perhaps be seen more as the outcome of socially determined (and thus manipulable) forces rather than the fearless description of how the world actually is.

'Rationers for equity': an unnecessary professional group?

The third premise – of the need to 'ration for equity' – fades away if rationing itself is not considered necessary. Instead the question is how should resources be rationally distributed to fit with levels of need? Here the lack of research on the epidemiology of indications[14] creates a serious problem, and in principle the use of socioeconomic indicators as proxies for need has some merit. In practice there are difficulties with this approach. Many resource allocation formulae inadequately account for the full range of differences created by social circumstances[25] (although this has not limited the enthusiasm of some of those who recognised these difficulties when it came to contributing to the cottage industry of formulae production).[26]

Socioeconomic indicators and their relationship with need are complex. First, not only does the prevalence of specific health problems differ across socioeconomic groups, but also at any particular level of ill health, severity and multiplicity of the problems tend to be greater among those in worse social circumstances.[27] Thus, reported prevalence of disease does not take account of the added burden of increased severity among disadvantaged people. Second, much current work focuses on targeting healthcare resources on those who are most at risk, since these have most to gain from such treatments.[28] However, risk indicators use clinical measurements and do not take into account the added risk among those in less favourable social circumstances.

For example, guidelines for targeting the use of cholesterol lowering drugs are based on predicting an individual's level of risk for future catastrophic cardiovascular events using measurements of blood pressure, blood cholesterol, presence of diabetes, age, sex and smoking behaviour.[20] Given all these factors, people from worse social circumstances have a considerably higher level of cardiovascular risk than those from better off circumstances.[29]

Therefore, a rational approach would be to build social circumstances into such models which would automatically lead to greater targeting of treatment on the socially disadvantaged who have most to gain.

Conclusions

We consider that health services now have a substantial impact on population health, whether measured as quality of life or survival. This is likely to increase in the future. Therefore, adequate provision of health services to all social groups is a factor which will, increasingly, come to influence inequalities in health. However, we do not consider the evidence that it is impossible to meet the population demands for health services is reliable; rather such claims are based almost entirely on supposition and are supported by professional self-interest. A rationally planned health service could deliver on the basis of need. Social circumstances should be one indicator of need since adverse conditions can increase the degree of benefit from the medical care which will be received and therefore can improve the benefit:risk ratio. Further research on the epidemiology of indications for the major areas of healthcare provision is essential to evaluate the scale of potential need:demand mismatches. Returning to the principle of a national health service which delivers according to need, and not being constrained by the chimera of demands which cannot be met, is the best way of moving towards equity of health service provision, thereby increasing health equity.

References

[1] This commentary was produced in discussion of a paper at the Health Equity Network UK inaugural meeting, 20 March 2000 in London. The paper under discussion reiterated all three of these premises.

[2] Benzeval, N., Judge, K. and Whitehead, M. (1995) 'The role of the NHS', in N. Benzeval, K. Judge and M. Whitehead (eds) *Tackling inequalities in health: An agenda for action*, London: King's Fund.

[3] McKeown, T. (1976) *The role of medicine*, London: Nuffield Provincial Hospital Trust.

[4] Szreter, S. (1988) 'The importance of social intervention in Britain's mortality decline c. 1950-1914: a reinterpretation of the role of public health', *Social History of Medecine*, vol 1, pp 1-37.

[5] Johansson, S.R. (1994) 'Food for thought: rhetoric and reality in modern mortality history', *Historical Methods*, vol 27, pp 101-25.

[6] Bunker, J.P. (1995) 'Medicine matters after all', *Journal of the Royal College of Physicians of London*, vol 29, pp 105-12.

[7] Tunstall-Pedoe, H., Vanuzzo, D., Hobbs, M. et al (2000) 'Estimation of contribution of changes in coronary care to improving survival, event rates, and coronary heart disease mortality across the WHO MONICA Project populations', *Lancet*, vol 355, pp 688-700.

[8] Peto, R., Boreham, J., Clarke, M., Davies, C. and Beral, V. (2000) 'UK and USA breast cancer deaths down 25% in year 2000 at ages 20-69 years', *Lancet*, vol 355, p 1822.

[9] **Davey Smith, G., Dorling, D., Gordon, D. and Shaw, D. (1999) 'The widening health gap: what are the solutions?', *Critical Public Health*, vol 9, pp 151-70.**

[10] Blatchford, O. and Capewell, S. (1997) 'Emergency medical admissions: taking stock and planning for winter', *British Medical Journal*, vol 315, pp 1322-3.

[11] Morgan, K., Prothero, D. and Frankel, S. (1999) 'The rise in emergency admissions – crisis or artefact? Temporal analysis of health service data', *British Medical Journal*, vol 319, pp 158-9.

[12] Office for National Statistics (1997) *Living in Britain: Results from the General Household Survey 1995*, London: The Stationery Office.

[13] DoH (Department of Health) (2000) *Shaping the future NHS: Long-term planning for hospitals and related services*, London: DoH.

[14] Frankel, S. (1991) 'The epidemiology of indications', *Journal of Epidemiology and Community Health*, vol 45, pp 257-9.

[15] Frankel, S., Pearson, J., Greenwood, R. et al (1999) 'Population requirements for primary hip-replacement surgery: a cross-sectional study', *Lancet*, vol 353, pp 1304-9.

[16] Hopper, C., Frost, N.A., Peters, T.J., Sparrow, J.M., Durant, J.S. and Frankel, S. (1999) 'Population requirements for cataract surgery', *Journal of Epidemiology and Community Health*, vol 53, p 661.

[17] Thomas, H.F., Darvell, R.H.J. and Hicks, C. (1989) '"Operation Cataract": a means of reducing waiting lists for cataract operations', *British Medical Journal*, vol 299, pp 961-3.

[18] DoH (2000) 'The new NHS – 1999 reference costs', London: DoH.

[19] Frankel, S., Ebrahim, S. and Davey Smith, G. (2000) 'The limits to demand', *British Medical Journal*, vol 321, pp 40-5.

[20] Wallis, E.J., Ramsay, L.E., Haq, I.U., Ghahramani, P., Jackson, P.R., Rowland-Yeo, K. and Yeo, W.W. (2000) 'Coronary and cardiovascular risk estimation for primary prevention: validation of a new Sheffield table in the 1995 Scottish health survey population', *British Medical Journal*, vol 320, pp 671-6.

[21] Davey Smith, G., Song, F. and Sheldon, T.A. (1993) 'Cholesterol lowering and mortality: the importance of considering initial level of risk', *British Medical Journal*, vol 306, pp 1367-73.

[22] 'Cholesterol reducer Simvastol' (1999) *Indian Express*, 10 January, p 3.

[23] Ebrahim, S., Davey Smith, G., McCabe C., Payne N., Pickin, M., Sheldon, T.A., Lampe, F., Sampson, F., Ward, S. and Wannamthee, G., (1998) 'Cholesterol and coronary heart disease: screening and treatment', *Quality in Health Care*, vol 7, pp 232-9.

[24] Wood, D., Durrington, P., Poulter, N., McInnes, G., Rees, A. and Wray, R. (1998) 'Joint British recommendations on prevention of coronary heart disease in clinical practice', *Heart*, vol 80, suppl 2, pp S1-S29.

[25] Sheldon, T.A., Davey Smith, G. and Bevan, G. (1993) 'Weighting in the dark: resource allocation in the new NHS', *British Medical Journal*, vol 306, pp 835-9.

[26] Smith, P., Sheldon, T., Carr-Hill, R., Martin, S., Peacock, S. and Hardman, G. (1994) 'Allocating resources to health authorities: results and policy implications of small area analysis of use of in-patient services', *British Medical Journal*, vol 309, pp 1050-4.

[27] Eachus, J., Chan, P., Pearson, N., Propper, C. and Davey Smith, G. (1999) 'An additional dimension to health inequalities: disease severity and socioeconomic position', *Journal of Epidemiology and Community Health*, vol 53, pp 603-11.

[28] Davey Smith, G. and Egger, M. (1994) 'Who benefits from medical interventions?', *British Medical Journal*, vol 308, pp 72-4.

[29] **Davey Smith, G., Hart, C., Blane, D., Gillis, C. and Hawthorne, V. (1997) 'Lifetime socioeconomic position and mortality: prospective observational study', *British Medical Journal*, vol 314, pp 547-52.**

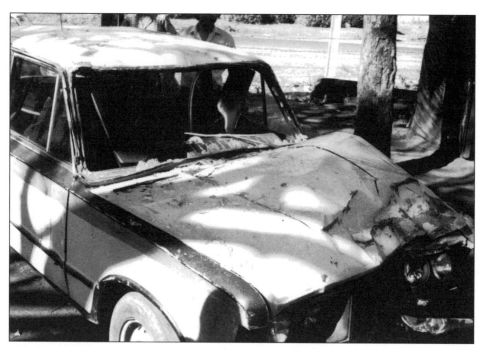

Photograph by Gerald Welsby

Afterword:
Still wanting to be James Dean

George Davey Smith

The strangest thing about flying through the air and then smashing through the windscreen of an oncoming car was the feeling that the glass sealed up behind me after I had passed through it. Apart from that the business was depressingly prosaic – I experienced neither a rapid religious conversion nor my life passing before my eyes. I was pulled out of the car through the broken windscreen, shouted insults in inappropriate English at the driver of the car, tried to hit him, and then collapsed. I came to while I was being shoved into the back of a van, followed by my pillion passenger, who I was relieved to see was alive. She was conscious but complained of pain in her abdomen and said she thought she was bleeding inside. By then I could see nothing as blood was running into my eyes and attempting to rub it away was ineffective as well as painful and it was miserable to feel the jelly mass that used to be my eyebrows.

At the time, in early 1989, I had been working for two months on a health services research programme in Nicaragua, and had been impressed at how the clinical services functioned in a country with a collapsing economy. But I was not convinced enough of their ability to deal with emergencies to have any desire to try them out. The general advice given by longer-term residents was that if you got sick insist on going to either the Lenin-Fonseca or Carlos Marx Hospitals, as they had large contingents of experienced Cuban, and (then) East German staff. I tried repeating these names to the driver of the van (a bypasser as it turned out) but it seemed he took them to be incantations of ideological commitment and we arrived at the emergency room of the Manolo Morales Hospital. As we were being carried in I kept repeating "I want to telephone", and ended up having to resist being examined, which continued until it was realised that I was going to cause trouble and cover the whole of the casualty department in blood if a telephone wasn't produced. I spoke to a friend, another doctor – but like me an epidemiologist with no recent

British Medical Journal, 1991, vol 303, p 528

clinical experience – asking him to come quickly and check out whether my passenger was bleeding internally. After that my memory became hazy, probably thankfully as my face and head were being sutured.

Friends arrived and I was helped into a chair. Things remained confused but at some stage I remember my watch being removed, never to reappear. I was graced with a turban, which fell off after 20 minutes, a lump of dressings stuck at random over my face, and ripped, blood soaked clothing. Thus I was ideally dressed for the observation room and attracted no attention at all. Suddenly I found myself weeping uncontrollably. I had heard about delayed grief reactions, but to experience one was bizarre. I didn't feel shock or panic, I could continue to think rationally, and I realised that the behaviour was inappropriate – but I couldn't stop crying. The driver of the car arrived and tried to persuade one of my friends not to involve the police, which managed to make things seem even more wretched. As suddenly as I'd started I stopped sobbing, to discover that my friend was receiving an injection of dexamethasone "to stop the brain swelling". This seemed inappropriate for a patient who had not been unconscious and who had not had a skull x-ray examination, and for a health service in a country which found it impossible to pay for essential antibiotics.

I had only seen two crash helmets in Nicaragua and had not driven to Costa Rica to buy one. The irony of a professional preventive medicine apparatchik failing to engage in health protective behaviour was increased by the fact that I had recently participated in the examination of a Nicaraguan epidemiology student's degree thesis on a case-control study of serious road traffic accidents. I displayed most of the risk factors detected by that study, the conclusion of which was that not all accidents were caused by the military (a popular perception) and that deterrents should be made more harsh. The family of the other driver certainly seemed concerned about the latter, and sums of money were being mentioned in return for non-prosecution. Then a policeman arrived, asked me two questions, and removed the car driver to prison.

Our party trooped into the x-ray examination room to be greeted by a well fed brown mouse. During the examinations, from an ancient high dose machine, the supervisor wore a protective apron while a large array of spectators fried. We returned to the observation room, where relatives and friends were standing around other patients who were lying on the benches or, if lucky, beds. My friend's drip was barely running, and when we pointed this out the whole system was fiddled with, resulting in no increase in speed but a mixture of air and saline passing through it. It was clear that I'd been finished with, so I was taken home where I tried to get out of my clothes. On removing the remains of my trousers a plug of cotton and congealed blood was pulled out from a gaping hole over my shin and I started bleeding impressively. I was taken back to the hospital where the permanent large crowd locked outside the doors (for what purpose I never discovered) parted, as an obvious member of the wounded approached. I was admonished for not having taken off my trousers earlier and sutured. It was only days later that I remembered the teaching I'd received about wound suturing, and began to worry both about the thick silk stitches in my face and the poorly vascularised area of my shin.

We were told that my friend had four fractures of her pelvis and would be kept for another four hours and then discharged home for bed rest. This seemed somewhat premature, as she was complaining of increasing pain in her abdomen and chest. As someone who had always been critical of high technology medical interventions, I was disturbed to find myself fantasising about aortic grafts, balloon pumps, and computed tomography. I started wishing I'd paid more attention in the lectures on cardiac tamponade, and was relieved that we had medical insurance. We were eventually flown, accompanied, to London and taken to King's College Hospital. My friend recovered rapidly, and caused trouble for those trying to ensure that the requisite period of bed rest was observed. A few months later, out nightclubbing, she was dancing long after the rest of us had given up.

With an economy that had been ruined by US backed Contra aggression, and with the concentration of public spending on defence that the war entailed, it was remarkable that Nicaragua could sustain a hospital system at all. The position now, after the defeat of the Sandinistas and the election of a government committed to privatisation, is almost certainly worse. Many hospitals are in disarray as the government uses inflation as a means of cutting the hospital workers' wages. But back in the Manolo Morales Hospital, as I hobbled off to find someone to do something with the defunct drip, I spotted a cockroach, and realised that perhaps British and Nicaraguan hospitals weren't that different after all.

INDEX TO THE ARTICLES

References to figures and tables are in *italics*.